Praise for *The Fat of the Land*

"An entertaining, intelligent and comprehensive book . . . Fumento unleashes a surprising deluge of studies, carefully measured arguments and puckish quips to overwhelm Americans' emotional resistance to embracing the rigors—and joys—of meaningful weight loss. This good book is as convincing as it is (excuse the term) digestible."
   —*The Detroit News*

"Putting theories to test and shysters to shame, the book is worth reading for its lively look at the confusing ideas out there."
   —*San Diego Union-Tribune*

"At last, here is a book that exposes the cherished but faulty beliefs and assumptions of obesity researchers, the obese, and those who make money off the obese. This is a *must read* for everyone concerned about obesity."
   —G. Ken Goodrich, Ph.D., Baylor College of Medicine, and co-author of *Living Without Dieting*

"There is much to relish in *The Fat of the Land*. . . . a call to action and sermon to the heavy-set . . . This is sage counsel."
   —*The Wall Street Journal*

"Anyone who's trying to lose weight can surely benefit from this simple, humorous, educational, no-nonsense volume. . . . This book is bulging with information, heavy on the humor and spiced with stories of profiteers and pushy peddlers in the diet industry. . . . If you want to lose weight, do what Fumento recommends—count calories and get off your duff. And do what I recommend—read this book."
   —*The Virginian-Pilot*

"Skewers fat-acceptance myths . . . debunks much of the phony advice."
   —*The Philadelphia Inquirer*

"Finally a smart book for the person who knows successful weight management involves more than dieting: It is about thinking about how to change your life and develop the behavioral skills to enjoy portion-controlled, good-tasting food that is low in fat and high in fiber—namely, rich fruits and vegetables."
>—George Blackburn, M.D., Ph.D., Director of the Center for the study of Nutrition and Medicine, Beth Israel Deaconess Hospital and Harvard Medical School

"Pound for pound, more fascinating information than any book I've consumed in the past year."
>—*The Weekly Standard*

"Fumento . . . has the guts to say that the emperor's clothes don't fit because the emperor is too fat. He debunks a lot of the myths about fat, dieting, exercise, and the industries that feed on them."
>—*San Antonio Express-News*

"*The Fat of the Land* has the research of a doctoral dissertation, yet reads like a compelling novel. People who need this book include anyone who is overweight, who loves someone who is overweight, or who is aghast at the needless deaths of 300,000 Americans a year. Even after losing 185 pounds and keeping it off, I can't begin to say how much I've learned from this book."
>—Rosemary Green, author of *Diary of a Fat Housewife*

"This medical journalist has a knack for debunking popular beliefs and revealing the true state of things. While this candid approach incited controversy before, the author's tone here is too likable to provoke the ire even of those groups he is most critical of. . . . It's hard to doubt the author's conclusions. . . . Fumento is a rational man but that doesn't mean he's dry. In fact, he's a sharp and witty writer who isn't afraid to joke around."
>—*Publishers Weekly* (starred)

"Highly recommended."
>—*Library Journal* (starred)

PENGUIN BOOKS

THE FAT OF THE LAND

Michael Fumento is a medical journalist and a resident fellow at the American Enterprise Institute. He is also the author of *The Myth of Heterosexual AIDS*. He lives in Arlington, Virginia.

The
FAT
of the
LAND

OUR HEALTH CRISIS

AND HOW OVERWEIGHT

AMERICANS CAN HELP

THEMSELVES

Michael
Fumento

PENGUIN BOOKS

PENGUIN BOOKS
Published by the Penguin Group
Penguin Putnam Inc., 375 Hudson Street,
New York, New York 10014, U.S.A.
Penguin Books Ltd, 27 Wrights Lane,
London W8 5TZ, England
Penguin Books Australia Ltd, Ringwood,
Victoria, Australia
Penguin Books Canada Ltd, 10 Alcorn Avenue,
Toronto, Ontario, Canada M4V 3B2
Penguin Books (N.Z.) Ltd, 182–190 Wairau Road,
Auckland 10, New Zealand
Penguin India, 210 Chiranjiv Tower, 43 Nehru Place,
New Delhi 11009, India

Penguin Books Ltd, Registered Offices:
Harmondsworth, Middlesex, England

First published in the United States of America by Viking Penguin,
a member of Penguin Putnam Inc. 1997
Published in Penguin Books 1998

10   9   8   7   6   5   4   3   2   1

THE LIBRARY OF CONGRESS HAS CATALOGUED THE HARDCOVER AS FOLLOWS:
Fumento, Michael.
The fat of the land: the obesity epidemic and how overweight Americans
can help themselves/by Michael Fumento.
p.   cm.
Includes index.
ISBN 0-670-87059-5 (hc.)
ISBN 0 14 02.6144 3 (pbk.)
1. Obesity—United States.   2. Weight loss.   I. Title.
RC628.F86 1997
616.3′98′00973—dc21   97–7173

Set in New Baskerville
Designed by Kathryn Parise

For my brothers:

David, Andrew, and

Matthew

Foreword

Obesity is an escalating epidemic of alarming proportions in the United States, and a serious health crisis looms on our horizon. Recent data from a national survey indicate that one third of adult Americans can be classified as obese, as compared with one quarter a decade earlier. This translates to 58 million American adults (32 million women and 26 million men) who are obese and at risk for obesity-related health problems. Americans have gained an average of 8 pounds per person (an aggregate gain of nearly 2 billion pounds of fat tissue) in the past ten years. Children and adolescents in the United States and much of the Western world are also heavier than ever. At the same time, tomes of research now attest to the serious health risks of excess weight. The medical evidence is compelling, and undebatable, that obesity leads to high blood pressure, adult-onset diabetes, abnormal cholesterol levels, and heart disease. Overweight also contributes to the risk of stroke, certain cancers (particularly of the colon, breast, prostate, and uterus), gallstones, certain forms of arthritis, reduced quality of life, and premature death. In our research in the Harvard Nurses' Health Study, we found that nearly one quarter of all deaths in nonsmoking women were attributable to overweight, supporting the national estimate of 300,000 obesity-related deaths in the United States each year. Even modest weight loss among the overweight (a magnitude of 5 to 10 percent weight reduction) can confer important health benefits. It is clear that our nation can no longer afford to be complacent about the obesity epidemic.

The growing girth of Americans is replete with paradox. This is a nation obsessed with thinness. Increasing body weights in the United States, ironically, have paralleled the increasing preoccupation with weight and dieting, as well as the increasing frequency of weight-loss efforts. As many as 40 percent of women and 24 percent of men are trying to lose weight at any given time. What's wrong with this picture? Whatever we're doing, it's clearly not working. Our nation is only getting fatter. At least 60 percent of us are sedentary and most are overeating. The more we seem to "diet," the more weight we seem to gain. The laws of thermodynamics have lost all relevance in the process. The American public is bombarded with mixed messages, confusing research results, and "quick fix" solutions. The most recent exploitation is a spate of books telling the public what the authors think they want to hear: that obesity is healthy and weight loss is not only unnecessary but dangerous. A new set of myths is being promulgated to confuse and appease the American public.

Michael Fumento's *The Fat of the Land* rescues us from this chaos and finally sets the record straight. With incisive wit, clarity of thought, and scholarly synthesis of the medical literature, Fumento exposes the deceptions and scams that are rampant in many of the popular books on this subject. Unlike so many previous books that selectively review the scientific literature, Fumento critically examines and synthesizes the full range of scientific evidence on weight and health. In this fascinating and lively compendium, he "tells it like it is," finding more consistency than controversy in the science. Despite its humor, this book couldn't be more serious. This myth-busting book challenges recent claims that heredity is destiny when it comes to our weight, that lower body fat is "good fat" that protects against heart disease, that weight is unrelated to fitness or health, that calories don't count, and other misguided "feel good" theories. Fumento gets it straight, separating fact from fiction, truth from hype, and explodes a number of common myths about our weight and our health in the process. His common-sense approach to maintaining healthy weight, through a balanced reduced-calorie diet and regular exercise, is refreshingly straightforward. This book is a "must read" for anyone seeking reliable information about fitness, weight, diet, and health, and frustrated by the mixed messages and counter-intuitive theories bombarding us daily on these subjects. Nearly all Americans and the better part of the global population should find it helpful.

JoAnn E. Manson, M.D., Dr.P.H.
Director of Endocrinology and
Co-Director of Women's Health,
DIVISION OF PREVENTIVE MEDICINE,
BRIGHAM AND WOMEN'S HOSPITAL,
and ASSOCIATE PROFESSOR OF MEDICINE,
HARVARD MEDICAL SCHOOL

Acknowledgments

I must first acknowledge the countless hours of help provided by my research assistant, Mary Oliver, who, like any good research assistant, let me pawn off much of the tedious, boring stuff on her so I could do the more exciting work. Matt Kaufman was an editorial consultant and sounding board for the entire manuscript. I also take this opportunity to thank him for graciously editing my weekly column over the past two years and often enough coming up with "my" best lines. Robert Whelan was my United Kingdom correspondent for this book, as with myriad other projects over the last nine years. Miss J. J. Green read the entire book in manuscript form and in galleys, finding errors each time. (If she finds any in the final book, I don't want to hear it.) Joe Millan was my New York correspondent, spending numerous hours pulling articles from the New York Public Library. Medical journal articles, which Miss Oliver couldn't find, were fastidiously tracked down by Dr. Barbara Rapp of the National Center for Biotechnology Information. Dr. Bruce Ames of the University of California at Berkeley kept me appraised of much of the latest obesity research. Dixie D'Souza provided valuable criticism. Billy Richards was always there for me when I needed him.

I commend my friends and agents Glen Hartley and Lynn Chu for not letting their startling success of the past few years go to their heads and for continuing to make time for non-million-buck writers like myself. My editor at Viking, Cathy Hemming, showed unusual courage (and soundness of mind, I like to think!) in acquiring, pushing, and editing this project. Carolyn Carlson, along with Erin Boyle, greased the skids.

Generous support for this project came from the William H. Donner Foundation and from *Reason* magazine. I specifically thank Donner's William Alpert and *Reason*'s editor Virginia Postrel.

Though I didn't contact her until late in the project, Rosemary Green put some hard questions to me and was a source of inspiration and encouragement—not to mention a blast to talk to on the phone.

I hereby submit the standard disclaimer that the views expressed herein are my own, as are any of the mistakes. I also take full responsibility for any jokes that fall flat. That said, numerous obesity researchers have given me invaluable aid, including though not limited to Drs. John P. Foreyt and G. Ken Goodrick of Baylor College of Medicine in Houston; Dr. Steven Heymsfield at St. Luke's–Roosevelt Hospital in New York; and Drs. JoAnn Manson and Walter Willett at Harvard.

And finally to a big, burly sweetheart of a guy from half a lifetime ago, Mike Virella. Though he was only in his twenties, he was the first friend I lost to obesity. May he be the last. Mike, this one's for you.

Contents

Foreword *by JoAnn E. Manson, M.D., Dr.P.H.*   vii

Acknowledgments   xi

Introduction   xv

  1. The Perils of Poundage   1

  2. One Nation, Overweight   27

  3. The Low-Fat Myth   56

  4. Give Us This Day Our Daily Half Pound of Sugar   82

  5. Big Fat Myths That Make Us Fatter   93

  6. The Profiteers   131

  7. Diets Don't Work—Except When They Do   164

  8. The Fiber Factor   187

9. Exercise: Move It and Lose It 206

10. Pill Talk 229

11. Defatting the Land 253

Notes 273

Index 323

Introduction

"But wait a bit," the Oysters cried,
"Before we have our chat;
 For some of us are out of breath,
 And all of us are fat!"
                   —LEWIS CARROLL,
                   Through the Looking Glass

It is the most common chronic health problem in America. Its incidence is skyrocketing and the number of illnesses it appears to cause is increasing. Though individuals obsess over it as a personal problem, it is given little attention as a medical problem on a national level. Indeed, as one prominent doctor put it a couple of years ago, "With any other condition it would be called an epidemic."[1] The problem is obesity, and it kills an estimated 300,000 Americans a year.[2] It boggles my mind to think that in the two years I took to write this book, 600,000 of my countrymen have had their lives cut short by this disease.

A third of American adults are now classified as obese, defined as being at least 20 percent fatter than they should be.[3] A quarter of our children are obese.[4] Both of these numbers represent huge increases from just a few years ago. According to the Institute of Medicine of the National Academy of Sciences, about two thirds of us are too heavy for optimum health.[5]

Perhaps worst of all, there is no end in sight to this epidemic. The AIDS epidemic, like all infectious disease epidemics before it, has followed a bell-shaped curve and is now in decline. But there is no such natural constraint on obesity. It is the one disease that can just keep getting worse and worse.

My interest in the American obesity problem began a few years ago. I was traveling in Europe and noticed that no matter what country I was in, the Europeans were considerably thinner than Americans. In fact, you can usually identify Americans in Europe just on the basis of their size. (Also their tendency to wear tennis shoes.) I even joked about writing a book called *The European Weight-Loss Plan.*

On Zaandvoort Beach near Amsterdam, instead of ogling all the topless young women (well, maybe I did ogle a bit), I was more intrigued to see Dutch mothers in their thirties who clearly hadn't put on an ounce since college. In Rome my girlfriend and I expected to see only "roly-poly" types, befitting the image Americans have of Italians. We would have expected it all the more had we any idea how wonderful real Italian food is. Instead, Italy boasts some of the leanest, handsomest men and women we've ever seen.

On some Greek islands (though interestingly not on others) we saw many obese people, but even they could not begin to compare with Americans. In Bavarian beer halls some huge Teutons downed mugs of *Brau* so big I calculated each glass was the equivalent of 3.4 trips to the bathroom. And despite the image perpetuated by the labels of St. Pauli Girl beer, which always depict thin beautiful women with huge breasts, we've never seen a beer-hall maiden who wasn't fat—though they did have large breasts. But outside the beer halls, truly fat Germans appeared to be a rarity and outside of Bavaria rarer still.

Interestingly, many Americans are unaware that we are so much fatter than the rest of the world. But Europeans will readily volunteer that they are alternatively aghast and amused at this peculiar American problem.

The most startling aspect of the weight differences between Americans and Europeans is that according to the advice regularly doled out by American experts, the Europeans are doing everything wrong. They had no diet sodas until just a few years ago and most that are now consumed appear to be purchased by Americans. Many of their stores don't even sell skim milk. Low- and no-fat bread and desserts are almost non-existent. They haven't the least idea what a SnackWell's is. They don't have the benefit of the tens of millions of diet books sold in the United States each year. The very word "diet" is a rarity in Europe, hence diet Coke is labeled "Coca-Cola Light" in most countries and Diet Pepsi is called "Pepsi Max" or "Pepsi Light." The Dutch bicycle a lot, but aerobic exercise, whether in dance classes or on equipment, is fairly rare. European women's magazines rarely discuss weight loss per se, though cellulite seems to be a hot topic. Instead, they prefer more mundane topics like sex, makeup, movie stars, and royalty.

So I wondered: Why haven't all these ingenious Yankee schemes helped us in our battle with obesity? Could it even be that they're hurting? And why, with the constant media bombardment telling us not to eat fat, does it seem that residents of many European countries are eating so much more fat than we are and "getting away with it." The Dutch appeared to be the thinnest Europeans I saw, yet their favorite snack is a cone of French fries with a mayonnaise-based sauce glopped all over them. Yech! The French are far thinner than Americans, but my girlfriend and I couldn't even stomach much of the restaurant food because it was so fatty. By the time you cut the visible fat off it, what remained was about the size of a postage stamp.

To answer this puzzle, I consulted some of those American diet books. Dozens of them. But none of their authors mentioned the European-U.S. difference. Indeed, diet books seem cognizant of little more than P. T. Barnum's dictum about a sucker being born every minute. (The earth's population having increased by several times since he said that, I'm confident the rate has increased considerably.) Oh sure, most talked about their findings being based on all the latest medical literature, on hundreds, even thousands of studies. But if so, how come they never seemed to mention more than three or four of those studies?

It was clear I was not going to find my answers to the American weight problem in the popular literature. So I consulted the medical literature. Foolishly, I thought I might find a few hundred articles. Instead, by the time my assistant and I were through pulling articles, I found I had a stack of papers so high that a pair of bald eagles built a nest on the top. (OK, I'm kidding but I did break my toe running into one of the many boxes that held the material.) Later I read a medical journal editorial noting that, as of 1995, "34,894 publications related to obesity have accumulated since 1966, with 4,785 related to treatment."[6] *Now they tell me!*

What I found in that mountain of paper shocked even me. Much of the conventional wisdom on weight loss is either unsupported by the voluminous research data on obesity or clearly contradicts them. The question was then no longer "Why are Americans so much heavier than before and so much heavier than Europeans?" but rather "Why aren't we even *heavier* than we are?" The short, sad answer appears to be that we're getting there—fast.

At the same time, it's true that obesity is a universal phenomenon. Even among European nations there are marked differences, and many Europeans, while glad they're lightweights compared to Americans, are nonetheless distressed by the growing problem of obesity within their own ranks. They perceive, correctly, they are starting down a path already blazoned by the United States.

Now it's confession time. (No, nothing about sex or murder or anything juicy like that.) I've told you one reason I wrote this book: despair for my country. But the other was despair for myself. For years I've fought against the twenty-five extra pounds I'd put on since I was eighteen. I read the best-selling diet books, I read the magazines filled with "tips" and "fifty-two ways to lose weight," and I watched the infomercials. I did the fad diets. One, I recall, comprised nothing but low-fat buttermilk and sugar-free Jell-O. (I hope you're laughing with me, and not *at* me.) As it happens, as with most fad diets, I did lose weight on this bizarre regimen. And as with all fad diets, I found I could not sustain it, and quickly all the weight roared back with a vengeance.

I finally realized that if I were ever to succeed I would have to comb through the medical literature myself; no one was going to do it for me. As this book progressed, the weight fell off. I have now lost that twenty-five pounds and then some, maintaining the lowest weight I've been as an adult. I've gone from borderline obese to being deep within the safe zone. No, I haven't been asked to model underwear, but hope springs eternal. And while I know that keeping it off will always require a degree of vigilance, I also do not live in fear that my weight will uncontrollably go back up as it always did after the fad diets. Not incidentally, my editor also lost weight as my work progressed and I shared my findings with her. So I know that what I have found is useful not only to me; indeed, it should be useful to everyone. It has clearly been the case here that, as a medieval German poet put it, "He who helps in the saving of others, saves himself as well."[7]

Like any good convert, I'm standing on the rooftop and shouting my message to the people. And from that rooftop, I'm watching those people get bigger by the year. When I wrote most of this book I was in Colorado, which, statistics say, has the lowest incidence of obesity in this country.[8] Indeed, in 1990 when I moved to Colorado and lay out by my apartment complex's swimming pool studying my German, almost all my fellow sunbathers were thin. Six years later I moved back, still studying my German (it's a hard language, damn it), and now most of the sunbathers are fat. Every day, in this thinnest of states, I saw such sad specimens of humanity, huffing and puffing after even a short walk, sweat dripping down their faces even in Colorado's dry climate.

Most people probably know they are cutting their lives short. They know their weight is damaging their quality of life, by interfering with their ability to play sports, play with their children, or just with getting the mail. Many would be delighted if they were only twenty-five pounds overweight, as I formerly was. But most people, as was the case with me, have no idea what to do. They know they're on a conveyor belt straight to obesity, but have no idea how to get off. We are deluged with so much wrong and useless information that even when we hear or read something scientifically based, we have no idea whether it's accurate or just the same old nonsense.

Saddest of all, we see our own children growing up fat. We suspect (correctly) that our children are on the path to a lifetime of obesity, ill health, and premature death. Unlike me, though, few people know how to read a medical journal article. They don't know how to track down and interview the top experts in the field. That was my job.

In sum, I have accomplished one goal: I'm thin again and I love it. It will always be one of my life's biggest accomplishments. As to my second goal, I cannot yet say. I have painstakingly brought together the best that science has yet to offer the obese and slapped it between two covers. Most of the studies from which I've drawn were a heck of a lot less exciting to read than—to use a comparison that appeals to us male types—the *Sports Illustrated* swimsuit edition. I have, however, done my darnedest to make the science interesting—even fun.

Still, can a book that tells the truth about losing weight compete with hundreds of books that tell readers what they want to hear but leave them as fat or fatter than ever? In a sea of books selling nothing but gimmicks, can you sell one that has as its gimmick that all the gimmicks are wrong? I think so. Much of the public has realized that if the first fifteen fad books didn't work, there's not much hope that number sixteen will, either. Tens of millions of Americans have been betrayed by fad-diet books and many darned well know it.

I know I can get individuals off that conveyor belt to obesity. I hope I can reach enough people to get the country as a whole to recognize how truly serious obesity—as a personal problem and as a national epidemic—really is. All I know is, somebody has to try to start a groundswell of change. Somebody has to start crying, "Slam the 'emergency stop' button!" Otherwise, 300,000 people will fall off the end of the belt each year. Permanently.

Michael Fumento
Arlington, Virginia

1

The Perils

of Poundage

"I realized after treating the obese for several years that I had been treating the wrong diseases," Jerry Darm, M.D., told me in an interview. Darm, the director of Weight Control Services at Providence Milwaukie Hospital in Portland, Oregon, is physician to the author of *Diary of a Fat Housewife*, Rosemary Green. She insisted that I talk to him.

"What do you mean?" I asked him. "It was like a religious conversion," he said. "I suddenly realized that hypertension, heart disease, and diabetes are the symptoms of the disease. The disease is obesity."

As with cigarette smoking, the belief that obesity is harmful long predates modern epidemiology. Indeed, at least since Greco-Roman times, obesity has been seen as a health hazard. The Hippocratic texts state that "sudden death is more common in those who are naturally fat than in the lean."[1] Founding Father Benjamin Franklin observed in his *Poor Richard's Almanack*: "To lengthen thy life, lessen thy meals."[2]

How does obesity kill and cripple? Let me count the ways.

Since 1959, data began to confirm earlier suspicions that obesity is harmful. That's when the first Build and Blood Pressure Study appeared. Conducted by the Metropolitan Life Insurance Company of Chicago, it found that using what would be called the

1959 Metropolitan Life Standards as its baseline, the fatter the person, the more likely the person was to die prematurely. By the time one reached 30 percent over recommended weight, there was a 42 percent greater chance of dying early.[3] (As to how much earlier, this will be discussed presently.)

The second Build and Blood Pressure Study came out twenty years later and confirmed the findings of the first. Death rates increased steadily as weight increased, and went up steeply as the percentage over ideal weight increased. The 1979 study found that those least likely to die before their time were from 5 to 15 percent *under*weight.[4]

The American Cancer Society (ACS) conducted a prospective study of 750,000 men and women, meaning the people were enrolled and then their sickness and death rates were observed and compared to their obesity. Reporting in 1986, it found that on the whole, men and women who were 40 percent overweight or more were just short of twice as likely to have died as non-overweight persons. These people were found to suffer excessive diabetes, heart disease, and digestive diseases.[5]

The chart below, from the ACS data, shows a clear correlation between increasing obesity and increasing likelihood of dying during the study period. Thus, for example, persons in the heaviest category (40 percent or more above average weight) had an 87 percent greater chance of dying than those of average weight.

VARIATIONS IN MORTALITY BY WEIGHT AND HEALTH STATUS IN HEALTHY PERSONS IN THE ACS STUDY

Percentage Above Average Weight	*Increased Likelihood of Dying*	
	MALE	**FEMALE**
10%–19%	15%	17%
20%–29%	27%	29%
30%–39%	46%	46%
40%–49%	87%	87%

Source: Adapted from *Annals of Internal Medicine*.[6]

Overseas studies from the Netherlands and Sweden,[7] among other countries, have produced similar findings. A Danish study found obesity was already causing death in men in their twenties and thirties.[8] Scary stuff. In Norway they found that the lowest death rates for men was below the Body Mass Index (BMI) 25 level, while for women it was a 27 BMI.[9]

Let me explain this BMI stuff right now, because you're going to hear about it repeatedly in this book. To calculate your BMI, get your trusty calculator and multiply your weight in pounds by 705. Divide this by your height in inches. Divide this again by your height in inches. Your BMI will be somewhere in the twenties, unless you're extremely overweight or quite thin. If you come up with a BMI of something like 11 or 126, do your calculations again. I'll give you one example to show you how this is done, then you're on your own. Say you're five feet seven inches and weigh 140 pounds. Multiply 140 by 705, which gives you 98,700. Divide this by your height, which is 67 inches. This gives you about 1473. Divide again by 67, which gives you a BMI of 22. This probably won't qualify you for the cast of *Baywatch*, and if you want to model for *Vogue* or *Glamour* you'll have to be below a BMI of 20—and have excellent teeth. But from a health perspective you're in great shape.

THE "20 PERCENT" MYTH

Traditionally obesity has been defined as 20 percent overweight, because it was thought you had to be carrying around that much extra poundage before health problems kicked in.[10] This belief has now been shot to pieces by two major studies, one of Harvard male alumni that appeared in 1993 and one of female nurses that appeared in 1995. Both have much to teach us.

The Harvard study, while declining to opine on whether it's possible to be too rich, made it clear that unless you are affecting your immediate health (such as some anorexics do) one cannot be too thin. It looked at almost 20,000 male Harvard University alumni who graduated between 1916 and 1950. By 1988, almost 4,500 had died. The less the men weighed when they filled out questionnaires (either in 1962 or 1966), the less likely they were to be among the dead when the researchers did their evaluation. The study found that a five-foot-ten-inch man seeking to live as long as possible should weigh no more than 157 pounds, 20 percent less than the average American male of that height. Men in the thinnest fifth were 60 percent less likely to die of heart disease as men in the heaviest fifth.[11]

The Harvard study finally shattered the myth that being somewhat underweight, compared to the average person, is as detrimental to long-term health as being overweight. Why had people believed this? As William Castelli, M.D., director of the Framingham Heart Study, put it, "The lowest-weight group keeps getting contaminated by people who lose weight because they have a chronic illness, usually cancer."[12] Often these people's cancer was smoking-related. So when researchers excluded smokers from their study, and people who therefore died within the first few years of the study (and who were therefore presumably already ill when the study began), they found that the correlation between thinness and premature death disappeared.

The Nurses' Health Study, directed by endocrinologist JoAnn Manson, M.D., of Brigham and Women's Hospital in Boston, was much larger than the study of Harvard men. It comprised 115,000 women and, for the reason I just gave, excluded smokers. It looked at two issues. First, it observed the risks of being heavier than the leanest women. It found that women who weighed about 15 percent less than the average American woman of the same height were least likely to die during the study. Risk did not increase appreciably until the women's BMI surpassed 25, however. Since the average American woman is five feet five inches tall and weighs 150 to 160 pounds, the study indicates that the average woman weighs 30 pounds too many to have a full life expectancy. Those women in the lightest category (120 pounds or less) had the lowest death rates, though Manson emphasizes that these women were not suffering from anorexia.[13] Making yourself little but skin and bones is not healthy; being below average weight in a country where most people are overweight *is* healthy.

Nurses' Health Study

Weight Category (Avg. Ht. 5' 5")	Excess Chance of Death During Study Period
120–149 lbs.	20%
150–160 lbs.	30%
161–175 lbs.	60%
176–195 lbs.	110%
196 lbs. or more	120%

Source: Nurses' Health Study, *New England Journal of Medicine*.[14]

Second, the study looked at the effects of gaining weight (twenty-two pounds or more) after the age of eighteen. It did so because from 1990 to 1996, government weight guidelines allowed persons over the age of thirty-five to weigh twenty pounds more than those under thirty-five. There was little scientific reason for this; rather it appeared to be a mere concession to the reality that persons over thirty-five tend to keep gaining weight. A moment's reflection leads to the realization that this excess weight is not muscle or bone—and therefore it must be fat. Adding fat at any age is just not going to be good for you. The revised government standard was severely criticized,[15] and Manson's findings were the final straw. She found that moderate weight gain (greater than or equal to twenty pounds) after the age of eighteen was harmful.[16] Finally, in 1996 the government bowed to science and abolished the laxer standard for those above 35.[17]

Manson said she was astonished to discover that nearly one third of the deaths from cancer in the nonsmoking women in her study—especially those of the breast, colon, and endometrium—appeared to correlate to obesity.[18] Overall, based on her study and the Harvard male alumni one, Manson said that about 300,000 deaths a year in this country can be attributed to people being overweight. If you do me the honor of finishing this book in a single day, during that time 822 Americans will have succumbed to their fat. This figure may even be a conservative estimate, she said, since the women and men being studied are better educated, more affluent, and presumably more health conscious than average Americans, and therefore likely to have lower death rates.[19] Among controllable causes of deaths, only tobacco smoking takes more lives—an estimated 400,000 annually. By comparison, alcohol claims 100,000 and microbial agents 90,000.[20] But, if current trends continue, says Manson, "it won't be long before obesity surpasses cigarette smoking as a cause of death in this country. We can no longer afford to be complacent about the epidemic of obesity in America."[21]

DUELING WEIGHT CHARTS: WHAT IS AN IDEAL WEIGHT?

The generally accepted standard for appropriate weight is the 1983 Metropolitan Life Table. Yet some people, such as those at the Center for Science in the Public Interest, advocate sticking to the 1959 chart, which allows considerably less weight for height. "It is folly to tell Americans it's OK to weigh more when the people who meet the ideal weights in the old 1959 Metropolitan Life Table do the best," says Castelli, Framingham study director. Agreeing is Meir Stampfer, M.D., professor of Epidemiology and Nutrition at the Harvard School of Public Health. "The lowest mortality rate is not where they say it is," he says of the 1983 table.[22] Indeed, a 1993 review of mortality data in the *International Journal of Obesity* found that the 1959 Metropolitan Life Table probably remains the closest indicator of truly healthy weight, though the authors did grant that in light of today's burgeoning bellies it might seem a bit unrealistic.[23]

METROPOLITAN LIFE TABLES, 1983 AND 1959

Measurements are in bare feet and without clothes. The numbers in bold and parentheses are for the 1959 table.

MEN

Height	Small Frame	Medium Frame	Large Frame
5'1"	123–129 (107–115)	126–136 (113–124)	133–145 (121–136)
5'2"	125–131 (110–118)	128–138 (116–128)	135–148 (124–139)
5'3"	127–133 (113–121)	130–140 (119–131)	137–151 (127–143)
5'4"	129–135 (116–124)	132–143 (122–134)	139–155 (131–147)
5'5"	131–137 (119–128)	134–146 (125–138)	141–159 (133–151)
5'6"	133–140 (123–132)	137–149 (129–142)	145–163 (137–159)
5'7"	135–143 (127–136)	140–152 (133–147)	147–167 (142–161)
5'8"	137–145 (131–140)	143–155 (137–151)	150–171 (146–165)
5'9"	139–149 (135–145)	146–158 (141–155)	153–175 (150–169)
5'10"	141–152 (139–149)	149–161 (145–160)	156–179 (154–174)
5'11"	144–155 (143–153)	152–165 (149–165)	159–183 (159–179)
6'	147–159 (147–157)	155–169 (153–170)	163–187 (163–184)
6'1"	150–163 (151–162)	159–173 (157–175)	167–197 (168–189)
6'2"	153–167 (155–166)	162–177 (162–180)	171–202 (173–194)
6'3"	157–171 (159–170)	166–182 (167–185)	176–202 (177–199)

WOMEN

Height	Small Frame	Medium Frame	Large Frame
4'9"	99–108 (89–95)	106–118 (93–104)	115–128 (101–116)
4'10"	100–110 (91–98)	108–120 (95–107)	117–131 (103–119)
4'11"	101–112 (93–101)	110–123 (98–110)	119–134 (106–122)

METROPOLITAN LIFE TABLES, 1983 AND 1959 *(cont'd.)*

WOMEN

Height	Small Frame	Medium Frame	Large Frame
5'	103–115 (96–104)	112–126 (101–113)	122–137 (109–125)
5'1"	105–118 (99–107)	116–129 (104–116)	125–140 (112–128)
5'2"	108–121 (102–110)	118–132 (107–119)	128–144 (115–131)
5'3"	111–124 (105–113)	121–135 (110–123)	131–148 (118–133)
5'4"	114–127 (108–116)	124–138 (113–127)	134–152 (122–139)
5'5"	117–130 (111–120)	127–141 (117–132)	137–156 (126–143)
5'6"	120–133 (115–124)	130–144 (121–136)	140–160 (130–147)
5'7"	123–136 (119–128)	133–147 (125–140)	143–164 (134–151)
5'8"	126–139 (123–132)	136–150 (129–144)	146–167 (138–155)
5'9"	129–142 (127–137)	139–153 (133–148)	149–170 (142–160)
5'10"	132–145 (131–141)	142–156 (137–152)	152–173 (146–165)
5'11"	135–148 (135–145)	145–159 (141–156)	155–176 (150–170)

Source: Metropolitan Life Insurance Company.

Still, weight tables are just a tool. If you're a weight lifter, it's only natural that you will exceed the table margins. If you're a model, you're probably going to want to be below; that's not for reasons of health but rather the demands of your job.

Certainly there are other means of measuring excess fat, some of them better. One is the aforementioned BMI. Remember that if you're over a 25 BMI (unless you're quite muscular), you're probably putting yourself at risk. The higher the BMI, the higher the risk.

Another method of determining fat, which I don't recommend you do yourself, is using calipers. If somebody knows how to use them on you, fine. But if they're not placed in just the right position, your results are meaningless.

More sophisticated methods of body-fat measurement can only be done at clinics or health clubs. These include both being submerged in a pool of water for five seconds while your underwater weight is measured on a scale, and having a painless electrical charge sent through your body. The latest innovation is called the Bod Pod. It's a unit you sit inside that's egg-shaped—though not to worry since it's cholesterol-free.[24]

John Foreyt, director of the Nutrition Research Clinic at Baylor College of Medicine in Houston, recommends choosing as a target the lowest weight you've been able to maintain for a year as an adult while exercising regularly and eating healthily.[25] Of course, if there was no year in your adulthood where you exercised regularly and ate healthily, start now and use one of the other methods I've discussed above. All this said, there are going to be some people who will never be lean by any of these standards. They won't make the top level of the 1983 chart, much less the 1959 one. I'm convinced very few such people are out there, but the advice for them is to at least lose *something*. If you're 300 pounds now and think you'll probably never be able to sustain yourself at 150, you're probably right. But if you can get down to 250 you'll feel better, look better, and probably live longer.

Inevitably to tell people they should be thin is to suffer accusations that you're encouraging anorexia nervosa, a disorder in which women—and occasionally men—greatly undereat and sometimes even starve themselves to death. America's favorite tabloid in magazine format, *People*, had a 1996 cover story telling us "How Media Images of Celebrities Teach Kids to Hate Their Bodies."[26] (Never mind that *People* leads the way in showing these media images; in that very issue, aside from advertising, it portrayed twenty-seven exceptionally thin actresses and models, two overweight ones, and one average-weight one.) If we stopped worrying about being so thin, we are told, we wouldn't have these problems.

But charging that telling people to be thin is encouraging anorexia is like saying that telling people they should wash their hands frequently is encouraging the obsessive compulsive anxiety disorder in which people may wash their hands hundreds of times a day. Both anorexia and compulsive hand-washing are mental illnesses, not just the extreme end of a spectrum.

The way to deal with these problems is to treat the underlying disorder, not to tell people it's OK to be fat and to have filthy hands.

How Does Obesity Kill?

That obesity is a tremendous cause of premature death is simply beyond doubt. There is some room for speculation, though, as to *how* it kills. The following is the latest medical science has been able to come up with, broken down by disease category.

HEART DISEASE

The major risk of death from obesity is from heart disease. There may be independent factors such as high cholesterol, diabetes, and hypertension. Studies associating obesity with heart disease and death include the Framingham Study, the Coronary Heart Mortality Risk Study, the Honolulu Heart Study, the Paris Prospective Study, and the Study of Men Born in 1913.[27] Some of these studies found that obesity was an independent risk of disease while others found it had to be associated with high cholesterol or other health problems that themselves contribute to heart disease.[28] The development of drugs to treat high cholesterol and other heart-related problems has no doubt contributed greatly to the seeming paradox of a national decline in heart-disease deaths even while the population gets fatter by the year.

Unfortunately, some wishful people have latched onto this decline in heart-disease deaths, claiming it as evidence that obesity isn't harmful. For example, Dale Atrens, in his book *Don't Diet*, claims, "The fact that, as a species, humans continue to get fatter and healthier at the same time suggests that perhaps we are not so blighted after all."[29] Actually, what he means is simply that we're living longer. But that's like saying that AIDS must not be killing anyone because the year before the epidemic began, 1980, American life expectancy at birth was 73.7 years and by 1993, at the height of the AIDS epidemic, it was 75.5 years.[30] Medical advances elsewhere have offset deaths from obesity, that's all.

HYPERTENSION

High blood pressure greatly increases the risk of stroke, a condition that is debilitating and often fatal. High blood pressure is also a risk factor for heart attacks. As one review of studies put it, "There is overwhelming theoretical, epidemiological and experimental evidence for an association between obesity (especially upper body obesity) and high blood pressure."[31] For example, according to one study of Americans aged 20 to 75, overweight people were three times more likely to have high blood pressure.[32] True, a host of blood pressure–lowering medicines are available, but even these are less effective with obese than non-obese persons.[33]

In 1997 the Nurses' Health Study directly tied stroke to obesity. The more weight gained, the greater the risk. Women who gained more than 44 pounds were two and one half times more at risk of a blood clot–related stroke, the most common kind. Each year, more than twice as many women die of stroke than of breast cancer.[34]

DIABETES

About 15 million Americans have Type II diabetes, or what used to be called adult-onset or non-insulin-dependent diabetes. Insulin is the pancreatic hormone that regulates transport of glucose (blood sugar) into cells. Unlike Type I diabetes, in which the body fails to produce insulin, Type II diabetes is characterized by adequate amounts of insulin, at least at first. But the body develops a resistance to insulin's actions. Type II diabetes disproportionately afflicts nonwhites. It occurs in blacks about twice as often as in whites. Among Hispanics, the rate is two to three times that for whites, and in Native Americans it is five to six times the white rate. While Type II diabetes afflicted less than 1 percent of the population in 1958, that figure has more than tripled to about 3 percent, with the rate continuing to rise. The disease and its complications now account for as much as 15 percent of health-care costs. Each year, 24,000 Americans develop kidney failure and 54,000 have to have a leg amputated because their diabetes wasn't properly controlled. At any age, people with diabetes have twice the normal death rate. Most of the blame for this increase in the incidence of diabetes goes to obesity.[35] Despite the claims of fat activists that "obesity by itself is not a risk factor" in high blood pressure, high cholesterol level, or adult-onset diabetes,[36] the link between diabetes and obesity has long been regarded as a clear and present danger. For example, in a Scandinavian study that followed subjects over a period of ten years, *moderate* obesity was associated with a *tenfold* increased chance of diabetes while the rate rose much higher with severe obesity.[37] According to the Nurses'

Health Study, a weight loss of eleven to forty-four pounds can reduce the risk of diabetes in just four years.[38] One study estimated that half of all non-insulin-dependent diabetes could be prevented by controlling obesity,[39] while another said that three fourths of persons with Type II diabetes would benefit from weight loss.[40]

CHOLESTEROL

High levels of cholesterol are often associated with obesity. In the National Health and Nutrition Examination Survey conducted from 1976 to 1980 (NHANES II) obese persons had a 50 percent higher risk of high cholesterol than lean ones.[41] A fairly recent analysis of white men found that the higher the BMI, the higher the men's level of triglycerides (blood fat) and total cholesterol levels. Likewise, the higher the BMI, the lower the level of high-density lipoprotein (HDL), the so-called good cholesterol.[42] Data for women is sketchier, though there's no intrinsic reason to think that they are different in this regard than men. So obesity increases the bad stuff and decreases the good stuff.

CANCER

In his 1996 book advocating fat acceptance, *Big Fat Lies*, Glenn Gaesser tells readers that many studies show a link between obesity and *lower* rates of lung cancer and premenopausal breast cancer.[43] He doesn't mention that premenopausal breast cancer is fairly rare, nor does he talk about any other types of cancer. That could be because they don't support his conclusions. The aforementioned ACS study found that death from cancer overall was 33 percent higher for men and 53 percent higher for women whose weight was 40 percent, or more, above average.[44] Overweight men had a significantly higher chance of dying of colon and rectal cancer and prostate cancer than men at the healthiest weights. Overweight women had significantly higher rates of endometrial, gallbladder, cervical, ovarian, and breast cancer (post- and pre-menopausal combined).[45]

The more researchers look for links between obesity and cancer, the more links they find. Thus a 1995 study in the *Journal of the National Cancer Institute* documented that the heaviest men it considered had three times the risk of contracting cancer of the esophagus as the lightest ones.[46] A 1994 study found that weight

gain in women by age thirty of even ten or twenty pounds may substantially increase the risk of breast cancer later in life. The study,
from the H. Lee Moffitt Cancer Center and Research Institute
in Tampa, Florida, found that at age thirty, the women who later
got breast cancer weighed an average of 131 pounds while the
comparison group weighed 120. By age forty, the women who
got breast cancer weighed 139 pounds, compared to 128 for the
healthy women.[47] Similarly, Harvard researcher Walter Willett,
M.D., in an as yet unpublished evaluation of the Nurses' Health
Study, found a steady correlation between obesity and breast cancer
in postmenopausal women. Women just forty-four pounds over
ideal weight fully doubled their risk of breast cancer. He also found
this had nothing to do with their fat intake; rather, the correlation
was to the fat they were carrying around on their bodies.[48] If that's
not bad enough, yet another study has found that overweight
women who detected breast tumors as a result of self-examination
generally caught the lumps at a later—and more dangerous stage—
than leaner women.[49] All that extra fleshy tissue just makes it that
much harder to find small lumps.

ARTHRITIS

As one would guess, extra weight on the knee joints can lead to
arthritis, and it's not for nothing that one sees a lot of severely
obese people using canes or even wheelchairs. Then the lack of
walking makes them even fatter, in a vicious cycle. One study of a
thousand London women showed that the heaviest women it
looked at were six times more likely to have osteoarthritis of the
knee than the lightest ones. It also found other joint problems.[50]

GALLBLADDER DISEASE

Formation of gallstones has been associated with obesity for many
years. It's been reported that 29 to 45 percent of extremely obese
persons have gallbladder disease[51] and that gallstones occur three
or four times more often in obese persons than in lean ones.[52]

SURGERY

Putting it bluntly, after a certain point, the fatter you are the less
likely you are to survive an operation, which is why some doctors
tell their patients they won't even do surgery until the patient loses

weight. A survey of women undergoing hysterectomies for cancer found that an amazing 20 percent of women 300 pounds and over did not survive the operation. For women 250 to 299 pounds, this dropped way down to about a 5 percent chance of death, while for those 200 to 249 it fell to a 1.5 percent chance of dying during the operation.[53]

TRAUMA

Each year, there are about 19 million injuries to Americans that are at least temporarily disabling. Ninety-two thousand die. The obese are no more likely to be injured, aside from such instances as the 300-pound young man I know of who leaned against the rail on his second-floor balcony and broke through, falling to the ground and breaking numerous bones. But they are considerably more likely to die of their injuries. Again, death rates increase dramatically as weight goes up. One study of persons admitted to a Virginia hospital for blunt trauma found that severely overweight patients (a BMI of 31 or greater) were more than eight times as likely to die of their injuries as those in the lean group (average BMI less than 27). Those with a BMI between 27 and 31 were 38 percent more likely to die. Deaths were most likely to be the result of lung difficulties, particularly pneumonia.[54]

GOUT

As obesity increases, so too does the risk of gout. One study found that obese women had more than twice the chance of developing this painful but not life-threatening disease.[55] The risk appears to be even higher for men.[56]

BLINDNESS

Cataracts are the leading cause of blindness worldwide and cost Medicare (meaning you and me as taxpayers) an estimated $3.4 billion in 1991. A recent study found that obese Americans (using as its definition a BMI of 27.8 or higher) have twice the chance of developing cataracts as lean ones.[57]

BURNS

This is a new area of study and the information is limited but suggestive. A study of fifteen obese burn patients carefully matched with fifteen non-obese patients found that the obese ones were eight times more likely to have a spread of bacteria in the bloodstream, twice as likely to have their wounds become infected, and twice as likely to develop pneumonia. They also required antibiotics for twice as long. Fortunately their conditions were generally treated successfully, and only six of the obese patients died compared with five of the non-obese ones.[58]

BIRTH DEFECTS

A pair of 1996 studies found that obese women are at least twice as likely as thinner women to have babies with debilitating birth defects. The problems involved so-called neural-tube defects including spina bifida (an incomplete closure of the spinal column that often results in paralysis), and anencephaly (in which most of the brain is missing). The increased likelihood of these defects was found in the offspring of women who were obese at the time of conception, not in women who just gained too much weight during their pregnancies. Further, the studies found that while consuming enough of a B vitamin called folic acid can reduce the incidence of these defects in thinner women, it did nothing for the babies of the obese women.[59] Thus we now know that for a woman, reducing her weight can save not only her own life but that of her future children.

BAD SEX LIVES, MARRIAGES, AND SOCIAL LIVES

Weight loss can also save your marriage. Persons who have lost weight and the spouses of these people report an increase in the frequency of sexual relations, and the spouses think of their thinner partners as being more sexually attractive. Obese people are less valued as potential marital partners. Obese persons have a more difficult time arranging dates and establishing intimate relationships, marry later, and their mates tend to be less desirable than spouses of thinner people.[60]

SUFFER THE LITTLE CHILDREN

Many adults think chubby children are cute. That's a matter of personal preference. What's not a matter of opinion is that fat children may be looking at a lifetime of trouble, and a shorter lifetime at that.

An ongoing study of 14,000 people in Bogalusa, Louisiana (one of the fattest states in the country), finds that heart disease clearly begins in childhood. "We have evidence of fatty streaks in the arteries of overweight children as young as three years old, and high blood pressure in children as young as five years old," said Gerald Berenson, M.D., principal investigator of the Bogalusa Heart Study and director of the Tulane Center for Cardiovascular Disease in New Orleans. "Those fatty streaks begin to turn into fibrous plaque, the kind of lesion that can ultimately lead to a heart attack."[61] One doctor recently estimated that of the 80 million children in the United States today, 30 million will die of heart disease, because even if they lose their extra weight later, they are causing irreversible damage to their hearts.[62]

Obesity is the most common cause of high blood pressure in children. One study showed that of 309 children classified as obese, 114 suffered from hypertension.[63] Obese children also have higher risk factors for other causes of heart disease, including high cholesterol.[64] Childhood obesity is also associated with numerous non-life-threatening diseases, such as skin irritations caused by skin rubbing against skin.[65]

But the most dangerous aspect of childhood obesity is that it makes adult obesity and early death all the more likely.[66] One review of studies found that about half of the obese preschool children became obese adults, and that for all children of all ages the obese child is about twice as likely to become an obese adult as a thin child.[67] The older the obese child, the more likely that child is to become an obese adult. Another study review found that "The prediction [that an obese child will be obese at age thirty-five] is excellent at age eighteen years, good at thirteen years, but only moderate at ages younger than thirteen years."[68]

The good news is that fat babies apparently usually don't stay fat. One group of 203 British infants were followed, of whom initially 14 percent were obese and another 26 percent were overweight. But by age five, only 2.5 percent were obese and 11 percent overweight.[69] This also helps dispel the notion that fat adults were born that way. Obese people are made, not hatched. In any case, the lesson for parents appears to be that if you have a fat baby, don't worry about it. Don't put skim milk in your baby's bottle and don't put your two-year-old on a diet. But by the time the child is in school, if he or she is still fat it's time to start doing something.

A Harvard study of 508 people ages thirteen to eighteen who were enrolled from 1922 to 1935 found that "overweight in adolescence predicted a broad range of adverse health effects that were independent of adult weight after fifty-five years of follow-up." In other words, regardless of whether they became thin later in life, being obese as adolescents left them with permanent risks. Among these risks were premature death in general, coronary heart disease, hardening of the arteries, colon and rectal cancer, and gout.[70] Other studies in the United States and elsewhere have found similar results.[71]

As one team of researchers put it, "Because body-mass index appears to be programmed early in life, the prevention of overweight in childhood and adolescence may be the most effective means of decreasing the associated mortality and morbidity in adults."[72]

But the flip side of the problem of fat children becoming fat adults is that if you can stop the problem in childhood, you can greatly reduce the nation's adult obesity problem. "Obesity could be eliminated in a few generations if our children were raised to know and practice prudent eating and exercise habits," stated John Foreyt and his colleague at the Baylor College of Medicine in Houston, G. Ken Goodrick, in an editorial in the British medical journal *The Lancet*.[73] An editorial in a different journal echoed that sentiment, declaring, "The solution of the [obesity problem in general] requires improvement in life styles from early childhood on. . . ."[74]

Obese children may also be set up for psychological problems later in life. Children can be cruel—intentionally or otherwise—to overweight kids. One researcher asked children to rate individuals as potential playmates based on questionnaires and photographs. He found that a child will choose a playmate with a major physical handicap or one in a wheelchair over one who is obese.[75]

CHILD SEE, CHILD DO

One day while sitting in a doctor's office I caught an installment of Leeza Gibbons's show, *Leeza*. I swear, I do not watch talk shows unless I'm a captive audience. This show featured three mothers and their obese children.[76] One of the mothers wasn't particularly concerned about her child's problem, and in truth her child appeared to be the least fat. The other two wrung their hands in desperation over their children's habit of overeating. Perhaps because everybody in the audience was as fat as the mothers, nobody bothered to point out that both of these mothers were terribly obese themselves. But how can a mother expect her child to not overeat when she, the prime role model, does? How can a mother expect a thin child when she presents an example of obesity?

The number one thing parents can do to keep their children from becoming overweight is to keep their own weight down. As if we needed them, studies show a direct correlation between the eating habits of mothers and their children.[77] Says Rockefeller University's Michael Rosenbaum, M.D., "Often when I tell parents to get the potato chips out of the house, I'll hear, 'I can't; my husband loves them.' " But, he says, "It's just not realistic to expect a child to make restrictions in his diet if everyone around him isn't."[78] Parental obesity has also been associated with having children who are less active.[79] Likewise, less-active parents, who are often obese, tend to have less-active children.[80]

In 1996 Leonard Epstein released four studies that began with obese children ages eight to twelve and followed them for ten years. The studies "provide the first indication that children can make changes in eating and exercise behaviors resulting in long-term improvement in relative body weight," he concluded. The key? Getting the parents to not only help and encourage the children but to change *their* habits, too.[81] Again, it comes down to child-see, child-do. As two researchers, Alexander Leung and William Robson of the University of Calgary in Canada, recommended, "All family members should alter their eating habits to conform to the child's needs, because a double standard at the family table undermines the child's efforts."[82]

As always, dealing with the problem requires that people recognize it. And clearly we're not there yet. Childhood obesity is rarely mentioned by politicians, the media, or health-care workers, and so apparently this problem will very likely continue to grow worse and affect our society for decades to come.

THE "NOT AN INDEPENDENT CAUSE" FALLACY

One argument fat acceptance people make that drives obesity researchers and nutritionists to slam their heads against the nearest wall is the claim that, as Glenn Gaesser puts it in *Big Fat Lies*, "No study yet has convincingly shown that weight is an independent *cause* [his emphasis] of health problems."[83] First, when you see "convincingly" used like that, it usually means "they haven't convinced *me* yet"—and it's implicit that they never will.

More to the point, Gaesser is conceding that, yes, there certainly does seem to be a connection between obesity and certain health problems; it's just not necessarily causal. Then the way the game works is to argue that "If you just eliminate the excess hypertension and coronary disease and cancer among this group, you find that their death rate is no higher than that of the thinner people." And essentially this is correct. Likewise, you could argue that the heavy, sharp blade of Madame Guillotine was not the actual cause of death of France's King Louis XVI. Rather, it was the severing of his vertebrae, the cutting of all the blood vessels in his neck, and the slicing of his windpipe. Add to that the trauma caused by his head dropping several feet into a wicker basket. But for some reason, historians don't usually make this point.

"IT'S OK, I'M A 'PEAR,' RIGHT?" WRONG.

You've probably heard that being an "apple"—that is, having your excess fat concentrated in the abdominal region—is worse for you than being a "pear," which is when the excess fat concentrates in the lower body. Medically, this is expressed as a matter of waist-to-hip ratios. If you have a high ratio, you're an apple; if you have a low one, you're a pear. If you watch too much television, you become a vegetable, but that's discussed in a later chapter. You have no doubt read that if you are a pear, you have little to worry about. Some have even gone so far as to proclaim lower-body (also called noncentral) fat as being good. Gaesser has a chapter on it called "Good Body Fat, Bad Body Fat." In it he writes, "It's not how much body fat you have but where you have it that is important."[84] *Newsweek* magazine, in an April 1997 cover story titled "Does It Matter What You Weigh?," based heavily on Gaesser's claims and those of fat acceptance journalist Laura Fraser, says, "Fat hips and thighs, which give you that much-maligned pear shape, may injure only the ego."[85]

But while I fully encourage you to buy apples and pears, please don't buy into the apple-pear mythology. "Noncentral obesity is not metabolically benign," concluded a recent report in the *Journal of the American Medical Association.* Instead, the researchers found that among the more than 2,300 Canadians whom they studied, BMI, a measurement that makes no distinction as to where fat is located, "tends to be the stronger predictor" of conditions that can cause illness and death such as high blood pressure and high cholesterol. It specifically warned against the belief that people who are overweight but carry the fat below the waist are at no risk.[86] This study notwithstanding, it could still be true that "Dunlap's disease" (in which the gut "done laps" over the belt) does carry a higher risk than Thunder Thighs or Bubble Butts. But to equate lower risk with no risk, much less being "good," is terribly irresponsible.

Let's go further to consider the case of an acquaintance of Gaesser's, "Lucy," a thirty-year-old woman who despite being 206 pounds at only five feet five inches "has excellent levels of cholesterol, blood sugar, and blood pressure." How can this be? "Lucy, like a lot of women, carries the body fat on her hips and thighs," Gaesser points out.[87] But at age thirty, Lucy would be in no real danger of heart disease no matter what these various indicators showed. (Unless, of course, she had some rare condition that made these indicators absolutely astronomical.) Only about 1,100 American women between the ages of twenty-five and thirty-four die of heart disease each year. It's only after menopause, which usually takes place around the late forties or early fifties, that a woman's risk of dying of heart disease starts to go up.[88] About 8,100 American women between the ages of thirty-five and forty-four die each year of heart disease, and more than 22,000 women die between forty-five and fifty-four.[89]

But guess what else happens after menopause? Estrogen levels drop drastically and a woman's body fat to a great extent shifts up above the waist.[90] "In the Nurses' Health Study," Manson told me, "we saw a trend towards higher waist-to-hip ratio with age."[91] Just when Lucy least wants that shape, she'll get it anyway. It's proof once again that life isn't fair. It's also proof that telling women it's okay to be pear-shaped is potentially deadly advice.

The other problem with Gaesser's dictum is that "how much body fat you have" can determine "where you have it." Once a woman reaches a certain level of obesity, invariably she's carrying much of it above the belt. One ramification of this is that as the population fattens we are also seeing a shift from pears to apples.

THE BOTTOM LINE ON OUR GROWING BOTTOMS

Obesity hurts us all when physical problems strike us or our loved ones. But obesity hurts us all in another way: our pocketbooks, courtesy of federally-funded national insurance programs like Medicare, Medicaid, and Social Security Income. Harvard researcher Graham A. Colditz, writing in the *American Journal of Clinical Nutrition* in 1992, calculated the costs to the nation of obesity as of 1986. At that time, about 34 million U.S. adults were considered obese. Breaking down health problems by category, he found that Type II diabetes cost $11.3 billion; cardiovascular disease, $22.2 billion; gallbladder disease, $1.5 billion; hypertension, $1.5 billion; and breast and colon cancer, $1.9 billion. Together these came to $39.3 billion, or 5.5 percent of the costs of all illnesses in that year. But, he said, adding in the costs of obesity-induced or aggravated musculoskeletal diseases, like arthritis, would raise that to 7.8 percent of costs.[92] In 1994 he updated that number to $68.8 billion.[93] The Institute of Medicine (a branch of the National Academy of Sciences) in a report released in December 1994, *Weighing the Options*, adapted Colditz's figure and estimated that additional expenditures on obesity, such as for diet programs, devices, and foods, was $30 billion, putting the national cost of obesity at a nice round $100 billion per year.[94]

CAN THE HEALTH EFFECTS
OF OBESITY BE REVERSED?

In Charles Dickens's classic *A Christmas Carol*, a repentant and terrified Ebenzer Scrooge implores the Ghost of Christmas Yet to Come, "Why show me this, if I am past all hope!" Says Scrooge, "Assure me that I yet may change these shadows you have shown me, by an altered life!"[95] The overweight reader may well now ask the same of me. And the answer is that for you, like Scrooge, it is not too late. Sure, the best thing is not to have become overweight in the first place. Like smoking or using illicit drugs, it's a heck of a lot easier not to do it originally than to quit. I hope I've provided some nice incentive for lean persons to stay that way. But for the overweight, as with old Ebenezer, there is hope of redemption. (Unlike with the spirits, however, it can't all be done in one night.)

"Indirect evidence suggests strongly that weight loss does reverse almost all the health hazards of obesity," says John Garrow, M.D., the dean of British obesity researchers. "Life insurance data show that people who were impaired solely on account of obesity have normal insurance risks after losing weight[96] and all the risk factors for coronary heart disease—blood pressure, cholesterol, triglyceride, uric acid, and fasting glucose concentrations; forced vital capacity—also improve with weight loss.[97] The obese patient who loses weight is likely to improve greatly with respect to infertility[98] and osteoarthritis of the knees."[99] The only real disadvantage of weight loss, he says, is that during the loss itself cholesterol trapped in fatty tissues is released into the bloodstream and raises cholesterol levels. But that is a scant added risk for a short time in exchange for a lifetime of lessened risk.[100] A review of numerous studies in the *International Journal of Obesity* in 1992 also bore this out, finding that even modest weight loss was beneficial, but that naturally the more weight lost, the better.[101]

"I'm amazed," says Jerry Darm. "Sometimes within weeks [of a patient beginning a weight-loss regimen] I see problems go away. I've seen diabetics normalize with a few weeks of weight loss."[102]

Would you like some more good news? Just as obesity is "contagious" in the sense that people tend to fatten up to the level of the persons around them, losing weight also appears to be contagious within a family. A Swedish study looked at forty-seven family members of ninety-two patients in long-term obesity treatment and found that thirty-seven lost weight—a considerable thirteen pounds on average.[103] So when you lose weight, you may not just be doing it for yourself. And if you want your child to lose weight, look to thine own self first.

CAN EXERCISE MAKE UP FOR OBESITY?

One thing the fat acceptance groups and their outside supporters are very keen on is the idea that somehow exercise can make up for obesity. "It has become abundantly clear to me that in terms of health and longevity, your fitness level is far more important than your weight," Steven Blair of the Cooper Institute for Aerobics Research writes in his foreword to Glenn Gaesser's book. He emphasizes that "if the height-weight charts say you are five pounds too heavy, or even fifty or more pounds too heavy, it is of little or no consequence healthwise—*as long as you are physically fit*" [emphasis his]. Gaesser makes the same point throughout the book, with one chapter titled "Exercise for Metabolic Fitness: Shaping Up Without Necessarily Changing Shape."[104] This really gives self-deceiving obese people something to hide behind, because they can (and do) assure themselves that while, yes, they burst through the ceiling of the height-weight charts long ago, they "feel like" or "just know" they're in damned good condition.

Of course, exercise can make you less obese, but that's not what Gaesser is talking about. It's also better to be obese and exercise than to be obese and not exercise. The question is: Can exercise actually make up for the health effects of obesity? And the answer is: No.

One group of doctors in 1995 looked at precisely this issue. They compared groups of middle-aged and older men on a nine-month moderate weight-loss regimen who eventually lost an average of twenty-one pounds with those who remained obese but engaged in regular aerobic exercise. In every measured risk factor for heart disease except for one, the study found the benefits of weight loss outweighed those of exercise. In that one study, decreased insulin levels, the two groups came out the same. Conclusion? "These results suggest that weight loss is the preferred treatment to improve coronary artery disease risk factors in overweight, middle-aged and older men."[105] There's simply no substitute for dropping excess pounds.

By great coincidence, both Gaesser and Blair work in the exercise field. (Gaesser is an associate professor of exercise physiology.) Likewise, it's common to see those in the nutrition area (such as weight-loss clinics) downplay or dismiss exercise, while those who tout weight-loss drugs will sometimes downplay both diet and exercise. Parochialism is a common vice among people. But when you're dealing with other people's health and lives, you do have a responsibility to try to rise above it. Gaesser and Blair have not.

THE FOUNTAIN OF OLDNESS

Since long before Ponce de León's travels, men and women have sought a simple potion to make them look younger and live longer. As I write this, the only class of allegedly nonfiction books outselling the diet ones are those promising longevity by popping a pill or other such nonsense. Yet if lab animals are any indication, we as a nation, by getting fatter every year, are doing just the opposite of what we should be doing to live longer. Study after study has found that undernourishment (as opposed to malnourishment) makes creatures live longer and stay in better shape while they're alive. "We've known for years that if you feed laboratory rats and mice less food they can live longer," says George Roth of the National Institute on Aging in Baltimore.[106] There's just not enough human data to say this would also be true for us, but it certainly is intriguing research.

It's also interesting to note what happens to overfed rodents. A 1995 newspaper article showed starkly the consequences of animal obesity. These rats and mice weren't fattened as part of an obesity study but just became so as a result of being allowed to eat too much. In some labs, one common strain of rat has almost doubled its average weight over the last twenty-five years. "They're just blobs of fat with legs," said a researcher.

The animals are used to test various chemicals for toxicity and carcinogenicity, but the health problems caused by their obesity made it "hard to interpret the results of studies that are designed to tell whether a chemical is deadly or safe," the article said. It quoted one researcher saying, "It was a joke in our laboratory—although not a very funny one—that the most toxic substance we've tested in our laboratory over the past twenty years was the food." The article quoted an FDA official saying that a middle-aged lab rat that's allowed to eat its fill "tends to have rough hair, it's yellowish in color, it has horrible-looking teeth, it just looks horrible." In contrast, a rat on a restricted diet "looks young, healthy, slim, shiny, more active," he said.[107]

Yes, I know you have better things to worry about than the appearance of overfed lab rats. But there's clearly a message for us here. Animals—rodents or primates, including humans—were not meant to sit around all day long, whether in a cage or in an office or living room, and eat. Overeating kills. Sure, you can buy nice fashionable clothing that helps hide your obesity. You can blame your genes. You can join a fat rights group. You can stuff your face with only fat-free, "guilt-free," "sin-free" foods. But as the saying goes, you can't fool Mother Nature. We don't have to worry about our fur going yellow, but we are as a nation well on our way to becoming "fat blobs with legs."

My point in this chapter isn't to get everyone to live as long as Methuselah. Rather, it's to try to drive home just how terribly dangerous our growing national obesity problem—and individual obesity problems—are. Life is longer when you're thinner. *And* it's better. Sure, it's amazing what people *won't* do to protect their health. In his book *The Thin Game: Dietary Scams and Dietary Sense*, Edwin Bayrd recounts a story of a Mayo Clinic physician who diagnosed a grossly obese patient with a slow-growing cancer of the colon that required surgery, but said that surgery was out of the question until the patient lost 100 of his 430 pounds. The patient was given a nutritionally balanced, low-calorie diet plan to follow, and was released with a stern warning that his life depended on his ability to lose the weight. In the course of the year, relates Bayrd, "the patient evidently decided that life without the calories to which he had grown accustomed was not worth living, for he returned to the clinic as corpulent as before, and was sent home without the needed operation. Two years later his slothful cancer caught up with him and put an end to his heedless gluttony."[108]

Such inability or refusal to change habits is hardly confined to obesity. In their book *Treatment Adherence*, Donald Meichenbaum and Dennis Turk describe a study on the serious but very treatable eye disease glaucoma. Patients who were diagnosed with glaucoma were told that "they must use eyedrops three times per day or they would go blind." Yet only 42 percent of these patients used the eyedrops frequently enough to avoid permanent damage to their vision. Even of those whose sight had deteriorated to blindness in one eye, only about a fourth took action to avoid further loss.[109]

If I may be allowed to return to my Dickens analogy, I will spend much of the rest of this book in the role of the three spirits. I will do my very best to show you the way. But as with Scrooge, everything is ultimately up to you. I'm no spirit and regrettably possess no magical powers. But I've got one thing going for me that the spirits didn't have: empathy. I've been there. I've been fat. And though that's no longer the case, I still share the American culture, with its weaknesses and temptations. I just happen to have learned a few things others haven't. Come, take hold of my garment (OK, enough of the *Christmas Carol* stuff) and let's see what I've found.

2

One Nation,

Overweight

If you listen carefully, you can almost hear it. It's the sound of zippers tearing, of buttons popping, of spandex stretching. The world is getting fatter by the day. And the United States is leading the way. It was perhaps a sign that within a three-month period in 1996, two different Americans, both living in the same New York City borough of Brooklyn, had to be cut out of their homes and taken to hospitals on stretchers normally used to carry small whales. Both weighed nearly 1,000 pounds.[1]

Just how many of us are obese? I've said one third, but we can't say exactly because researchers always take several years to analyze the data and American waistlines are expanding so fast the statisticians have trouble keeping up. At this writing, the latest data available was from 1988 to 1994. At that time, the government considered over 71 million Americans to be obese. To determine obesity, the government uses the Body Mass Index (BMI), a formula comparing weight to height. In exceptional cases such as bodybuilders, BMI is not an accurate measurement, but for most of us it is accurate, and it certainly is accurate when studying the population in general. Traditionally, the definition of obesity has been 20 percent higher than the maximum healthy level.[2] This is a BMI of about 28. Unfortunately, the government data can be confusing because the government uses the term "overweight" only for those

20 percent overweight or more. In other words, it uses "overweight" for "obese." Thus a *Wall Street Journal* reporter recently tried to reassure her readers that a third of us aren't really obese, just overweight.[3] No, at least a third of us really *are* obese.

For all racial and ethnic groups combined, 31 percent of adult men (twenty years or over) were obese between 1988 and 1991, as were 35 percent of women. This, however, varied greatly by race and ethnicity, especially in the women's category. For white men, the percentage who were obese was about 32; for black men, 31 (the lowest category overall); for Mexican-American men, about 39. For white women, the obesity percentage was about 32, essentially the same as white men and black men. But black women came in at the heaviest at 48.5 percent, while Mexican-American women were close at about 47 percent.[4] The problem is actually probably worse than this, though, because these data rely on people's own word for their height and weight. Nobody actually puts them on a scale. And studies show that people routinely understate their weight and overstate their height.[5]

Young Americans are also plagued by obesity. "Generation X" is well on its way to becoming Generation X-Large. There appear to be no national data on obesity on small children, but what there are on older ones tells a frightening story. Twenty-one percent of adolescents aged twelve to nineteen were obese (20 percent male, 22 percent female) in the measuring period 1988 to 1991, according to 1994 figures. In the previous measuring period, 1976 to 1980, it was only 15 percent. Thus, adolescent obesity jumped by forty percent in the course of a little over a decade[6] while adult obesity went up "only" by a fourth.[7] A separate recent survey of American servicemen and women found that a fifth of those below the age of twenty-one were overweight. "To a degree that often startles visitors to U.S. military bases and even the halls of the Pentagon," commented a *New York Times* writer, "many of the nation's men and women in uniform are seriously out of shape."[8]

While Americans as a whole clearly have a problem, just as clearly that problem is greatest among minorities and especially minority women. The government surveys from which the data is drawn do not, unfortunately, look at other ethnic groups such as Asian-Americans and Hispanic-Americans who are not Mexican.

FATTENING OF THE LAND:
INCREASING AMERICAN OBESITY SINCE 1960

	1960–1962	1971–1974	1976–1980	1988–1994
All	24.3	25.0	25.4	34.9
White Men	23.0	23.8	24.2	33.7
White Women	23.6	24.0	24.4	33.5
Black Men	22.1	23.9	23.9	33.3
Black Women	41.6	43.1	44.5	50.1

Source: *Journal of the American Medical Association.*[9]
*Numbers given represent the percentage of the population within the group.

What is really scary, though, is the trend. For blacks and whites we have good data, going back to the first government survey at the beginning of the 1960s, and the data show obesity is exploding. From the 1960 to 1962 survey period to the 1976 to 1980 period, there was only a slight increase, from 24.3 percent obese to 25.4. But in the ten-year period from then until the 1988 to 1994 survey the number skyrocketed to 34.9 percent.[10] So while ten years earlier, about one fourth of Americans were obese, by 1994 over a third were. If that trend continues, by the turn of the century, 44 percent of Americans will be obese. But remember that the trend is increasing, not just continuing. If it continues to increase as it has, it is possible that by century's end fully one half of us will be obese.

And it gets even worse. So far, the standard I've been using is obesity, which you'll recall is 20 percent overweight or more. But as I explained in the previous chapter, 20 percent is actually an old standard dating from the time when doctors thought you had to be that much overweight before serious health problems began kicking in. As we shall see in the next chapter, that is no longer the case. The Institute of Medicine (IOM) released a report in 1995 in which it determined that for the most part adverse health effects begin at a BMI of 25 or above, not the traditional government standard of about 28. Using data collected from 1989 to 1991, the IOM found that of Americans over the age of thirty-five, *59 percent* are over the healthy limit.[11]

As I've discussed, another way of determining healthy weight is to look at the Metropolitan Life height and weight charts. These were released in 1959 and 1983, based on the findings of the Metropolitan Life Insurance Company as to which of their policyholders were living longest. The firm of Louis Harris & Associates does a poll each year in which it asks people their weight and height and compares these figures to the 1983 Metropolitan Life table. And almost every year, Harris finds Americans are heavier. In its latest poll, released under the title "Americans Get Fatter, and Fatter, and Fatter," *three fourths* of us were too fat for our health.

HARRIS POLL TRENDS

Year	*Percent Overweight*
1983	58
1984	56
1985	62
1986	59
1987	59
1988	64
1989	61
1990	64
1991	63
1992	66
1994	69
1995	71
1996	74

Source: Louis Harris and Associates, Inc.[12]
*No poll was done in 1993.

Note how closely the Harris data match the IOM data. IOM found 59 percent of us at an unhealthy weight between 1988 and

1991, while Harris found it was a little over 60 percent at that time. So IOM's data back up Harris's, meaning that the figure of 74 percent of Americans being at an unhealthy weight in 1996 was probably right on target. So instead of talking about a third of Americans being at risk because of being overweight, we really should be talking about somewhere around *three fourths*.

Now how about mitigating factors to explain the epidemic? For example, when people quit smoking they tend to gain weight, and a lot of us have quit smoking in recent years.[13] This has been a factor but a small one, accounting for perhaps a quarter of the weight gain among women and a sixth of that among men.[14] And now that the decline in smoking appears to have leveled off,[15] no new growth in obesity can be attributed to "kicking the habit."

How about the aging of the population? This, too, is only a small factor. The population has been getting older for decades now, not just in the last ten years. In any case, the government breaks down the data by five age categories, and in all categories weight has inexorably climbed.

No, there's no avoiding the fact that more of us are fatter. And there's no end in sight.

A VERY AMERICAN PROBLEM

Despite numerous trips overseas, I never cease to be amazed at how thin other people are compared to Americans. For example, during a three-day visit to Vienna I saw only two people that could be considered extremely obese, a fraction of the number I would see in any WalMart in America. During a four-day stay in Hong Kong I saw no Chinese of Buddha-esque proportions, although potbellied men and overweight women were somewhat in evidence. But during the next four days in Beijing, in which I had the opportunity to observe enough Chinese to wear out a high-quality electronic calculator, I observed not only no obese natives but also practically no one I could even rate as overweight. I did see two terribly obese persons. One was an American man in my group. The other was an American woman holed up in the McDonald's in which I myself had taken refuge after seeing too many menus with items such as goose feet, fish lips, and dog. (I also saw bottles of liquor in stores that had large snakes coiled up in them and street hawkers selling—I don't kid about such things—duck fetuses on a stick.)

As the table below shows, Americans are the fattest people in the Western world.

THE GIRTH OF A NATION

Average weight of men and women, in pounds, based on an assumed height of five feet four inches:

North America	162
Southern Europe	156
Eastern Europe	150
Western and Central Europe	147
Northern Europe	146
South and Central America	145
Africa	137
Asia	128

Source: Per Björntorp and Bernard N. Brodoff, eds., *Obesity*.[16]

What truly amazes visitors to the United States, though, is not the number of fat people but that the fat people are so very, awfully, terribly fat. "Arriving in America for the first time," James Langton observed in the *Sunday Telegraph* of London, "can be like entering the doors of a freak show. You watch, slack-jawed, as a succession of ever more tremendous backsides parade down Main Street. And then you realize: nobody else even notices." He goes on to describe the "summer uniform of the all-American behemoth: single vest and long baggy shorts to the knees, vast sneakers, like Spanish galleons, supporting tree-trunk calves. These are clothes for comfort, clothes for eating."[17]

Europeans I've interviewed say similar things. "Particularly if you go to a resort like Disney World," says a friend of mine from London. "You come across these amazing characters. They look like Macy's Thanksgiving Day Parade balloons come down to earth without the guide ropes."[18]

How Much Are Americans Really Eating?

Yet, there are those who claim counterintuitively that Americans are eating no more than ever—or perhaps even less. They base this on survey data in which people are asked to recall what they've been eating. One problem with these data is they go back only to 1965, but here are the caloric totals since then.

Historical Caloric Intake (Recall Data)

Years	Total Calories
1965	2,422
1977–78	1,854
1987–88	1,785
1998–91	1,839
1993	1,854
1994	1,949

Source: U.S. Department of Agriculture, Agricultural Research Service.[19]

Some writers have looked at these figures, especially the 1965 one, and concluded that we must be eating far less than we used to; therefore, it can't be additional calories that are making us fatter. In fact, the real explanation for this anomaly is that people don't tell the truth about what they eat.

One indication of this is that the amounts people confess to eating aren't enough to sustain their sizes. For example, for women aged nineteen to twenty-two, average energy intakes in 1987 to 1988 were reported at about 1,500 calories—though it was calculated they really needed to be taking in at least 2,200 calories to sustain their weights.[20] "I don't believe the [consumption] data," says Marion Nestle (no accent over the "e" and no relation to the chocolate company), head of the New York University Department of Nutrition. "We know people are fudging. Average caloric intake on data sets is 1,800 to 2,000 and if that's all people were eating, people would be losing [weight] and not gaining."[21]

Nestle calls this recall bias "the central dilemma of the entire field of nutrition." She says, "The research is very clear that people can't tell what they're eating, whether it's conscious or unconscious," adding, "People tend to overreport consumption of foods that they think are good for them and underreport foods that are bad for them. It's human nature."[22]

For example, a 1991 study comparing what people said they ate to their actual energy intake found that more than half underreported consumption by 20 percent.[23] Another study that year found that 81 percent of subjects surveyed underestimated their food consumption—by an average of 565 calories a day. It also found that the less people reported eating, the more likely they were to be underestimating. The report concluded that "The results of this study, if they can be generalized, will have a substantial impact on the interpretation of our national survey data. . . ."[24]

Who authored the study? Why, the Agricultural Research Service of the Department of Agriculture, the same nice folks who provided the data in the above table. If they don't trust their own numbers, neither should we.

Unfortunately, the incorrect consumption data has led to all sorts of half-cocked theories and studies and diet books purporting to show the "secret" of why Americans are so obese despite eating less. "I've seen absolutely atrocious studies basing their conclusions on dietary intake recall data," says Steven Heymsfield, M.D., an obesity researcher at St. Luke's–Roosevelt Hospital in New York.[25]

Another way of measuring what people might be eating is called "disappearance data." To come up with this, the Department of Agriculture considers all the food available to the American public (meaning that exports are taken into account), and simply divides it by the number of people in the country. These numbers are hard and fast and unaffected by recall bias. They show that we are producing more food per American than ever. Throughout the 1930s and 1940s it was 3,200 to 3,300 calories per person. It actually dipped a little after that but by the 1970s it was up to 3,400 calories and by 1990 had reached 3,700, where it remains today.[26]

The problem with disappearance data is they don't take into account waste—food that never makes it from the farm to the store, from the store to you, or from your refrigerator or pantry into your stomach. Still, Nestle thinks the disappearance data are fairly accurate. "I like disappearance data a lot," she told me. "There's only two places for the food to go, in your garbage and in your stomach. [People argue a lot] goes in the garbage," she said, "but I don't believe it."[27] Indeed, food packaging and preservation techniques are improving all the time, so it's really hard to conceive that we must be dumping more.

"What's wrong with Americans, and I'm one of them, is we just eat too much," says Judith Hallfrisch, a leading carbohydrate researcher with the Department of Agriculture's Human Nutrition Research Center in Beltsville, Maryland.[28]

It's not just that we're eating more, but drinking more as well. And it ain't tap water. "One of the most striking changes in food consumption patterns in the past two decades is the increased consumption of soft drinks, citrus juices, beer, and wine," noted a National Research Council report.[29] The council went on to make its case by using disappearance data. It gave the same warnings on this that I gave you, that a certain amount is lost due to spillage and whatnot, but the steady increase in beverages produced is so stark as to be undeniable. In 1965, Americans each bought an average of 117 gallons. This rose steadily until the last year for which I have data, 1994. That year 167 gallons were available per American—a 43 percent increase since 1965. Only nine of those 160 gallons were bottled water.[30] The most amazing increase was in carbonated soft drink consumption, which has increased more than 140 percent since 1965, from about 19 gallons per person to over 52 gallons in 1994.[31] Carbonated soft drink sales in 1993 were about $49 billion, about the same as the entire Gross Domestic Product of Ireland or New Zealand.[32]

GALLONS OF BEVERAGES AVAILABLE IN FOOD
SUPPLY PER PERSON: 1965–1993

1965	1975	1980	1985	1990	1991	1992	1993	1994
117.3	142.9	142.9	149.8	166.4	167	161.1	162.1	166.8

Source: U.S. Department of Agriculture, Economic Research Service.[33]

AMERICA LEADS THE WAY

But world obesity is also on the rise. Consider it an American export. "It's looming as a large problem," says K. Dun Gifford, president of the Olways Preservation and Exchange Trust, a Boston-based non-profit organization dedicated to promoting traditional foods of many cultures. Europeans are eating "more calories, more meat and more American-style fast food. American fast food combined with a sedentary lifestyle is making the citizens of the world fat."[34]

OBESITY: A GROWING WORLD PROBLEM

Country	Obesity Definition (BMI Greater Than . . .)	Year	Ages	Men %	Women %
Australia	All (men and women): 25	1980	25–64	48	22*
		1986		49	29
Brazil	All: 30	1974–75	18+	2.5	6.9
		1989		4.8	11.7
Canada	All: 27	1985	25–64	20	14
		1991		30	20
England	All: 30	1980	16–64	6	8
		1991		13	15
Germany	All: 30	1985	25–69	15.1	16.5
		1990		17.2	19.3

Country	Obesity Definition (BMI Greater Than . . .)	Year	Ages	Men %	Women %
Netherlands	All: 30	1981	20+	3.9	6.2
		1988		4.6	6.8
Sweden	Men: 30/ Women: 28.6	1980–81	16–84	4.9	8.7
		1988–89		5.3	9.1
United States	All: 30	1988–91		18	24
United States (whites)	Men: 28.8/ Women: 27.3	1960–62	20–74	23.0	23.6
		1988–91		32.0	33.5
United States (blacks)	Men: 27.8/ Women: 27.3	1960–62	20–74	22.1	41.6
		1988–91		31.8	49.2

*Women aged <50 years.

Source: *International Journal of Obesity*,[35] Robert Kuczmarski.[36]

Since at least the end of the Second World War, American culture has had a profound effect on the rest of the world. All indicators are that obesity is part of this package. But if that's any comfort to the average American, consider this: No matter how fat we get, if we keep going the way we are, we will always be that much fatter than everyone else.

OBSESSED WITH THINNESS?

We are constantly told that American culture is obsessed with thinness. This is strange, because usually someone obsessed with something does it a lot. You don't see too many people obsessed with cleanliness who walk about dirty. It is true that when it comes to thinness, we certainly like to talk about it a lot, but talk is usually as far as it gets. For example, we always hear about how many of us are dieting. Dieting is supposedly more common now than brushing your teeth and having sex combined. (I said "combined," not "at the same time.") For example, Glenn Gaesser in *Big Fat Lies* says he's calculated from government figures that "close to one quarter of the entire U.S. population [is] dieting at any one time. . . ."[37] But this doesn't mean anything since "dieting" isn't defined. To some people it means following part of a strict regimen of reduced calories, but to other people at other times it means eating as much as ever but just feeling a bit more guilty about it.

In one *USA Today* article warning about eating disorders in children as a result of dieting attempts, the only study the reporter cited showed that the difference between the children who claimed to be trying to lose weight and those who said they weren't was all of 40 calories a day.[38] Some eating disorder! In fact, the share of Americans who say they "eat pretty much whatever I want" is on the upswing. In 1977 it was 45 percent; in 1987, 52 percent; by 1994, 64 percent.[39]

A 1995 survey by the American Dietetic Association found that only 35 percent of Americans claim to be doing all they can to eat a balanced diet, down from 44 percent in 1991 and 39 percent in 1993—this though 79 percent of those polled said they recognized the value of good nutrition.[40] Health club memberships are down and superindulgent foods like high-fat ice cream are more popular than ever. As one British newspaper reporter put it, "After a decade characterized by the near-obsessive pursuit of health and fitness, after Jane Fonda and Dr. Pritikin, after the optimistic embrace of every slimming and shaping fad from low-cal linguine to liposuction, America is fatter than ever. The populace is literally splitting at the seams, billowing over its belt, and busting out of its buttons."[41]

O FAT NEW WORLD

It would be wrong to conclude that America isn't doing anything about its obesity problem. In fact, as stomachs have stretched and butts have bulged, industry and society have come to the rescue. No, they're not making us any thinner, to be sure. They're just making it a lot easier to be fat.

For example, we've built up a whole lexicon of euphemisms to replace nasty-sounding words like "obese" and "fat" and even the old euphemisms like "big boned" and "heavyset." Now we talk of "people of size," "abundant," "ample," "full," and "supersized." Observed *Time* magazine, "More and more Americans are couching their excess in euphemism these days, and they're not necessarily ashamed of it." It quoted a twenty-six-year-old woman saying, " 'Obviously I don't care,' while gesturing to her 'ample figure and equally ample lunch.' 'I don't care because I find most men I go out with like a woman with some meat on her body.' "[42]

Another sign of the times is the increasing number of fat activist groups, like the National Association for the Advancement of Fat Acceptance (NAAFA), though their combined memberships remain small as yet. They say they're mad as hell and aren't going to take it anymore. But if it's fat acceptance they want, they doth complain too much. For year by year, they're getting their wish more and more. Europeans may be aghast at how large Americans have become, but to Americans being overweight has become normal. Consider:

- Every year, the NPD Group, a market research company in Park Ridge, Illinois, asks how respondents feel about overweight people. In 1985 some 55 percent said being overweight was unattractive. By 1994, that was down to only 36 percent.[43]
- In 1993 *Playboy* proclaimed its first obese Playmate of the Year, Anna Nicole Smith. She was also named the Guess? jeans model that year. She eventually ballooned to 250 pounds.
- A Tampa, Florida, woman, upon having a ninety-one-pound cyst removed, later exclaimed, "All my life they told me I was just obese. I wasn't!" Her weight *after* the tumor was removed? Two hundred and fifteen pounds.[44]
- During the 1996 Summer Olympic games CNN did a short feature on how excess food from the cafeterias was being collected and given to the hungry. The word "hungry" was repeatedly used. But the only person they actually showed receiving the food was so obese that she could have lived off her adipose tissue until the Winter Olympics in 1998.

THIN ACCEPTANCE, ANYONE?

At the same time it's becoming more acceptable to be fat, under-standably it's becoming less acceptable to *not* be—at least if you're really quite thin. Talk show host Oprah Winfrey related the time when she was jogging and a passerby said to her, " 'You better quit losing weight, because you're going to make the rest of us feel bad.' What she really meant," Winfrey says, "was 'Listen, if you start looking better than I do, I'm not going to like you anymore.' "[45]

One extremely thin essayist for *Glamour* magazine related how a woman in a clothing store said to her in a loud and nasty voice: "I can't wait to see how much weight you gain when you have kids. You'll have to go on a diet like a real woman!" On another occa-sion a woman from a campus sorority saw her and whispered to another sorority sister, "Well, I just hope she starves herself to death. It would serve her right!"[46]

Noting that we are being taught that we shouldn't make moral assumptions about people who are overweight, the *Glamour* writer observed, "But we still assume that thin people are narcissistic or emotionally disturbed, and we feel free to express our envy, our suspicion and our contempt in their presence." Indeed, as our society fattens and thin people become more and more the rarity, perhaps it is thin people who will require the protection of our civil rights laws.[47] Still, at a 1996 NAAFA convention, an advisory board member, Michael Loewy, addressed the faithful, telling them, "I have a daughter whom I adore. She is not fat. Nonethe-less, I adore her."[48] (Ah, love conquers all!)

TENT CITY

For those who are fat but want to try to look chic, their choices are growing almost as fast as their bellies and thighs. Sales of large-size women's clothes are growing twice as fast as sales of other apparel, increasing to $16.6 billion by 1994, according to Michael Hand, a vice president at the NPD Group.[49] The market for "big and tall" men, while considerably smaller, is growing faster—22 percent from 1992 to 1993 and 12 percent from 1993 to 1994.[50]

The biggest seller of large clothing is Lane Bryant, whose sales in 1995 reached $1 billion. "We find that women right now are accepting themselves. They love who they are and they're accepting who they are," says one Lane Bryant representative.[51] Yet Lane Bryant is getting more and more competition. Many stores now carry separate lines of clothing for extremely obese women, while some new chains with names like August Max Woman and Modern Woman have also sprung up. In 1991 Saks Fifth Avenue opened a department for obese women, Salon Z. In 1995 it opened an entire floor in its new Beverly Hills store for Salon Z.[52] To make their patrons feel better about themselves, stores employ a variety of Orwellian euphemisms, the most popular of which are "plus" or simply "woman." This makes obesity sound like the standard.

Likewise, it's becoming more difficult for lean people to buy clothes. Increasingly pants, especially jeans, are being sold as "relaxed fit" or "loose fit." "Relaxed" generally means there's more room for a bigger butt and thicker thighs, while "loose" means the actual waist size is bigger. This allows you to wear a size 32 like you did in high school when in fact your waist has since ballooned to thirty-five inches. As "mainstream" stores shift their inventories toward fat people, there does seem to be more catering, specifically to the new outcasts, but even then what does it mean when I walk into a store called Petite Sophisticate and find it sells size 16 outfits?

Women's clothing makers cater to vanity much more often. According to the Institute for Standards Research in Philadelphia, the average size 8 dress in 1942 had a twenty-three-and-a-half-inch waist and thirty-four-and-a-half-inch hips. Today that size 8 has a twenty-seven-inch waist and thirty-seven-and-a-half-inch hips. In her humor column, the late Erma Bombeck observed, "Size 8s are really size 10s; size 10s are really 12, and if there were a shred of truth to advertising, my slacks with the elastic waistband would have a flag attached and be labeled 'Wide Load.' " She continued, "It's been noted that Calvin Klein is a 'forgiving' designer. His size 8s fit bodies that haven't seen a size 8 since they were in grade school. He's not only forgiving, but downright compassionate." She concludes, "Women's dresses and suits are the only clothes that aren't standardized. Downsizing is dishonest. It's misleading. It's downright sleazy. I hope it's a trend that continues to grow."[53]

THE "GROWTH" IN ADVERTISING

As of 1980, a survey found that obese persons in television commercials of any type were virtually non-existent.[54] In the America of today, that's all changed. And while you'd think that advertisers would still shy from using fat people to sell food because of the obvious possible negative connotation, it appears to be in food commercials that they are the most common. "Fat people are visible on American television in a way that would be unthinkable in Britain," commented a reporter for a London newspaper. "One current advertisement ends with a lingering shot of a clearly overweight child devouring a dripping slab of pizza." In Britain, he said, "it would be a turn-off. In America, the fat kid sells pizza."[55]

A better example is a television ad being used by both American and British stations. It features a terribly obese young man in a backwards baseball cap, tennis shoes, and a T-shirt hanging over baggy knee-length shorts. He's dancing to music. In the American version, he just dances. In the British version, however, the voiceover admonishes, "Listen to our station or next time he's naked." To Brits, the young man is a repulsive, slobbish swine. To Americans, he's supposed to be cute.

The Snapple company unabashedly used an extremely overweight representative, Wendy Kaufman, to pitch its product consisting of 220 calories of high fructose corn syrup, water, and a bit of tea in a sixteen-ounce bottle.[56] The commercials were among the most popular on television.[57] Meanwhile, another company specializing in fattening food and fat actors in commercials is the Wendy's hamburger chain. In one ad Wendy's founder, Dave Thomas, appeared as guest "speaker" at the Big Eaters Club, where he presented the Big Bacon Classic Combo, a burger with cheese and not two but THREE strips of bacon. Every member of the Big Eaters Club shown was obese. Since that advertisement, Wendy's has routinely featured obese people in its ads, sending a clear message to its customers: If our huge food makes you huge, that's quite all right.

Still, one commercial deserves a special award for chutzpah. It's a Purina television advertisement for low-fat dog food to reduce your pet's potbelly. The dog actually appears to be in fine shape. But the owner is obese! The message: Put your dog on a diet even if your own health is going to pot.

ADJUSTING TO OBESITY

There's nothing wrong with a fat woman wanting to wear fashionable clothes. Nobody wants a country of slobs. But what I've illustrated here is that as a nation we are making it both easier and more acceptable to be obese, indeed even to be huge. One woman told a newspaper that in the past the lack of stylish clothes for obese women made her watch her weight. But now that stylish clothes are readily available, that's no longer a problem. "I don't want to get any heavier, but I don't feel compelled to lose weight," she said.[58] When you make something easier and more acceptable, you get more of it. You relieve the pressure to deal with the problem. The United States is now effectively institutionalizing obesity, even as we obsess over minor health risks.

It is an irony typical of our times that the September 20, 1995, edition of *The New York Times* carried an article on page B6 gushing over the booming fashion market for the obese,[59] while on the facing page it carried an article by health reporter Jane Brody on the latest study confirming that 300,000 Americans die prematurely each year from obesity.[60] Just as one small company began marketing cigarettes with the cynical name "Death Cigarettes," it would be nice if a company advertised its line of clothing for obese women in terms of "Looking your best as they lay you to rest," or perhaps, "Great frocks for when they lay you in that oversized box!" The title of the Brody piece was "A New Study on Midlife Weight Gain Raises Concerns Among Millions of American Women." But while millions of women were becoming concerned, millions of others of equal or greater weight were too busy shopping at Lane Bryant and Salon Z to notice.

ATTACK OF THE GIANT KILLER FOOD

In 1977 America was struck by *The Attack of the Killer Tomatoes*. Fortunately, it was just a movie. But today the country is under siege by something far more insidious than gargantuan orange-red fruits. It's besieged by giant food.

I knew for sure we were under attack when I visited a Borders book store on the Santa Monica, California, promenade and found that their little pastry and coffee shop sold muffins virtually the size of a head of lettuce. They were worth a thousand calories if they were worth one. I was surprised the server wasn't required to wear a back support belt.

Portion sizes in the States are already fit for a velociraptor and will soon measure up to the expectations of even the largest *T. rex.* *The New York Times* ran a humorous essay on the subject. "In some restaurants," stated reporter Florence Fabricant, "it takes a salvage vessel to recover a fork that accidentally slips into a bowl of fish stew. There are tables set with wine glasses large enough to hold half a bottle." Meanwhile, "Mega-muffins have become the norm. A pretzel from a street vendor is as much food as five slices of bread, a simple cup of coffee has turned into a pint of latté, and beers are starting to come in twenty-two-ounce sizes. Chocolate truffles? Some are as big as hens' eggs."[61]

Four slices of Pizza Hut's recently introduced stuffed crust pizza contain more than 1,700 calories, enough to satisfy your requirements for a day. McDonald's started out with its humble hamburger, weighing in, bun and all, at 3.7 ounces. Then came the Quarter Pounder at 6 ounces and the Big Mac at 7.6. The newest addition, the Arch Deluxe, comes in at close to 9 ounces. In some parts of the country McDonald's sells a Double Big Mac that contains an amazing four beef patties. Sizzler restaurants offer Australian chicken, comprising half a chicken baked, then deep-fat fried. Denny's serves a Super Slam breakfast with three eggs, three pancakes, three sausage links, and three strips of bacon. It's enough breakfast for three persons or one grizzly bear, but is generally consumed by just one human.

A Macho meal at the popular Del Taco Mexican fast food chain weighs almost four pounds, with a pound and a quarter of that coming from just one burrito. But that's Lilliputian food compared to the Green Burrito's three-pound burrito, which compares in heft with a Webster's Collegiate Dictionary. A "medium" theater popcorn now contains sixteen cups.[62] In 1995 Hardee's rolled out its Big Hardee with cheese, which at 690 calories has 160 more than the next-biggest Hardee's sandwich. By one estimate, nearly 25 percent of the $97 billion American consumers spent on fast food in 1995 went for items promoted on the basis of larger size or extra ingredients.[63]

But it isn't just fast food. A chain known for its pasta and dessert dishes, the Cheesecake Factory, heaps food practically a foot high onto its plates and proudly serves up a twelve-ounce burger. Its sales increased by over a third in 1995.[64] The Claim Jumper chain offers a twenty-six-ounce prime rib. Even makers of Lean Cuisine have introduced hearty portions, with 50 percent more food.

More ominous yet is the tremendous upsurge in steakhouses. In 1995, two of the top twenty fastest-growing chains were steakhouses. Lone Star Steakhouse's sales increased by over 50 percent, while those of the Outback Steakhouse increased by almost as much. Steak Out sold almost a third more cow flesh in 1995 than the year before.[65] As I write this, the highest-calorie food at a fast food restaurant is Carl's Jr. Double Bacon Western Cheeseburger, which, including bun, weighs in at about twelve ounces. Yet steakhouses commonly sell porterhouses at twenty-eight ounces, not to mention the accompanying French fries or potato with sour cream. At a new Brazilian steakhouse called Rodizo's in Denver, you're not even limited to that. For $15.99 you can just keep eating meat brought around by several waiters until your belly button pops out and hits a busboy in the eye.

Without fail, the answer you always get from these places when a group like the Center for Science in the Public Interest accuses them of serving three days' worth of calories at a single meal is, "People don't come here every day. This is a special occasion for them." There's a nugget of truth to this. Just because a given person shouldn't be eating more than, say, four ounces of meat a day doesn't mean he or she can't splurge occasionally or perhaps have no meat one day and eight ounces the next. But as the sales growth figures for places such as steakhouses show, visits to such restaurants are becoming less and less special occasions and more and more part of a regular routine.

GIANT FOOD COMPARISONS

Item	Maker of Giant Size	Calories in Giant Size	Calories in Regular Size
Muffins	local shop	705	158
Steak & Fries	Outback Steakhouse	2,060	730
Cookie	local shop	493	65
Ice Cream Cone	local shop	625	160
Nachos	local shop	1,650	569
Cinnamon Bun	Cinnabon, Inc.	800	109
Hot Dog	Oscar Mayer	350	150
McDonald's Meal	McDonald's*	1,310	680

*Specialty meal comprising bacon double cheeseburger, super-size fries, thirty-two-ounce soda. Source: *Prevention* magazine.[66]

Drink sizes are also going up. Twenty-five years ago the size of a soft drink dispensed by machines in the United States was eight ounces. In Europe it's still about that size (not exactly, since they use metric measurements), while in the United States it increased to twelve ounces and then to twenty. A "large" soda fountain drink in Europe is often smaller than the "small" size sold here. Many quick-stop markets in the States now sell drinks in sixty-four-ounce cups (for example, 7-Eleven's Double Gulp), containing 800 calories. One is left wondering if the lids on the cups are to keep the contents from splashing out or the drinker from accidentally falling in. The Double Gulp is doing so well that the company is considering making an even larger size, which its spokeswoman describes as a "wading-pool-sized drink."[67]

In my quest to find out why Americans are so much fatter than Europeans, nothing has struck me as a more obvious reason than portion sizes. Consider my two favorite German candy bars, Ballisto and Lila Pause. Ballistos come two to a package, weighing a total of 41 grams. Lila Pause bars are 37 grams. Contrast that with the smallest individual-size American Butterfinger, which weighs

59.5 grams and has 280 calories. The Butterfinger "supersize" clocks in at a hefty 104 grams and 510 calories. This bar is so big that *Time* magazine picked on it to illustrate the unhealthy trend of growing portion sizes. Unabashed, the Nestlé company created yet a larger size Butterfinger, aptly named the "Beast." It's an amazing 141 grams of mostly fat and sugar containing almost a third of a day's calories, 680. At seven times the size of a Ballisto, it's so big you can club somebody to death with one.

Part of the problem is that Americans don't have any idea anymore what a portion *should* be. "It amazes me how many people who come to me can calculate every gram of fat," says registered dietitian Elyse Sosin, a nutritionist at Mt. Sinai Medical Center in New York. "But they are totally unaware of portion sizes."[68]

Yet there's another reason why humongous portions are so very American. Bigness has a quality all its own. This is perhaps especially true for men. One brand of extra-large TV dinners calls itself the "Man-Handlers." Recall Del Taco's huge "Macho Meal." Macho men eat huge meals; only wimps and girls eat small portions. The Krystals chain specializing in small square hamburgers advertises special "Power-paks" of eight, ten, or twelve, asking "How much power can you handle?" The more of their burgers I stuff down my craw, the more powerful a person I am. The message is more insidious if one knows that in inner-city black vernacular, "power" has a special appeal.*

"Bigness is addictive because bigness is about power," says Irma Zandl, a teen-marketing consultant. She says that while few teenage boys can actually finish a sixty-four-ounce Double Gulp, "it's empowering to hold one in your hand."[69]

Arby's is currently promoting its new Giant Beef 'n' Cheddar sandwich. A sign promoting the sandwich reads: "Bigger *Is* Better." Arby's billboards feature a sandwich stuffed with about a calf's worth of meat. The large letters next to the sandwich read simply: "Big Eats." Meanwhile the Borden food company introduced in 1996 something called simply The Big. Borden discovered the solution to a problem that somehow nobody had ever noticed before, that those slices of "pasteurized processed cheese food"

*Malt liquor (high-alcohol beer) has long been seen as a particular problem among inner-city blacks because it provides inebriation at a low cost. Some years ago one brand of malt liquor advertised itself with the jingle, "Olde English 800 is the power!"

don't quite reach to the edges of a standard slice of bread. Therefore it now makes slices 30 percent larger—and with 30 percent more calories.

But Big Food is harmful for several reasons. First, in and of itself it provides too many calories for one course or at one time. Second, it motivates other manufacturers and sellers to produce big food. Third, it distorts people's ability to tell what a healthy-size portion is. Someone confronted with a mass of giant hamburger sandwiches at every hamburger outlet may understandably conclude that a normal-size hamburger contains a third or a half pound of beef, and will start to make and consume such sandwiches at home as well as in restaurants. Someone who sees eight-ounce steaks labeled "small" at restaurants, with larger sizes ranging up to twenty ounces or greater, may have a difficult time understanding that his meat portions at home should only be three or four ounces. Finally, people feel obligated to eat everything on their plate, whether they really want it or not.

Just as we've gotten over the idea that bigger cars are better cars, we can kick the Big Food habit. For our nation's health, we absolutely must. And the first step is quite easy. Stop buying the damned stuff.

THE COUCH POTATO REPUBLIC

When it comes to accomplishing big things, nobody is more determined or energetic than Americans. The little things, however, are another story. Nobody dislikes expending energy during day-to-day life more than we do.

For example, I know this one guy. He works like a dog—twelve or more hours a day, often seven days a week. As industrious as they come. He also works out several hours a week. Strangely, though, all over his apartment were these black handprints on his walls. They looked like warning signs left behind by some death squad. The culprit, of course, was the guy himself. He read five newspapers a day and got ink on his hands. The ink was then transferred to walls throughout his apartment because he had a very bad habit of leaning every chance he got. Sometimes it was butt-to-counter, but often enough it was hand-to-wall. One day he realized how foolish it was to go to the gym for several hours each week, and then save a few calories here and there by leaning all the time. (Don't confuse me by asking how many calories he burned to wipe the stains off.)

You've probably guessed by now that the person I'm describing is yours truly. "Begin this chapter with something funny, perhaps self-deprecating," suggested my editor. And so I have. But when it comes to couch-potatoism, there's plenty of deprecation to go around.

For example, when I lived in Florida I noticed a common tactic to save a bit of energy was parking in the driving lane right next to the store, even if the parking lot was empty. One day my girlfriend watched in amazement as a police officer wrote out ticket after ticket to such people at a grocery store.

Still, pathological slothfulness exists everywhere in this country. The last time I went to a fast food restaurant, in Denver, there were five cars lined up at the drive-thru window. I got out of my car and walked into the lobby where I was the only customer. If the purpose of fast food is to be fast, I got mine about twelve minutes quicker than the driver of that last car in line. But apparently, saving the effort of getting out of the car and walking a few steps was worth it to him. Denver also has a drive-thru See's candy shop so, as a local paper put it, "Now you don't have to make that embarrassing waddle into the candy store for your mocha truffles or chocolate-covered cherries."[70]

No more pathetic example exists of American sloth than the increasing fraudulent use of handicapped parking placards. As a *USA Today* story heralded in 1996, "Handicapped Parking Abuse Mushrooms." It noted that in Massachusetts the number of handicapped placards grew 600 percent during a period when the state's population grew but one percent. In Texas it jumped 214 percent in a two-year period and in Illinois 130 percent over four years. Granted, this fraud may not always be inspired by laziness. In some major cities it's tough to find a parking spot even at stores, and there may be the temptation to grab one of those open blue spaces. On the other hand, during the three-plus years I lived in Colorado I never had a problem finding a parking space, yet that state saw a rise in handicapped placards of 56 percent during a time when the state's population grew only 9 percent.[71] That doesn't reflect busyness and it doesn't reflect a sudden influx of handicapped persons; it reflects people who can't bear the thought of walking a few extra yards while they run into the store for a box of fat-free Fig Newtons.

The Decline (and Fall?) of Exercise

In 1993 federal health officials called on all Americans to get at least thirty minutes of exercise a day. (Lots of luck.) According to the CDC's head of Chronic Disease Control and Community Intervention, nearly 60 percent of Americans in 1993 were "either completely inactive or irregularly active, meaning fewer [times] than twice a week."[72] Nearly a fourth of American adults, according to a 1996 survey, don't do any physical activity whatsoever during leisure time. Based on a National Center for Health Statistics survey of almost 10,000 men and women over the age of twenty, more women than men (27 percent to 17 percent) have no leisure physical activity.[73] Not surprisingly, there is a link between the physical activity of people in different states and their obesity levels. For example, Colorado, usually rated as one of the leanest states in the country, also has the most people who say they regularly get exercise. On the other hand, Mississippi, which regularly rates as one of the fattest states in America, has a "sloth index" rate of 38 percent. The worst state was West Virginia, in which 45 percent of the people admitted to no physical activity for the purpose of having exercise.[74]

Exercise among children is also declining. Already by 1986 a study for the President's Council on Physical Fitness and Sports found that teenage girls performed worse than a decade earlier in eight of nine fitness-related tasks such as sit-ups and the standing long jump.[75] Gregory Heath, M.D. at the federal Centers for Disease Control and Prevention in Atlanta did surveys in 1990 and 1994, finding that just over that short period of time there was a drop in formal exercise. He also found that the higher the school grade, the less exercise.[76] "It was disappointing to see that the pattern of activity dropped over grade levels," said Heath. "If indeed we are sowing a sedentary lifestyle, it will likely carry over into adulthood, and what we are going to reap are the effects, like an increase in diabetes, obesity, and heart disease."[77]

LABOR-SAVING DEVICES

Life is becoming ever more sedentary. Without moving from my (swivel) chair, I can make telephone calls, send and receive faxes, get stock market quotes, search reference books, practice a foreign language, read classic books (hundreds on a single CD-ROM), do research in libraries throughout the world, make travel plans, play musical CDs to soothe the savage breast, send and receive mail and articles, read my favorite newspapers and magazines, and look up the last two weeks' worth of Dilbert cartoons.

In the last hundred years there has been an absolute revolution in labor-saving devices. Many of these are wonderful, none more so probably than the indoor toilet that saves a trudge through cold and rain to the outhouse. But many do little more than save a bit of labor.

None of this denigrates the value of modern efficiency. Sure, annually cleaning an oven probably burns a lot of calories, but it's a nasty job. Ditto for washing clothes with a scrub board or beating them on a rock in a stream. But the upside to such sorry activities was that they were vigorous and, when added to a host of other backbreaking chores, could literally keep you in shape. The loss in exertion through labor-saving devices must be compensated for elsewhere, either through reduced calorie intake or more planned exercise.

Individually, labor-saving devices don't add up to much. But together they play an important role in the obesity problem. Consider that even fidgeting can be an important method of burning calories. One study in a respiratory chamber found that some people burned as many as 800 calories a day just by fiddling and fussing.[78] We have got to end our obsession with labor-saving devices that do nothing but save calories.

KING CAR

To some extent, Americans have a natural disadvantage compared to Europeans in that we live in a much larger, more spread-out country. We also have largely abandoned inner cities with their walkways for the suburbs where the car is king. We've spread out in great part because land is relatively cheap, but our move to the suburbs has hurt us in many ways. In cities where people still live and work, they often get around by foot, or by bicycle. In the United States, only 1 percent of workers get to work by bicycle. By comparison, a town surveyed in Japan had a 15 percent rate; one in the Netherlands, 50 percent; and one in China, 77 percent. "Walking is built into the lifestyle to a great extent," says University of Minnesota School of Public Health epidemiologist Lawrence Kushi. "You can see that when you visit Europe and Asia; not only is the public transportation built better, but there's more infrastructure support for people who bicycle or walk. The streets are so narrow that having a car is almost a hindrance."[79] In some European inner cities, such as Athens, cars are forbidden. While there are no data to prove this one way or the other, I have noticed that in the few places where Americans are encouraged to abandon their cars and take to their feet, such as Manhattan, people do seem to be considerably thinner.

Another mode of getting around in cities is mass transit. This can be important in preventing obesity, because mass transportation is inherently inefficient—a point that mass-transit opponents often make. The car usually takes you right from door to door. But getting to a bus and especially a rail station is probably going to take some walking. Even if you drive to a rail station and park, you'll have to walk once you get to the rail stop closest to your destination. Once you're within the system and have to make transfers, this inevitably requires walking. In some places, such as Barcelona, Spain, subway transfers are absolutely grueling. You'll walk for blocks at the closest connections. I spent five days navigating that wretched system and during the whole time I don't think I saw a single extremely fat person in the tunnels. They might have started out on the heavy side, but making transfers in the Barcelona subway will work the weight off faster than any NordicTrack device or Richard Simmons video.

TV, OR NOT TV: THAT IS THE QUESTION

In the movie *Home Alone 2*, Macaulay Culkin is asked if he's had any trouble getting a television to work. "I'm ten years old," comes the flat response. "Television is my *life.*"[80] Unfortunately, for many American children and adults that's not so much a joke as a simple statement of fact. According to one market research firm, Veronis, Suhler & Associates, Americans watched 1,539 hours of television and 51 hours of videos a year, and played 21 hours of video games in 1994. That's 4.4 hours per day, up from 4.2 hours just six years earlier. Surveys by the NPD Group Inc. find that the only thing Americans do more than watch TV is sleep and work. Reading comes in at a mere 43 minutes a day and exercise 15 minutes. Dining out, at 24 minutes, absorbs almost twice as much time for us as exercise.[81]

Television has suffered the blame for causing any number of social ills, ranging from violence to unwed pregnancies to bad table manners to just plain making us stupid. Suffice it to say that you don't need to have a husband who spends all Sunday afternoon guzzling beers, eating corn chips, and yelling at the tube to realize that TV has fallen far short of being the educational tool some had predicted it would be. But does it play a role in the country's ever-widening haunches, as well? "I place much of the blame for American obesity levels squarely on television," says Marion Nestle, of the New York University Department of Nutrition.[82] And the scientific literature indicates she's almost certainly right.

In a 1987 study, Larry Tucker, now with Brigham Young University, concluded that "the more television adolescent males watch, the poorer their health tends to be. In general, this study suggests that light television viewers tend to be more physically fit, emotionally stable, sensitive, imaginative, outgoing, physically active, self-controlled, intelligent, moralistic, college bound, church oriented, and more self-confident than their counterparts, especially heavy television viewers." He added that "light television viewers tend to be less troubled, frustrated, and shrewd, and use drugs less frequently, particularly alcohol. . . ."[83]

But what of TV's impact on obesity specifically? In 1985, pediatrician William Dietz, M.D., of the New England Medical Center in Boston and sociologist Steven Gortmaker of Harvard University, asked in the title of their landmark *Pediatrics* article, "Do We Fatten Our Children at the Television Set?"[84] They found that the more television a child watched the more likely the child was to be obese. At the time they could do little more than speculate that it was probably more likely that TV was causing the obesity than that obese children, being less comfortable with more physical activity, were more likely to spend their time watching TV. But it made sense that it was more the former than the latter. Yes, fat children—especially extremely fat ones—might be less likely to engage in certain activities that require a lot of exertion. But most children's activities even aside from TV don't involve exertion. The kids play with GI Joes or dolls or shoot a slingshot at the neighbor's cat or do other things that fat children can do just as well as thin ones. Even physical things like playing on swings or playing tag or cops and robbers can be done by fat children at a reduced pace. There just aren't that many more incentives for a fat child to retreat to the TV room than for a thin child.

In any case, by 1990 Dietz and Gortmaker were ready to conclude that "Our studies have indicated a strong casual connection between the amount of time children and youth spend watching television and the prevalence of obesity," citing both the inactivity that normally attends television watching and the "effectiveness of television commercials in reinforcing the consumption of high-calorie foods." In assessing a number of demographic and behavioral variables, they found that "television viewing was the best single correlate" to children's fatness. They recommended that "During the assessment of obese patients, questions should be asked about their television and accompanying eating habits," and suggested that "parents set limits to viewing, with one option being that any television viewing above that limit needs to be accompanied by stationary bicycling or other aerobic activity."[85]

TV watching naturally lends itself to eating at the same time. In fact, the commercials actually encourage this. One study found that more eating occurred among obese than lean adult subjects when they were exposed to a television program accompanied by food commercials.[86] But it's not just the commercials we need to worry about. A 1996 survey found that television shows glorify pigging out. Cornell University researchers logged 276 prime-time shows and found that 80 percent showed characters eating or drinking. Healthful foods were often portrayed as not well liked, while foods high in sugar and fat were shown more positively. Forty-one percent of the time the food eaten was a snack.[87]

Some studies have shown that the more time a child spends watching TV, the more likely a child is to request and receive foods influenced by television.[88] And according to a 1994 report from the University of Minnesota, "the diet presented on Saturday morning television is the antithesis of what is recommended." After viewing more than fifty hours of Saturday morning programs on ABC, CBS, NBC, Fox, and Nickelodeon that contained nearly 1,000 commercials, the creators of the report found that not one commercial advocated eating fruits and vegetables; less than 5 percent promoted milk. About half the advertised foods included candy, soft drinks, chocolate syrup, whipped topping, cookies, chips, cakes, pastries, and gelatin desserts. Some 30 percent of the ads were for sugar-coated cereals.

And how about computers? A 1996 survey found that the main thing Internet users did less of in order to have more computer time was watch TV, which is good. On the other hand, 12 percent said they did less work—which is not so good—and the same percentage said they exercised less and played sports less—which isn't good at all.[89] You don't need to be running a computer with the latest, fastest microprocessing chip to calculate that if we let them, computers and the Internet are among the emerging technologies that threaten to make us fatter than ever if we don't learn to adjust to them and work them into an active lifestyle with moderate eating. And no computer is going to save us from the terrible consequences awaiting us if we don't begin to change our habits.

3

The Low-Fat Myth

Don't try telling a dieter this, but the human capacity to store energy as fat is very much a blessing. Consider the case of the tree shrew, which can store so little energy that if it doesn't eat it will starve to death in a matter of hours. Thus it must spend virtually all its waking hours desperately searching for food and eating it. No television, no time to watch the play William Shakespeare wrote about them, no buying a new outfit at the shopping mall. And definitely no foreplay before sex. In fact, they probably often stop halfway during the act to grab a ham sandwich. Nothing but searching and eating.

For humans these days, fat seems to be nothing but a villain. You see, telling overweight people to eat less and exercise more might send them fleeing for the hills, so the diet book authors and women's magazines search valiantly for some aspect of eating to blame, some way of telling people they can stuff their faces—and still lose weight. They found such a culprit in fat. It seemed to make sense: the fat you eat becomes the fat you wear. And there even seemed to be some science behind it.

And so the fad was launched. In part the attack on fat is justified because of its extra energy-carrying capacity. After all, a gram of fat does have nine calories compared to only four for carbohydrates and protein. As we shall see, reducing fat intake *to reduce calories* can be a major factor in weight control. But the centerpiece of the attack against Demon Fat is that even on a calorie-for-calorie basis, there is something especially bad about those calories coming from fat. Cut the fat and the pounds just melt away; right? Wrong.

Among the books promoting the argument that dietary fat is a special or exclusive cause of body fatness are: Martin Katahn's number one best-seller *The T-Factor Diet*,[1] and its companion book *The T-Factor Fat Gram Counter*[2] (which spent more than three years on *The New York Times* best-seller list); Susan Powter's number one best-seller *Stop the Insanity!*;[3] Dean Ornish's best-seller *Eat More, Weigh Less*;[4] John McDougall's best-seller *The McDougall Plan for Super Health and Life-Long Weight Loss*[5] and *The Fat Counter*[6] (the paperback edition cover claims there are 2 million copies in print); *Fight Fat and Win*;[7] *Bodystat*;[8] *How to Become Naturally Thin by Eating More*;[9] *Dr. Bruce Lowell's Fat Percent Finder*;[10] *The Fat Tooth Fat-Gram Counter*;[11] *Controlling Your Fat Tooth*;[12] *Fat to Fit, Without Dieting*;[13] *Get the Fat Out*;[14] and *How to Lower Your Fat Thermostat*.[15]

Most of these books call for reducing your fat intake to at most 30 percent of calories consumed, while others insist you try to get it down to 10 percent (*Eat More, Weigh Less*, for example), and some call for the elimination of practically all fat from the diet, such as *The McDougall Plan for Super Health and Life-Long Weight Loss*.

Weight-loss guru Covert Bailey has a chapter in *The Fit or Fat Target Diet* entitled "Fat in the Diet: Number One Enemy."[16] Jamie Pope (co-author with Martin Katahn of *The T-Factor Fat Gram Counter*) tells readers in her *The Last Five Pounds*: "The truth is simple: We gain unwanted pounds not because we eat too much, but because we eat too much fat and get too little exercise."[17] The authors of the best-selling *Eater's Choice* have written a new book, *Choose to Lose*, in which they shout at the reader: "The key to Choose to Lose is FAT. FAT MAKES FAT. FAT is what you don't want to be and FAT is what you ate to become FAT. . . . Don't focus on total calories . . . or sugar . . . or starch. Focus on FAT"[18] [ellipses and emphasis are theirs].

"Your body does not manufacture fat," states Susan Powter authoritatively in *Stop the Insanity!* Rather, ". . . it comes from the end of your fork." If you avoid fat, she says, "You can eat whatever you want, whenever you want it, and however much of it you want."[19]

Meanwhile *The Fat Attack Plan*, authored by the same team who wrote that 2-million-selling *The Fat Counter*, asserts that "you don't have to count calories. *All you have to do is learn to identify foods containing fat and eat less of them* [emphasis in original]."[20] *The Fat Attack Plan* gives the green light to eating sugared cereals: "You may be surprised to learn that our answer is 'No, sugared cereals *won't* make you fat.' Not the ones without fat, that is."[21]

"Calories do not count," writes Debra Waterhouse in her best-selling 1993 *Outsmarting the Female Fat Cell.* "What counts is how you eat those calories and where they come from: carbohydrates, protein, or fat."[22] Art Ulene of the *Today* show doesn't go that far in his book *Take It Off! Keep It Off!* He writes that "it appears that while calories do count, they are not the most important issue for a weight-loss program; dietary fat is."[23] Similarly, Dean Ornish says calories are a factor but, "Simply put, eating fat makes you fat, even if you take in fewer calories."[24]

Clearly some in the popular media have also bought into the calories-don't-count, only-fat-does thesis, letting it guide their reporting. For example, an Associated Press (AP) article in March 1995 discussed a report of the Center for Science in the Public Interest (CSPI) focusing on deli sandwiches. AP's accompanying sidebar listed twelve sandwiches, providing data concerning grams of fat, grams of saturated fat, and milligrams of sodium. Even though calories were listed in the actual CSPI report, the AP didn't think they were important enough to mention.[25]

In 1995 the Center for Media and Public Affairs in Washington, D.C., monitored three months of news coverage from thirty-seven different local and national news outlets to see how they covered issues of food safety and nutrition. The center found that fat consumption attracted twice as much coverage as any other nutritional topic. "Nearly half of all media reports mentioned some aspect of the need to reduce dietary fat intake," it reported in its newsletter. The media warned against fat consumption four times as often as the overconsumption of calories.[26]

But at least as important as anything the media has done has been the government's proclamation, in a 1990 report endorsed by a coalition of thirty-eight federal agencies,[27] that we should reduce fat in our diet to 30 percent or less. That fat is especially detrimental to weight control is also incorporated into the labeling that the Food and Drug Administration requires on virtually all food products. (In Europe, incidentally, only the United Kingdom has such a law.) Right next to where you're given the number of calories, you're told which calories come from fat. The label also incorporates the 30 percent of calories from fat recommendation.

Has this bombardment affected American eating and shopping habits? (Did the Beatles and Frank Sinatra make young women scream and faint?) A joint Food Marketing Institute and *Prevention* magazine survey in 1996 found that 72 percent of those polled made decisions to buy food based on the fat content listed on the label, while only 9 percent treated calories the same way. In fact, sodium content was rated as more important than calories.[28] An American Dietetic Association survey in 1992 found that many people believe fat should be completely eliminated from the diet.[29] Yet that action would prove suicidal since a small amount of fat is needed to absorb certain vitamins and carry out other bodily functions. "America is in the grip of a fat fanaticism," declared *Newsweek* at the end of 1994, "obsessed with the furtive grams of fat that lurk in our food plotting hostile takeovers of our health and our waistlines."[30]

The lesson here? You *can* change Americans' worries and, potentially, their eating habits. The problem? All this Demon Fat propaganda is false. It has changed our eating habits for the worse, devastating our diets and causing scales across the country to creak and groan and beg for mercy under added weight.

How did the Demon Fat fad come about? To some extent in the same way any urban legend (also called "friend of a friend story") does. It's just accepted and retold, accepted and retold.

THE KATAHN CATASTROPHE

Still, every urban legend got its start somewhere. The history of blaming dietary fat for bodily fat goes back to the turn of the century, when it was wrongly hypothesized that dietary fat passed unchanged through the digestive tract directly to become body fat.[31] But it wasn't until 1989 that it swept the imagination of the American public. That year saw the publication of *The T-Factor Diet*, written by Martin Katahn, a psychologist at Vanderbilt University.

Three years earlier Katahn had published *The Rotation Diet*,[32] which stayed on *The New York Times* best-seller list for six months and rose to number one. Had it worked, the obesity problem would have been solved, and there would be no more need for diet books, now would there? But the Rotation Diet didn't work,[33] and so Katahn was ready with a new foolproof plan three years later. His new book also rose to number one on the *Times* list and sold an incredible 2 million copies, making Katahn an even richer man.

"YOU CAN'T GET FAT EXCEPT BY EATING FAT!" exclaims Katahn in *The T-Factor Diet* in the obnoxious way pitchmen like to put things in all capitals.[34] "You are not going to be cutting calories or counting them," he says. "Except for fat, you are going to be eating just about as much of everything as you want."[35] Still later he insists, again all in capitals, that magical line that almost automatically leads to best-sellerdom: "FORGET ABOUT CALORIES!"[36]

But a funny thing happens later in the book. In a chapter in which he propounds an especially speedy system of weight-loss called the "Quick Melt" (sounds like a fast food sandwich, doesn't it?), he offers a diet that provides "approximately 1,000 calories for a woman, and 1,500 for a man."[37] But wait a second. Didn't he tell us that "only fat makes you fat" and that we can "forget about calories"? So how come suddenly we're counting calories, and not just fat ones, but all calories? But how many readers make it to that point and really analyze what the author is stating, that if calories count to make you lose weight quickly, they must count to make you lose weight at all?

Will the real solution please stand up? Is it true that only fat makes you fat, or do calories count? The answer, as we shall see, is that ultimately all that counts is calories, and that fat-free food will not make you fat free.

THE MAGIC FORMULAS

Katahn's thesis was based on two different formulas that began in the medical journals and should have stayed there. Both appear to be scientifically valid, but simply have no relevance to weight loss. One, dietary fat converts more efficiently to body fat than does carbohydrate or protein. Two, carbohydrates, whatever the conversion ratio, rarely become body fat in any case. Rather, they are almost always burned off immediately as fuel.

Thus, Dean Ornish, M.D., in his best-selling *Eat More, Weigh Less* states: "One hundred fat calories can be stored as body fat by expending only 2.5 calories, whereas your body must spend 23 calories—almost ten times as much—to convert 100 calories of dietary protein or carbohydrates into body fat." That's Formula Number One: fat turns to fat more easily. He then goes on immediately to say that very little protein and carbohydrate actually is converted to fat. That's Formula Number Two.[38]

If you think about it a moment—which, alas, no one ever does—you see that the second formula cancels out the first. It doesn't really matter that carbohydrates convert less efficiently to body fat, since the conversion rarely takes place at all. Thus we can forget the first part of the formula entirely. But what about the second part? It turns out that in everyday life, it's not very important either. What this all means is that the body has priorities. It prefers to get its energy from carbohydrates and store fat as fat. But if you are gaining weight because you're eating too many calories, even if the number of calories from fat is relatively small, the excess dietary fat will all convert to body fat, rather than any of it being burned off as fuel. Indeed, if you really eat to excess, even much of the extra carbohydrates will become fat, too. On the other hand, if you're already overweight, you can be eating virtually no fat and still not lose weight because your body isn't involved in making new body fat, just maintaining the fat that's already there.

So how do you lose that body fat? Simple. You either cut your calories or increase your energy expenditure. If your daily intake of calories is too small, your system is forced to convert the fat you eat into fuel, just like it converts the carbohydrates. Your body doesn't want to use fat for fuel. "I fain would use carbohydrates, thank you very much," it says to you with all the politeness of Little Lord Fauntleroy. But by restricting your energy intake (your calories), you restrict its options. Your body *must* burn off not only the fat you're consuming but the fat you're carrying around. "OK, damn it," your body says, much peeved now, "I need energy and I need it immediately, and since you're not giving me enough carbohydrates [its first choice], or enough dietary fat [its second choice], I'm just going to have to burn body fat instead."

So the low-fat diet gurus have it absolutely backward. Calories aren't irrelevant; ultimately, they're all that matters.

The scientist whose work was so crucial to Katahn and remains so to the low-fat faddists is a soft-spoken professor of biochemistry at the University of Massachusetts named Jean-Pierre Flatt, M.D. He is the person who came up with the formula for the cost in carbohydrate and fat burning. Katahn specifically cites Flatt's work.[39] When I contacted Flatt by phone, it was, truth be known, to pick a fight. Imagine how I felt when I found out the poor man agreed completely with my own findings and had no idea of the misconceptions and deception to which his work has led. "Anybody who eats more calories than he burns is going to gain weight," he told me. "If somebody eats 4,000 calories and burns 2,000, they will retain more of the fat they eat."[40]

THE CLINICAL STUDIES:
NO EVIDENCE FOR THE LOW-FAT MYTH

In all fairness, it must be said that diet gurus aren't the only ones who have bought into the low-fat myth. Some medical researchers have as well. Some have even convinced themselves they have found evidence for it, just as Christopher Columbus felt he could "prove" he had reached Asia, and not some land mass in between. But a look at some of the same studies these scientists invoke— along with studies they sometimes ignore because they don't fit with preconceptions—show that for weight control purposes, yes, all calories are alike.

A few of these studies have been retrospective, looking back at what subjects have eaten, and they seem to find that fatter people eat more fat.[41] But these studies suffer from "recall bias," meaning the researcher is dependent on what the subjects *claim* to have eaten. As we have seen already and will see again, recall is notoriously inaccurate for measuring what people have eaten. The only reliable way of measuring is to do so at the time they're actually eating. The methodology is fairly simple. You take two or more groups of people and feed them the same amount of calories. But you vary the amount of fat from which those calories are coming. Then you compare the high-fat eaters with the low-fat eaters and see if there are any differences.

Of these studies, I have found only a few that might lead to the interpretation that eating less fat as a percentage of calories translates into less fat on the body. All show only slight differences, and in each case the reduction in fat intake was drastic. Had it been a mere 33 percent to 30 percent reduction, such as the government is trying to get us to make, the differences wouldn't have shown up at all.[42]

Further, none of this difference may have been due to different levels of fat consumed. The complicating factor is that decreasing fat intake almost necessarily means increasing fiber intake. The only study that recorded this difference gave the low-fat subjects almost twice the fiber as the high-fat ones.[43] Considering the weight-loss benefits of fiber (discussed in chapter eight), this may completely account for the difference between the two groups.[44]

Some studies on rats and mice seem to show that fat content makes a difference, but others do not.[45] But among humans, most of the studies show that persons eating a high-fat diet lost as much body fat as, or even more than, those on the low-fat one. One study, reported in the *American Journal of Clinical Nutrition* in 1996, compared obese Swiss patients on diets in which 26 percent of the calories came from fat (45 percent from carbohydrates) with those on diets in which 53 percent of the calories came from fat (15 percent from carbohydrates). In both groups, total calories were limited to 1,000. If the low-fat myth were no myth, those 53 percenters should have been rolling their way onto the scales. Instead both groups lost the same amount of weight in the same amount of time. The authors concluded it was only the caloric reduction that caused weight and fat loss.[46]

A study two years before that at the famed Mayo Clinic in Rochester, Minnesota, compared one group of women given 42 percent of calories as fat with those given meals having 27 percent fat. Their caloric intake was kept to what they had been consuming before treatment. When the study ended four weeks later, neither group had lost or gained weight.[47] A study at Rockefeller University in New York determined its subjects' caloric needs, which was given to patients in a liquid formula. But the formulas had dif-

fering amounts of fat, ranging from zero all the way up to 70 percent of total calories. The result? Once again there was simply no
difference between subjects, this time after a period averaging
thirty-three days.[48] "Metabolically, the difference between conversion of fat or any other food is so minute as to be largely irrelevant
to dieters," said the chief author of the study, as reported in *The
New York Times*. "A calorie is a calorie," he added.[49]

Indeed, at least two studies found that persons on a diet getting
a small percentage of calories from fat lost *less* weight than those
getting more calories from fat. One, for example, found that
women getting 45 percent of their 1,200 daily calories from fat lost
ten pounds of body fat during the course of the study while those
getting only 10 percent of their 1,200 daily calories from fat lost
just six pounds.[50]

Interestingly, one 1993 study directly challenged Martin
Katahn's thesis, namely, if you just cut the fat, don't sweat the calories. Indeed, it was conducted at Katahn's school, Vanderbilt University, and even listed Katahn as one of the authors. The glove was
thrown down. The subjects were divided into two groups. One
group was restricted to 1,200 calories with twenty-five grams of fat
a day; the other group was also restricted to twenty-five grams of
fat a day but had no restriction on calories beyond that. If Katahn's
thesis were correct, both groups would have lost the same amount
of weight. Instead, the low-fat group lost ten pounds over the
course of the study, while the one that also restricted calories lost
twice as much. True, the group that restricted fat alone did show
some weight loss, but that's because their fat restriction also ended
up curtailing the number of calories they consumed.[51] All these
subjects were consciously trying to lose weight.

Lawrence Kushi and some researchers at Harvard University
undertook a survey of non-American data and found no substantia-
tion for the belief that fewer fat calories mean less body fat. "In
Europe," they wrote, "southern populations with lower fat intakes
display more obesity than do northern populations with higher fat
intakes. In China, where fat intake ranges from five percent to
25 percent of calories, there also has been found no association
between percent of calories from fat and body weight."[52]

"The studies are clear," says Walter Willett, chairman of the
department of nutrition at the Harvard School of Public Health.

"It's a myth that it's just the fat in your diet that makes you fat. As far as body fat goes, it doesn't make any difference where your calories come from."[53]

FAT IN OTHER LANDS

As I stated in the introduction, I got the idea for this book by noting the terrible disparity between Europeans' waistlines and those of Americans. But I didn't just look at other people's bodies; I looked at what they were eating, as well. And what I found was that, through simple observation at least, they seemed to eat at least as much fat as we do.* That especially seemed true for the Dutch, whose favorite snack appeared to be greasy French fries with a mayonnaise sauce glopped all over them. High-fat food was not making them fat, so why should it be making us so? Indeed, international consumption data makes this very point.

FAT CONSUMPTION AS A PERCENTAGE
OF CALORIES BY NATION

Hungary	41.1
Finland	41
Belgium	40.3
Netherlands	38
New Zealand	38
Israel	36.6
France	36.5

*Data from the Calorie Control Council in Atlanta makes it appear that low-fat and low-calorie foods and beverages are fairly common in Europe. A chart the council published in 1992 showed that 48 percent of the people in France and 69 percent in Germany use such products, compared with 76 percent in the United States. The problem with the data is that they don't measure frequency of use. An American who stocks her entire refrigerator with low-fat and low-calorie foods counts the same as a German who drinks a Coca-Cola Light (diet Coke) or Pepsi Max (Diet Pepsi) once a year.

FAT CONSUMPTION AS A PERCENTAGE
OF CALORIES BY NATION *(cont'd.)*

Switzerland	35.8
United Kingdom	35.3
Australia	35
Norway	34.9
United States	**33.7**
Italy	33.4
Spain	32.9
China	19.4
Japan	18.7

Source: *American Journal of Clinical Nutrition;*[54] *Journal of the American Dietetic Association* (French data).[55]

AMERICANS ARE NOT EATING MORE FAT

Repeatedly we hear the "calories don't count" diet gurus quiz us with, as the authors of the *Fat Attack Plan* put it, "Did you know that even though Americans are eating fewer calories than in the past, average body weight has gone *up*? [emphasis in original]."[56] That myth was discarded in the previous chapter, but books like the *Fat Attack Plan* have used it to say that since we're not getting fatter from eating more calories, we must be getting fatter from eating more fat. In fact, we are often told just that, that as a nation we are eating more fat. Yet the federal government's own data show just the opposite.

The Department of Agriculture has determined that as of the years 1994 to 1996, fat comprised about 33 percent of total calories in the American diet. This showed a continuing decrease from 34 percent in 1989 to 91 and 40 percent in 1977 to 78.[57] Thus at the same time our consumption of fat as a percentage of calories was dropping—just as the government was telling us it must—our waistlines were exploding. Fat consumption dropped 17.5 percent as obesity increased by 25 percent. A longer look at fat consumption appeared in a medical journal, comprising studies dating back to the 1920s, showing that even though we're fatter than ever before, we're actually getting fewer of our calories from fat.

FAT INTAKE AS A PERCENTAGE OF CALORIES

Years	Number of Studies	Fat as a Percentage of Calories
1920–29	2	35.5
1930–39	2	41.2
1940–49	20	37.6
1950–59	46	40.5
1960–69	53	39.9
1970–79	53	37.8
1980–89	20	37.5

Source: *American Journal of Clinical Nutrition.*[58]

Noting that obesity was a growing problem worldwide, a Dutch epidemiologist writing in the *International Journal of Obesity* in 1995 pointed out that on an international scale, as populations got fewer of their calories from fat, their waistlines nonetheless continued to grow.[59]

PROVE IT YOURSELF

I have now shown in four different ways why it's wrong to say that fat calories are any more likely to cause obesity than any other type of calories, much less to say that only fat calories count. First, I showed that the underlying theory was false. Second, I showed that the controlled studies of people on equal-calorie diets but with different levels of fat found no difference in the amount of weight lost by the different groups. Third, I showed that even though Americans are the fattest Westerners, we have a diet that is lower in fat than that consumed in most European countries. Fourth, I showed that American fat consumption has been going down, even though our waistlines have been exploding. Even the most ardent skeptic from Missouri, the "Show Me" state, should be convinced by this point.

But if after years of having people like Susan Powter scream nonsense at you this isn't enough, here's my trump card. You are going to make yourself a guinea pig. Instead of squealing and gnawing on the bars of your cage, however, you're going to go to a health food store like GNC or to a drugstore and buy a can of weight-gain powder bodybuilders use. Make sure you buy only the stuff that's fat free. (There's one brand at GNC called Russian Bear, but I'm not pushing anybody's products.) Now, if Powter and Katahn are right, you can down this stuff by the keg and not an ounce will go to your waist or hips; it will all burn off. Measure out 4,000 calories' worth and drink it down with water. (Bizarrely, Russian Bear tells you to drink it with whole milk. Why would you possibly want to mix a fat-free powder with whole milk?) Continue eating as much food as you normally have been. This way you will be adding 4,000 fat-free calories daily to your diet. Do this every day. I guarantee that very soon you will notice yourself getting fatter at a rate of somewhere around a pound daily. Sure, I hate to advise you to do anything that will make you fatter, but if this is what it takes to finally divest yourself of all this fat-free lunacy, then a few added pounds in the beginning will be a good investment.

Fat and Heart Disease

Now, how about claims that we should reduce fat intake to 30 percent of calories in order to reduce heart disease? In 1995 British cardiologist Michael Oliver, professor emeritus at the National Heart and Lung Institute in London, released a shocking analysis at the First International Conference on Fats and Oils and Human Disease, held in New York. He concluded that studies of people whose diets achieve the 30 percent goal show that the diets had virtually no effect on cholesterol levels. More restrictive diets are effective, he said, but few healthy people comply with them for very long. He went on to say that large clinical trials conducted over the last two decades have failed to demonstrate that the national goal of a 30 percent fat diet has any effect on heart disease rates. "Studies of this low-fat, low-cholesterol diet are completely negative," Dr. Oliver said. "We should face up to the fact that the [30 percent] diet doesn't work. He added that "vast sums of money are being spent on nutritional programs, dietician advice, and nurse counseling in pursuance of diets which may be completely ineffectual."[60]

In his analysis, Oliver cited six large studies of people at high risk for heart disease. All the studies included low-fat diets along with other interventions, such as smoking cessation. Only two of the studies found a reduction in heart-disease rates or in death rates from heart disease or in deaths from all causes. One actually found the group following the low-fat diet had more deaths, including more from heart disease.

When *New York Times* reporter Gina Kolata heard these fighting words she tried to find experts who would disagree with this premise and apparently found she could not. Said Harvard's Walter Willett, "Oliver's point is well taken," and that public health specialists have been "very dogmatic" in their recommendations without having proof.

Other researchers said Oliver's point was essentially correct, but needed clarification. If you're at high risk of heart disease, a 30 percent fat diet is still too much. On the other hand, if you're at low risk, it's probably unnecessary to restrict fat to 30 percent of calories. Prescribed across the board for everyone, the 30 percent admonition probably does few people any good.[61]

This said, not all fats are created equal. From a caloric perspective, they are the same. All have nine calories per gram. But different types of fats have different effects on cholesterol levels and hardening of the arteries. If you want to know more about this, look up the note at the end of this sentence—this one.[62]

LOW-FAT FOODS TO THE RESCUE. NOT!

As we have seen, the low-fat craze is just that. Scientifically it's utterly bankrupt. But oh, what a craze it is! And until the common knowledge catches up with the science, the food industry will do everything in its power to flood our taste buds and pack our growing bellies with engineered low-fat foods. It does so with the encouragement of the government. The Department of Health and Human Services' *Healthy People 2000* publication urges that by the millennium there should be an increase to "at least 5,000 brand items [in] the availability of processed food products that are reduced in fat and saturated fat."[63]

There's probably not much more I can tell you about the onslaught of low-fat and no-fat foods than you already know, because you've seen the same transformation in the grocery stores that I have. It's impossible to walk down any food aisle other than the produce section without seeing banners proclaim: LOW FAT! REDUCED FAT! NO FAT! FAT FREE! LITE! AS ALWAYS, FAT FREE! and a dozen other variations. As one network news correspondent put it: "In a world fighting fat, fat-free has become the battle cry."[64] You can even find fruit drinks advertising themselves as fat free, as if a substance comprising nothing but water, sugar, artificial flavoring, and artificial color could possibly have fat in it. What's next? Fat-free toothpaste, fat-free mouthwash, fat-free bottled water, fat-free vitamins, fat-free ice cubes?

Grocery sales of all low-fat foods amounted to $18 billion in 1993, and have been estimated to grow to $30 billion by 1997.[65] The aforementioned Food Marketing Institute–*Prevention* magazine survey asked shoppers about nine types of food engineered to be lower in fat, ranging from salad dressing to cake. It found that for each category, Americans were eating more of the low-fat items in 1996 than in the year before.[66] Much of this growth has been in the snack food industry. The Snack Food Association reported in 1995 that nearly every company in the $15-billion industry is working on low-fat or reduced-fat products. That category produced less than 5 percent of the industry's total sales in 1994 but is expected to grow to a third of the market by 2000, according to the association.[67]

No label is more associated with the low-fat fad than Nabisco's SnackWell's line of low-fat and fat-free cookies and other snacks. Although it didn't even exist before 1992, by 1996 it was producing an amazing $600 million annually in revenues.[68] "I've never seen anything like it in the industry," proclaimed a self-satisfied Ray Verdon, president of Nabisco Foods, about the SnackWell's line.[69] In those four short years, SnackWell's became America's most popular cookie.

When SnackWell's Devil's Food Cookie Cakes first appeared, demand was so high that Nabisco had to ration them out to stores.[70] Women's groups formed to scout out the cookies, fights erupted in the stores over the boxes, and grocery store managers kept the snacks under lock and key.[71] These cookies are hardly noncaloric, with 100 calories in a measly little ounce. I've never met anybody who thought they tasted very good, with "Styrofoam" being the usual adjective attributed to them. But people are convinced that if the cakes have no fat they can't possibly make you fat, so they eat away.

Nabisco doesn't just rely on popular misconceptions to foster sales; it perpetuates those misconceptions. A woman in a Snack-Well's commercial attends a Snack Eaters Anonymous meeting and confesses her sins. "Yesterday I faltered," she says, grief-stricken. "I couldn't resist those cookies! I've ruined everything!" She is redeemed and happy at the end of the ad, though, when she realizes the cookies she ate were fat free and couldn't possibly hurt her.[72] Meanwhile, Healthy Choice puts the expression "Eat What You Like" on its line of low-fat cookies and other snacks. It's even trademarked it. It doesn't take a genius to figure out that a lot of people are going to read into that: "Eat as much as you like."

Far more blatant was an Orville Redenbacher ad for the company's reduced-fat popcorn. It went:

> *Eat & eat & eat & eat*
> *eat & eat & eat & eat*
> *eat & eat & eat & eat*
> *& not feel the least bit guilty.*[73]

Note the ad doesn't say the product won't make you fat. It just says you shouldn't feel guilty eating it. Have you noticed the proliferation of the term "guilt free" (and its cousin "sinless") to a point where it's actually worked into the name of some brands? Basically, it's a clever way around FDA labeling regulations. The FDA requires that formerly ambiguous terms like "reduced fat" and "light" or "lite" fulfill certain requirements. But "guilt free" can mean anything the manufacturer wants it to, including "pig out!"

Meanwhile, Hershey somehow manages to pawn off chocolate syrup as a health food. "Because it's virtually fat free, you can really pour it on," says one of its advertisements. Yes, and with 100 calories in just two tablespoons, you can virtually feel your pants ripping at the seams as you do so. Similarly, Hershey's premixed chocolate milk is sold in 15.5-ounce bottles that state in bold letters: "99 percent fat free." That small bottle of fat-free drink delivers 240 nice low-fat calories, so the wide-mouth bottle enables you to down more than a tenth of a day's calories in a matter of seconds.

Potato chips, too, have somehow become a health food. When Frito-Lay introduced its Baked Lay's Low Fat Original Potato Crisps, its salesmen and delivery men were waylaid by would-be customers. A state trooper even pulled over a salesman to ask where he could buy a bag.[74] (Shouldn't he have been pulling over a salesman of low-fat doughnuts?) Betty Crocker, meanwhile, actually labels one of its products—two thin fudge brownies with a slab of "ice cream" between them—as "Healthy Temptations." Healthy? Yes, though absolutely packed with sugar, it contains no measurable fat.[75] By that definition, a cyanide pill might also be labeled healthy.

The only fat-free product advertisement I really like is one that has appeared in women's magazines under the banner "Fat-free Dressing." It turns out to be Tide with bleach. The ad depicts seven fatty foods, and the copy reads: "Tide with Bleach Ultra 2 can help keep your clothes fat free," meaning stains from fatty foods.[76] It's very clever and much-needed comic relief. (The only problem I have with the ad is that it gives Tide's World Wide Web site. If you ever even consider visiting the Web site of a detergent, you are in serious need of getting a life.)

FAT FREE ... AND FATTER ALL THE TIME

Of course, the food industry rakes in megabucks from people thinking they can eat twice as much as they did before and not worry about gaining weight. But while industry counts its money, health professionals are horrified.

- "I think the greatest myth is that fat-free means calorie-free and that means I can eat all I want," says Robert Kushner, director of the University of Chicago Nutrition and Weight Control Clinic. "If people only pay attention to fat, they will drift to fat-free products that are high in calories."[77]

- "While people who want to drop weight have decreased dietary fat, they've also become volume eaters, giving in to a second or even a third bagel because they're using no-fat cream cheese," says registered dietician Cathy Nonas, director of the Theodore Van Itallie Center for Weight Control at St. Luke's–Roosevelt Hospital Center in Manhattan.[78]

- "I have so many people who come to me and say, 'I'm eating only healthy food. I've really cut out the fat, and I still can't lose weight,' " says Colleen Pierre, a Baltimore registered dietician and a spokeswoman for the American Dietetic Association. "Because we think only fat counts, we think that if food has no fat in it, it's OK to eat all you want."[79]

- Even Dean Ornish admits, "The week that Entenmann's rolled out its fat-free desserts, a number of our patients gained weight. They thought that as long as they were eating something fat-free, they could eat as much as they wanted."[80] Ornish asked one patient what he had done differently that might have made him gain weight and the man said, "Well, I had—I had some cake." Ornish asked, "Well, how much?" And the man said, "Two." "Two slices?" queried Ornish. "No, two cakes." That was a total of 2,400 calories.[81]

Some media folks are catching on, as well. "Aside from what they should eat," observed *U.S. News & World Report* in 1996, "Americans just plain eat too much . . . replacing fats with seconds and thirds of everything else. Book titles like the best-selling *Eat More, Weigh Less* don't help."[82]

Laboratory tests, as well as anecdotes, provide evidence that people eat more when told what they're eating is low in fat. In one test, Florence Caputo and Richard Mattes gave seventeen volunteers meals consisting of a variety of low-fat, low-calorie foods. When the subjects were told the meals were low fat and low calorie, they pigged out. When told they were eating high-fat and high-calorie foods, they carefully restricted what they ate. And these were persons who were selected because they hadn't dieted in at least the previous six months.[83] Dieters would presumably fare much worse because they are always looking for an excuse to eat.[84] A 1996 survey found a third of shoppers admitting that they felt it was OK to eat more of a food because it was low in fat or had no fat.[85] My guess is most of the other two thirds fibbed.

Aside from the pig-out factor, there are other problems with this increased intake of low-fat foods. One is that, as we have seen, low-fat or no-fat may be extremely high in calories. A fat-free eight-ounce glass of grape drink has a whopping 200 calories in it and can be downed in seconds. Many of the new foods engineered to be low fat or fat free have as many or almost as many calories as they replace. This is partly because the fat was only a small component anyway. Reduce a small part by a small part, and you really don't have much reduction. Further, manufacturers often pump up the sugar content to make up for the taste lost from the shortening. "People are basically substituting sugar for fat," says Marion Nestle. "As people focused on eliminating fat, food marketers came up with fat-free substitutes. But the substitutes they provided were equally as fattening."[86]

SnackWell's Devil's Food Cookie Cakes lists three of its first four ingredients as sugar. Thus, one calorically dense ingredient is simply swapped for another, with the result being an inferior-tasting product.

Here are a few examples in which fat-free means little in calorie reduction:

Item	Full-Fat Version	Reduced-Fat Version
Cracker Jack	120 calories in 28 grams	110 calories in 28 grams
Oreo cookies	160 calories in 32 grams	140 calories in 33 grams
Vic's Gourmet Popcorn	150 calories in 30 grams	130 calories in 30 grams
Skippy peanut butter	190 calories in 32 grams	180 calories in 35 grams

Kraft shredded cheese	110 calories	90 calories
	in 30 grams	in 31 grams

Sometimes the reduced-fat version has just as many or more calories as the original or the full-fat competitor. SnackWell's reduced-fat Chocolate Creme Sandwich Cookies have slightly fewer calories per gram than Oreos, but because they're slightly bigger they actually have more calories per cookie. The Sourdough Unsalted Hard Pretzels from Snyder's of Hanover, while fat free, actually have substantially more calories than the original.

Other times a product may be labeled "reduced fat" but it's a reduction from a massive amount to a not-quite-so-massive amount. The Cheesecake Factory's Lite Cheesecake contains less fat and fewer calories than the original version, but still packs 580 calories.[87] A "reduced-fat" yogurt drink I saw in a Manhattan deli nonetheless had an incredible 460 calories in just sixteen ounces. When you consider that even a sugar-sweetened soda has fewer than half that many calories per ounce and that artificially sweetened beverages and water have few or no calories, it seems hard to justify getting a fourth of a day's calories from a few swigs of a drink—a reduced-fat one, no less.

When the low-fat version of a food turns out to have about the same number of calories as the regular version, the manufacturers often just shrink the portion sizes to make them look less caloric. Nabisco's original Nilla wafers have 4.3 calories per gram, compared with 4.1 for the low-fat version. It's essentially the same. So the company calls thirty-two grams a "serving" for the original, while the low-fat "serving" is lowered to only twenty-nine grams.

Some "low-fat" foods aren't even low fat. One major company that got slapped for false advertising regarding fat content is Häagen-Dazs, an American firm with a Scandinavian-sounding name. The Federal Trade Commission (FTC) forced Häagen-Dazs to stop advertisements which represented some of their yogurt desserts as containing a twelfth of the fat they really have.[88]

Another problem, as Barbara Rolls of Pennsylvania State University puts it, is that "Some people eat low-fat foods as an excuse to eat other high-fat foods." She calls this "the diet Coke and doughnut strategy."[89] Adds Mattes, now at Purdue University, "People think they've saved fat and can indulge themselves later in the day with no adverse consequences.... But when they do that, they don't compensate very precisely, and they often end up overdoing it."[90] "We found a lot of people buy low-fat foods but balance them with high fat," says Tom Dybdahl of *Prevention* magazine, which polls shoppers in conjunction with the Food Marketing Institute. "They'll buy premium ice cream *and* non-fat salad dressing."[91]

Most important, though, low-fat and even low-calorie foods can destroy the most important principle in weight control—moderation. High-fat and high-calorie foods help teach moderation. You may feel like eating the whole bag of cookies but you tell yourself you dare not. So you eat only one or two and thoroughly enjoy each bite. But low-fat foods often teach exactly the opposite. They encourage you to, as the bow-tied popcorn magnate put it, "Eat & eat & eat & eat." With no-calorie drinks, you can consume all you want and "get away with it." For reduced-calorie foods, it's partly true. But the message of "Pig out!" then carries over to other foods. The moderation impulse is crippled and the people who overeat SnackWell's one day may be overeating their steak, French fries, and ice cream the next. There's just no way around it: low-fat and no-fat foods are a Siren call to gluttony.

Registered dietician and co-author of *Intuitive Eating: A Recovery Book for the Chronic Dieter* Evelyn Tribole agrees. "People are suddenly adding foods they wouldn't normally eat," she says. "Some people who don't normally have potato chips are now adding fat-free potato chips to their diet, or they're adding fat-free cookies. I've especially seen that . . . with the fat-free foods." She adds, ". . . The moderation thing is what really works for me."[92]

Interestingly, the very lady who launched the sale of 5 million low-fat recipe books (*In the Kitchen with Rosie*[93]), Oprah Winfrey, says she tried the low-fat-only route and found it didn't work. She reports that her chef, Rosie Daley, "had been with me for two years before I lost a few pounds, because I was still consuming too much food."[94]

In theory, reduced-fat foods, usually being also slightly reduced in calories, could help make a difference in weight control if you swapped exactly the same amounts of food. But even then it wouldn't be of much help. That's because the reduced-fat foods on the market today are almost exclusively what is known as "peripheral foods," or things you shouldn't be having much of anyway. Yes, if half your diet was potato chips and sandwich cookies, reduced-fat Lays and reduced-fat Oreos might help you lose weight if you swapped evenly chip for chip, cookie for cookie. But if half your intake is cookies and potato chips, you're in a lot of trouble one way or the other.

THE "30 PERCENT" OBSESSION

The American and British governments have told their citizens to reduce their calories from fat to no more than 30 percent. The resulting reaction has been something like a sick joke for the simple reason that the government doesn't say *how many* calories the fat should be 30 percent of. Thus, some people, bizarrely enough, have taken this to mean it's OK to eat more calories just in order to reduce the percentage from fat. Nutrition columnist Elaine Moquette-Magee's book *Fight Fat and Win* advises readers to add sugar calories to a fatty meal. She says that it's OK to order a fatty (and high-calorie) sandwich or side order at a fast-food restaurant so long as you drink enough orange juice along with it. She even provides a formula so you know how much OJ to scarf down to balance out the French fries.[95] But why stop there, Ms. Moquette-Magee? Why not tell us how much Kool-Aid we should drink so that we can eat three slabs of cheesecake? Or how many sugar cubes we should pop in our mouths to allow us to consume a fat-laden twenty-four-ounce porterhouse steak?

American newspapers have also run stories with headlines like "Fat Intake Dips but Not Pounds," and "Fatty Diets on Steady Decline."[96] Yet if you read them carefully you saw we were actually eating *more* fat than previously, just less as a percentage of calories. Only in America, with the 30 percent obsession, can eating more fat be a "steady decline."

American waistlines are staggering under the one-two punch of weight-loss quacks and the processed food industry. How much fatter will we have to get before we finally catch on?

THE REAL SECRET: LOW-DENSITY EATING

Having read this far, you may now be shocked to hear that eating a low-fat diet can actually be a tremendous boon to weight loss and control *if* you use it as a means to an end, and not an end in and of itself. That's because fat has more than twice as many calories, for the same amount of weight, as carbohydrates or protein. By swapping carbohydrates or protein for fat, you can reduce your calorie intake, and the reduced calorie intake will help you lose weight.

Here's the basic rule and probably the most important sentence in this chapter: *Don't reduce the percentage of the calories you're eating that are coming from fat: reduce the fat in your diet in order to reduce the number of calories you're eating.*

The way you do this is by eating foods that are naturally low in fat. By "naturally," I'm not making a case for organic foods or only buying your food at places with names like "Alfalfa's" or "Sprouts" or "Green Things." I mean foods that haven't been processed, and especially those that haven't been processed to be low-fat in order to replace higher fat products. The problem with most of those, as I've noted, is that they've used sugar to replace fat. Sugar, like fat, is calorically dense. You're just replacing one high-calorie item with another.

Consider, for example, an orange versus a glass of orange juice. The juice is an orange in processed form. It has about eighty calories in a six-ounce glass. Like any liquid, it has little satiating effect on hunger; in fact, you get as much satiation from a glass of water, which has no calories. But an average-size California Valencia orange in its unprocessed form, which is to say simply an orange, has just sixty calories and sits in your stomach a long time while your digestive system works to break it down and pass it through the intestines. Part of the satiating effect comes from the high amount of fiber in oranges. Most orange juice has had the fiber completely removed.

Consider corn versus corn oil. In kernel form, corn has 89 calories in half a cup. Processed into oil it has 120 calories in just a tablespoon. How about spuds? Potatoes are a naturally low-calorie, highly nutritious food. Many Irish used to live practically on potatoes alone. (Though admittedly not through choice.) A pound of unpeeled potatoes has only 289 calories. Processed into potato chips, one of the unhealthiest foods ever discovered, they have an incredible 2,400 in a single pound. Peanuts are high fat and high calorie in their natural form, but processing makes them that much worse. A half cup of raw peanuts has 430 calories, but processed into peanut butter a half cup has a whopping 780. Processed even further into peanut oil it has 960 calories in a half cup.

The more you process a food, the more bulk and fiber you take out of it and the more calories you leave. What you're left with is less satisfaction and satiety per calorie. Thus in one study, subjects either ingested whole apples, apple puree (which contained the same amount of fiber as a whole apple), or fiberless apple juice. The ones who ate the whole apples were most satisfied, while those who drank the juice were least satisfied.[97]

Converting to a natural, low-fat diet can make a huge difference in how many calories you consume. Demonstrating this was a Cornell University study in which three groups of women were given fairly similar food each having a different level of fat: 15 to 20 percent of calories from fat, 30 to 35 percent, and 45 to 50 percent. Those on the low-fat diet consumed an average of 2,087 calories daily, while those in the middle range consumed 2,352 daily, and the high-fat eaters ate 2,714 calories a day.[98]

And does eating fewer calories on a diet low in energy density translate into weight loss? Of course. *It has to.* The Pope is always Catholic and calories always count. They are *all* that count. Another Cornell study compared women on a high-energy dense diet with those on a low-energy dense one and allowed both to eat as much as they wanted of the foods allowed them. The second group ate far fewer calories and lost 5.5 pounds in eleven weeks, twice the weight loss of the women eating foods that had a high energy density.[99]

What are we to make of all this? Simply that it isn't just fat that's the bad boy in our diets; it's anything that has lots of calories relative to its bulk. Fresh fruit is good, but dried fruit is not so good because all the bulkiness provided by water has been squeezed out. White bread isn't as good as whole wheat because part of the bulk provided by fiber has been removed. A seventy-calorie cookie isn't as good as a seventy-calorie banana regardless of whether it's a fat-free cookie, because the banana is big and heavy and bulky and the cookie can be popped down your throat like nobody's business and followed quickly by another. Many of us, including your humble author, know what it's like to eat six or eight cookies in short order. At one time I probably kept a couple of Girl Scout troops operating just through my purchases. Have you ever tried to eat six bananas or pears in one sitting?

The foods that are highest in energy density contain no fat whatsoever. They are soft drinks and juices. A glass of water and a glass of a soft drink sweetened with sugar, such as Kool-Aid or soda pop, have exactly the same bulk. Each requires as much swallowing, as little chewing (none), and takes up as much space in the stomach as the other. Each empties from the stomach as quickly as the other. But while the glass of water contains no calories, the sugar-sweetened soft drink contains about 140 calories in a twelve-ounce glass. Furthermore, for most people soft drinks are more palatable than plain water (indeed, this is the entire reason they drink them), making it clear that soft drinks can play an important part in making you fat. This is not so important in countries such as those in Europe where standard soft drink sizes are around eight ounces. But in the United States where the smallest size in theaters is twenty ounces, where machines now dispense twenty-ounce sodas, and where mini-marts sell bathtubs containing sixty-four ounces of soda, soft drinks can play a key role in popping your britches.

At one time, "low fat" was essentially synonymous with "low calorie." It was nearly impossible to eat a low-fat diet that wasn't also low in calories. But since then we've managed to devise all sorts of foods that are extremely high in calories while still being low in fat. Within just the last few years, as a result of the low-fat fad, this menu has expanded tremendously, with huge new selections of no- and low-fat cookies, ice cream substitutes, cakes, and other sweets. The result is that we are now able to eat vast amounts of calories from a wide array of palatable foods, all of which are low in fat. And that's exactly what we're doing.

The food industry is constantly trying to fool consumers into thinking that their processed foods are simply more convenient versions of the real, healthier thing. For example, there's Smucker's Simply Fruit, also called "spreadable fruit" on the front label. It makes you think you're getting nothing but mashed strawberries or whatever type of fruit is in the jar. In fact, instead of using sugar or corn syrup, Smucker's has "simply" added white grape juice concentrate, which is "simply" sugar by any other name.[100] There's nothing magical about juice as a sweetener as opposed to sugar. To get the same amount of sweetness, the manufacturer has to add the same amount of calories.

Or there's the advertisement in health magazines like *Self* that says, "Funny how bananas can travel all the way from Ecuador, only to disintegrate in the exotic depths of your gym bag. Until now, that is." It then goes on to exhort the virtues of the banana-flavored PowerBar, essentially a candy bar that doesn't taste as good as a normal candy bar but contains added vitamins and minerals. It doesn't say that while the PowerBar packs a powerful 255 calories, a big, satisfying banana has less than 100.[101] Next time, pack your banana more carefully and leave the PowerBar on the store shelf.

This isn't to advocate eliminating all processed foods from your diet. I, for one, would consider life not worth living if peanut butter were not available. But recognize that processed foods that are dense in energy are bad actors. If you're eating a lot of them and are having trouble controlling your weight, don't wonder why. You must reduce the processed foods in your diet and replace high-processed ones with less-processed ones. Bread, for example, is processed. Nobody expects you to eat plain wheat. But you should eat bread in which the grain has been less processed, namely, that which is whole grain.

Every year Americans gobble up more processed low-fat foods, and every year they grow fatter. The low-fat fad must end now. More than that, we must end a way of thinking that says that engineered foods can completely take the place of moderate consumption. Until that happens, don't even bother to ask why our buttons keep popping, our seams keep tearing, and our shoes get harder and harder to see.

4

Give Us This Day Our Daily Half Pound of Sugar

Once upon a time, there was a very bad creature in our diet. It was called sugar. Everybody said to beware of sugar, that it hurt your teeth and made you fat. But then one day, a new monster appeared on the horizon: fat. It was fat that made you fat and did any number of other nasty things to the fair people of the kingdom. And the monster sugar was forgotten and its terrible deeds became the stuff of myth and legend.

Which is too bad, because sugar is as bad for us as ever, and no doubt plays an important role in the obesity epidemic, even if it now bores so many researchers and newspaper reporters. The heyday of the attack on sugar was the 1970s. One respected nutritionist declared before a U.S. Senate committee in 1977 that "if the food industry were to propose the introduction of refined sugar as a new rather than as an existing additive, it would surely be enjoined from doing so."[1] The Royal College of Physicians in its 1983 report on obesity stated: "Sugar is an unnecessary source of energy in a community with such a widespread problem of overweight."[2] The 1977 *Dietary Goals for the United States*, also known as the (George) McGovern Report, came to much the same conclusion.[3]

Meanwhile, the 1975 book *Sugar Blues*, which declared that "refined sugar is lethal when ingested by humans," sold over 1.5 million copies.[4] Among other things, author William Dufty blamed "sugar in our bloodstreams [for attracting] mosquitos, microbes, and parasites,"[5] for causing freckles,[6] for being the actual cause of death for the millions of Europeans swept away by the bubonic plague,[7] and even for the fragmentation of the American family.[8] He didn't blame it for the Vietnam War, but perhaps that was edited out. All of this, along with much of his book, was nonsense of course.

Yet today, there is practically no public consciousness that sugar is anything more than bad for your teeth. And with the widespread use of fluoridation, even tooth decay is not the big deal it once was. Readers of women's magazines are told that it's not the sugar in candy that's bad for them; it's just the fat, and so if they have fat-free candies they can eat to their hearts' content. Indeed, the negative role of sugar has been so forgotten that one brand of shredded wheat carries on the front and back a large banner blaring NATURALLY LOW IN FAT, while on the side it states:

- Naturally low fat
- Naturally cholesterol free
- No artificial flavors
- No artificial colors

Only by reading the FDA-required label can one discern that it also happens to have no sugar in it!

Yet sugar is as bad for us now as it was in the 1970s, the difference being that now we're eating so much more of it. In 1970, Americans consumed an average of 121 pounds of sugar and corn sweeteners. By 1992 that had shot up to 142 pounds, almost half a pound for each of us a day. This occurred even though artificial sweetener use quadrupled in the same period of time. That extra 21 pounds of sugar and corn sweeteners provides 35,721 calories and converts to almost ten pounds of fat on the body. Of course, it doesn't quite work that way, since no doubt Americans are to some extent substituting sugar for some other foods. But it would be foolish to think that the addition of 21 pounds of sugar to our diets yearly is not a major player in the obesity epidemic. The federal government and the diet gurus have labored mightily to get us to restrict our fat intakes, even as they've ignored sugar. And apparently it's having an impact. While the percentage of Americans who say they've tried to reduce their fat intake has increased from

44 percent to 56 percent from 1992 to 1996, the number concerned with reducing sugar intake has dropped from a low 19 percent to an even lower 12 percent.⁹ A nation of fat-gram counters,
we've also become a nation of sweetener addicts.

SWEETENER CONSUMPTION*

Year	Sugar and Corn Sweeteners	Saccharin and Aspartame
1970	121.1	5.8
1975	116.6	6.1
1980	122.6	7.7
1985	129.9	18.1
1990	139.1	22.2
1991	140.3	24.3
1992	141.9	NA

*In pounds, per capita.

Source: U.S. Department of Agriculture, Economic Research Service.¹⁰

The average American—according to food surveys, at least—
gets 18 percent of his or her calories from total sugars (minus that
in milk) compared with 15.2 percent in the European Union
countries.¹¹ Nevertheless, if one accepts that Americans are substantially underreporting their calorie intake in general, then
they're certainly underreporting their sugar consumption by at
least as much.

Probably one reason sugar is getting a free ride these days is
that it is a form of carbohydrate, and dieticians and nutritionists
say carbohydrates are the way to go. But there are two classes of
carbohydrates, simple and complex—and the difference between
them is huge. Sugar is not calorically any more dense per gram
than any other carbohydrate. That is, all carbohydrates contain
four calories per gram. But unlike complex carbohydrates, such as
in breads, pasta, vegetables, and fruits, refined sugar has virtually
no bulk. Basically, it has had everything stripped from it but calo-

ries and sweetness. A sixteen-ounce bottle of tea sweetened with 220 calories of sugar is just as easy to consume as sixteen ounces of unsweetened tea. Likewise, when flour is sweetened with sugar—as in cakes, cookies, and pastries—the chewing required is increased little if at all.

Sugar is sugar. It all contains four calories per gram, no matter what the origin. So products that boast of being better for you because they are sweetened not with cane sugar but with sugar from fruit juice, such as Frookie cookies and certain jams and jellies, are a rip-off. They all contain added sugar and your body couldn't care less whether it is from cane stalks in Florida or Haiti or grapes from California or Chile. Unfortunately, some people in the media have aided the food industry's deceptive advertising. For example, an article in one woman's magazine advised replacing sugar whenever possible with all-fruit preserves or frozen apple or orange juice concentrates.[12] There is also nothing magical about the sugar naturally present in foods that makes it less harmful; it's all a matter of the concentration. Juice with a high sugar content, such as grape, has as many or more calories as soft drinks sweetened with cane sugar, such as Kool-Aid.

The difference between sugar in processed foods and unprocessed ones is simply a matter of concentration. Grapes have sugar, but grape juice has far more because all the bulk of the grape has been stripped away. Oats have a little sugar in them; oatmeal cookies have lots. There's no doubt that humans have always craved sugar, but for primitive people the bulky, fibrous nature of sweet-tasting fruits and roots made consuming sugar a slow and laborious process. If the stores at which you shop ever sell sugarcane, buy a piece and chomp on it for awhile. Your jaws will lock up in pain long before you get a sugar fix equal to that in a can of soda or a candy bar. Honey was the only naturally occurring source of sugar to most humans but was hard to find and literally a pain in the butt (and everywhere else on the body) to harvest. It was only the invention of technology that made it possible to extract and dry sugar that the stuff could be added to processed foods and rapidly and frequently consumed.

It has been shown in experiments that volunteers eating most of their carbohydrates as refined sugars often felt hungry; whereas, when they ate the same amount of carbohydrates as vegetables and partly or wholly unrefined cereal foods, they complained of being "stuffed."[13]

It is sugar, and not fat, that is the ultimate calorically-dense food. This also brings up sugar's stealth factor. Candy bars, ice cream, and glazed doughnuts are not inconsequential contributors to the obesity problem. In 1982 the average American ate almost seventeen pounds of confectionary products, excluding chewing gum. By 1993 the amount increased to twenty-two pounds, according to the National Confectioners Association.[14] Still, these are but the tip of the sugar iceberg. It can be downright hard to buy products that don't have sugar added. Who would think that a Healthy Choice Chicken Broccoli Alfredo frozen dinner would have seven and a half teaspoons of sugar, and that its sugar would outweigh its protein? Or that a product calling itself Ultra Slim-Fast Chocolate Fudge would have six teaspoons of sugar, just less than a can of Nestlé Sweet Success diet plan? Or that the tomato ketchup made by Weight Watchers' parent company, Heinz, would get 100 percent of its calories from sugar?

HIDDEN SUGAR

Product	Total Calories	Sugar Content	% Calories from Sugar
1 SnackWell's Devil's Food Cookie Cake	50	9 grams, or 2 tsp.	72
8-oz. Dannon Light nonfat cappuccino yogurt	100	13 grams, or 2 ¾ tsp.	52
8-oz. Dannon Fruit on the Bottom low-fat apple-cinnamon yogurt, "99% fat free"	240	45 grams, or 9 ½ tsp.	75
8-oz. Snapple All Natural Peach-Flavored Iced Tea	110	26 grams, or 5 ½ tsp.	95
1 Weight Watchers Breakfast-on-the-Go blueberry muffin	190	22 grams, or 4 ¾ tsp.	46

Product	Total Calories	Sugar Content	% Calories from Sugar
1 Healthy Choice Chicken Broccoli Alfredo frozen dinner	370	35 grams, or 7 1/2 tsp.	38
1 Quaker Banana Crunch Rice Cake	50	5 grams, or 1 tsp.	40
1 can Pepsi	150	41 grams, or 8 3/4 tsp.	100
11-oz. Ultra Slim-Fast Chocolate Fudge	220	28 grams, or 6 tsp.	51
4.5-oz. Ragu Chicken Tonight Light Honey Mustard sauce	60	8 grams, or 1 3/4 tsp.	53
1 10-oz. can Nestlé Sweet Success diet plan	200	30 grams, or 6 1/2 tsp.	60
2 fat-free Fig Newtons	100	15 grams, or 3 tsp.	60

Source: *Self,* February 1995.[15]

Sugar also plays a major role in the excess consumption of the other food high in calorie density—fat. One reason we can eat so much fat is that fat is often made more palatable by adding sugar. Try eating pure butter and see how much you can stomach. But butter combined with sugar is the basis for the modern dessert. Cookies, cakes, ice cream, brownies, candy bars—all are mere variations of the fat-and-sugar combination. To blame only sugar, as was formerly done, was wrong. To blame only the fat, as is now done, is equally wrong.

But it gets more insidious yet. Sugar is also addictive in the sense that sugary foods tend to squeeze out the nonsugary ones. An article in the medical journal *Appetite* observed, ". . . animals of most species will readily accept and ingest a large quantity of sugar solution." It noted that "a number of investigators have found that rats given free access to both a sugar solution and standard laboratory chow consumed approximately 60 percent of their calories as carbohydrates, overate, and became obese."[16] One study found rats that were given free access to a sugar solution and chow significantly increased their calorie intake and took in as much as 86 percent of their calories as carbohydrates.[17] Considering this, we humans could be doing a lot worse. But with us, as with rats, we allow sugar to take the place of more healthful nutrients in our diet.

A native of a country with little processed sugar might find a sugarless bran muffin to be quite palatable. The average American, however, would spit it out. When I first tried European pastries I thought they were bitter and unpalatable, because those pastries contain so much less sugar than ours. So American bran muffin makers pack their product with sugar to sweeten it to the point that Americans find the bran taste tolerable, whereupon they eat the muffin and congratulate themselves for consuming such healthy food. But these muffins ought to be labeled "bran-flavored sugar muffins."

As we add sugar to our foods we find ourselves adding ever more sugar, because our sweetness threshold keeps going up. The amount of sugar needed to make that muffin palatable ten years ago is no longer enough. This helps explain why artificial sweeteners, against all expectations, don't seem to help much if at all in weight reduction. Despite containing no sugar themselves, they maintain the high sweetness threshold, thereby encouraging consumption of products that do contain sugar.

There is some debate over whether sugar consumption causes obesity beyond the actual intake of the calories themselves. Under one theory, sugar consumption leads to more sugar consumption or more food consumption in general. According to this belief, when sugar is a small part of a product, such as starches and most fruits, it slowly enters the bloodstream, and the pancreas releases enough insulin to break it down. But when sugars enters the body quickly, as happens with sugared drinks or candy or pastries, the pancreas thinks the sudden onslaught is just the forerunner. It panics. Beads of sweat build up on the pancreas's forehead. There's no time to call the Psychic Hotline for advice. Instead, the pancreas errs on the side of caution and injects far more insulin than is needed, causing an excess in the system, or a hypoglycemic state. To deal with the excess insulin, the body gets a craving for more sugar. If the person consumes more sugar to satisfy the craving, the cycle can repeat.[18] This scenario seems to make sense, but actually scientific evidence for it is lacking.[19] I don't know in which direction I lean, except to say that the damage done by sugar calories alone is enough.

Strangely enough, some have argued that high sugar consumption is actually associated with leanness.[20] The problem with such studies is, as has been previously noted, that people consistently understate their consumption of things they know they shouldn't be eating. "The big suspicion in the dietary literature is that people overestimate foods [they eat] that are healthy and underestimate the unhealthy ones," says Marion Nestle.[21] Obese people know that they're not supposed to be consuming much added sugar; hence, they will tend to underestimate and underreport their sugar intake. Lean people will suffer no such compunctions. Thus studies that simply take people's word for it will naturally find that fat people consumed less sugar than thin ones.

BY ANY OTHER NAME

Manufacturers are nonetheless aware that some consumers do look for sugar listings on labels, which is one reason they use any number of words instead, including: dextrose, sucrose, glucose, honey, corn sweetener, brown sugar, fructose, dextrin, high-fructose corn syrup, lactose, modified cornstarch, maltodextrin, maltose, malt, fruit juice concentrates, molasses, mannitol, maple syrup, turbinado sugar, sorghum, xylitol, and sorbitol. I probably left out a few, but you get the idea. Some of these represent sugar from sources other than cane but with all the same ill effects. Some are just components of cane sugar. By breaking down sugar into components, food makers can comply with the labeling law that says ingredients must be listed from greatest to least, yet still have something other than sugar appear as the first ingredient when it *is* actually the first ingredient. That is, if they used the term "sugar" for the ingredient list of a brownie, sugar would appear first and flour second. But by breaking down the sugar (verbally, not chemically) into sucrose and glucose, the brownie maker gets to list flour first, with sucrose and glucose second and third.[22] Sneaky, huh?

Further, while we are often admonished by the government that no more than 30 percent of our calories should come from fat, the government's advice has no upper limit on sugar. Presumably one could eat a diet with 80 percent of the calories from sugar and not incur the wrath of Uncle Sam. Going to the other extreme, the World Health Organization has said processed sugar should be eliminated completely from our diets.[23]

A happy medium, according to Franca Alphin, nutrition director at Duke University Diet and Fitness Center, is that sugar should comprise no more than 10 percent of carbohydrate calories. If you get the recommended 55 percent of your calories from carbohydrates and consume 1,800 calories daily, that would be 99 calories from sugar—less than in a can of soda.[24] That's about a fourth of what the average American currently consumes. If that's impossible for you, then at least follow another rule: Eat and drink less sugar than you used to.

Do Artificial Sweeteners Make You Fat?

Americans have increasingly turned to artificial sweeteners to decrease their sugar intake. These include such chemicals as cyclamates (which has since been banned because it was a rodent carcinogen), saccharin, and aspartame (commonly known as NutraSweet). There are also many new such sweeteners at various stages of testing. Sometimes they're also called noncaloric sweeteners, which is something of a misnomer since they all have calories, though perhaps so few that in the course of drinking a single beverage you may not consume so much as one calorie. A better term is "intense sweeteners." Intense sweeteners must be distinguished from artificial sweeteners such as xylitol and sorbitol. These two sweeteners are artificial, yet they provide as many calories as sugar. Nonetheless, they may be preferable for diabetics because they don't prompt the same insulin response.

Paradoxically, we continue to eat more sugar even as we eat more intense sweeteners and as the range of foods containing those sweeteners broadens. In 1970 Americans ate 5.8 pounds of saccharin per person. Saccharin usage rose steadily and was joined by aspartame in the 1980s. By 1991 Americans were eating 7.3

pounds of saccharin and 17 pounds of aspartame a year. Could it be that somehow the sweeteners themselves are making us hungrier and therefore causing us to eat more?

Apparently so, concluded a highly publicized 1986 study in which two researchers fed aspartame or water with glucose or plain water to groups of male and female students and then gauged their hunger. The doses of glucose were reported to decrease self-rated motivation to eat and to increase self-rated fullness. Aspartame, conversely, was reported to increase the motivation to eat and to decrease the feeling of fullness.[25] The study was criticized, however, because the students were never actually fed anything; therefore it was impossible to judge whether they really did act as if they felt more or less full.[26]

Barbara Rolls, of the University of Pennsylvania, who specializes in intense sweetener use, did a review of these myriad studies in the April 1991 *American Journal of Clinical Nutrition*. She concluded that if the substitution of aspartame is substantial "there will be some reduction in energy intake." She adds that "if intense sweeteners are part of a weight-control program, they could aid calorie control by providing palatable foods with reduced energy. It needs to be stressed that there are no data suggesting that consumption of foods and drinks with intense sweeteners promotes food intake and weight gain in dieters."[27] More recent studies appear to bear her out. For example, one showed that compared to sugar water and just plain water, neither aspartame nor saccharin increased feelings of hunger or the amount of food the volunteers later ate.[28]

So why is it, then, that after this massive influx of artificial sweeteners we are fatter than ever? Simple. As Barbara Rolls explained in her paper, the ability of an intense sweetener to reduce caloric intake depends on one's motivation. "If the individual uses the consumption of a low-calorie food as an excuse to eat a high-calorie food . . . daily energy intake may remain unchanged."[29] But that's putting it mildly. Americans have convinced themselves that if they can save 120 calories by drinking a diet drink rather than one with sugar, they can splurge and eat an extra 200 or 300 calories elsewhere. It's not the intense sweetener itself inducing excess food consumption; the problem lies in the American psyche. Once again, there is just no substitute for eating and drinking in moderation. Swap a diet soda for a regular soda and change your diet in no other way and you come out ahead of the game because you've saved anywhere from 120 to 200 calories. Use the diet soda as an excuse to pig out on other foods and you're still pigging out. Don't blame the guys who make aspartame or diet Coke or Diet Pepsi when the results show up on your waist and hips.

It saddens, even frustrates, me when I see an overweight person drinking sugar-sweetened soft drinks. A few days before I wrote this I saw a grossly overweight woman load eight 24-can cases of sugar-sweetened sodas into her tiny car, which sagged under the weight of the cans. Such drinks account for a quarter of all the sugar we consume.[30] If you're thin and don't have a cavity problem, drink up. But if you're overweight and want to drink soda, please make the switch to diet ones. At first they'll taste a bit bland, but soon enough you'll try a sugar-sweetened soda and find it's too sweet for you. I drink about one can of diet soda a day and find I cannot stomach soda with sugar in it. Over a long enough period of time, a person who drinks a lot of sodas—as apparently the woman I saw at the store does—can go from obese to fat or fat to lean just through quitting the sugared-soda habit, so long as he or she doesn't add other foods or drinks to compensate for the calories.

To broaden that advice, the average American could lose a substantial amount of weight just through moderate reductions in sugar consumptions. You don't have to agree with the author of *Sugar Blues*, who stated that refined sugar breaks up families and killed millions of Europeans in the fourteenth century, to know that getting the sugar monkey to loosen its grip on your back is a good idea.

5

Big Fat Myths That Make Us Fatter

Americans in the 1990s have become fascinated with genes. More and more we find that they influence not just looks but also health and numerous aspects of behavior. Unfortunately, this interest in genes has led many to simplistically blame the national obesity problem on them. After all, it seems as though scientists can find genes that explain everything else. A 1995 study by the Center for Media and Public Affairs in Washington, D.C., found that most discussions of the causes of obesity targeted neither food intake nor exercise but genetic predisposition, the result of heavy media coverage of the "fat gene."[1]

The desire on the part of fat people and their doctors to blame genes has a lengthy history. At the turn of the century obesity was considered the result of excess eating and laziness, but in the 1920s and 1930s scientists came to consider it a genetic problem. Still later in the 1930s scientists announced they did not find lower metabolisms in fat people. Thus the stigma began to return. Today the discovery of obesity genes, heavily promoted by the media, has swung the pendulum back. Once again it is fashionable to blame obesity on factors supposedly beyond our control. As a short *Time* magazine article title put it (though it was contradicted by the text): "Chubby? Blame Those Genes."[2]

TWIN STUDIES

The best evidence that there is some genetic component to obesity comes from studies of twins. In one study, Canadian researchers led by Claude Bouchard overfed (by 1,000 calories a day) twelve pairs of identical twins for six days a week over a 100-day period. They gained on average about eighteen pounds (two thirds of which was fat; one third, muscle). This wasn't remarkable. What *was* remarkable was that the range of weight gain varied from slightly over nine pounds to almost twenty-nine pounds. They also found that more often than not, brothers tended to gain weight along the same line as their twins. There were six times more variance between pairs than within them.[3]

Most twin studies, though, focus on twins raised separately so as to factor out the environmental component. The grandmaster of such studies is Dr. Albert Stunkard of the University of Pennsylvania. He has found repeatedly that twins reared apart from each other ended up with body-mass indices (BMIs) much closer to each other than to the families with whom they were raised.[4] (Remember that BMI is a calculation based on your weight and height.) While most studies have looked only at whites, at least one study on blacks had the same result.[5] As far as how often the tendency toward obesity is inherited, Claude Bouchard has estimated the frequency to be as low as 25 percent.[6]

Two Danish researchers have noted, however, that such studies "rely on BMI and provide more support for the inheritance of frame size or fat-free mass than for the inheritance of obesity." In other words, identical twins tend to have the same size bones and the same tendency to grow muscle, both of which, along with fat, go into BMI. A measurement of the twins' actual fat content would have been much more helpful.[7]

Stunkard himself has written, "Although there now seems to be little doubt about the role of genes in human obesity, the environmental causes are as important, as evidenced by the great variation in its occurrence over time both in individuals and populations."[8] Likewise, the National Academy of Science's Institute of Medicine says in its 1995 report *Weighing the Options*: "Although it is clear that genetics has a modest influence on obesity on a population basis, by far the largest amount of the variance in body weight is due to environmental influences."[9] Environmental influences are what you eat, how much you eat, and how sedentary you are.

Arlen Price, a geneticist at the University of Pennsylvania, also worked on some twin studies and found what Stunkard did: if one twin is overweight, the other is considerably more likely to be overweight, even when they were raised separately. "But," he cautioned, "there is great variation in the degree of overweight of twin siblings. One brother might only be 20 percent overweight, while his identical is 40 percent overweight."[10] The implication is that, even if you are genetically inclined toward being fatter, you still have control over your own body. It's not like height or eye color. Similarly, two Danish researchers who did twin studies have acknowledged that genes do play a role in obesity, nonetheless this does "not mean that obesity is determined at conception, but that subjects with the genetically determined predisposition become obese when they are exposed to a particular range of environmental conditions. This implies that the heritable tendencies may be prevented and that they are potentially reversible."[11]

One 1996 study showed just that. Paul Williams and his colleagues at the Berkeley National Laboratory combed through a database of 55,000 runners to identify all those with identical twins. They then contacted them to find out how many of them had as their twin somebody who was basically a couch potato. "None of the runners having overweight sedentary twins were themselves overweight," Williams told me. "This suggests to us that running may mitigate or even nullify the genetic predisposition to gaining weight."[12] There's no reason to think this doesn't apply to other exercise, as well.

HIDING BEHIND GENE DISCOVERIES

In December 1994, researchers in a report in *Nature* magazine rocked the world with their findings of a human genetic mutation that appears to disrupt the body's energy metabolism and appetite control center, the mechanism that tells the brain one has eaten enough. If you have a flaw in this gene, you keep on eating past a point where other people would be satiated.[13] It was instantly dubbed "*the* obesity gene" and heralded by heavy people everywhere. *The New York Times* led off its front-page "obesity gene" article with "Lending new support to the theory that obese people are not made but, rather, born that way. . . ."[14]

Reacting to another gene discovery, National Association for the Advancement of Fat Acceptance (NAAFA) president Sally Smith editorialized, "This study [in the March 9, 1995, *New England Journal of Medicine*] is significant in that it shores up the movement's argument that the dieting process, not the dieter, is to blame for the failure of the weight-loss process." She concluded that, "once again we are faced with research that, on the surface, validates our experience as fat people and supports long-held theories of the size acceptance movement."[15] Meanwhile, National Public Radio's fat defender Daniel Pinkwater wrote in an essay, "The recent announcement of a 'fat rat gene' suggests what we knew all the time—fatness is hereditary."[16]

Oh, yeah? Let's take a few seconds out of our busy schedules and think about this. Can genes explain the explosion of obesity we've been seeing in the United States? George Bray, M.D., editor of the journal *Obesity Research*, states the obvious when he says, "Our genes haven't changed in the past ten years."[17] Can genes explain why I can walk around some European cities for days and not see anyone as fat as Sally Smith, but if I went to an American buffet (which I never do anymore), I'd see half a dozen persons rivaling her in size? "Compared to us . . . most Irish, Chinese and Italians seem petite, if not downright scrawny," observed an editorial in the Louisville, Kentucky, *Courier-Journal.* "Does that mean all the fat genes crossed the ocean to take up residence in our bountiful land?"[18] Very clever of those genes, huh?

In August 1995, scientists pinpointed another human gene they said appeared related to obesity. Again, the fat acceptance groups cheered and again newspapers portrayed it as absolving fat people of responsibility. "Reassuring the overweight that obesity is more than a matter of sloth and gluttony . . ." began the Associated Press story.[19] But if you had the patience to read down far enough, you'd learn that "many skinny people have the [gene in question], and many fat people do not." The article also noted that in the part of the study conducted in France, the persons with the flawed gene average 147 pounds, while those without it were 112.[20] That's a huge difference, but remember from chapter two that in the

Nurses' Health Study, the average American woman is between 150 and 160.[21] The average American man is heavier yet. So even French people with a copy of the obesity gene were thinner than most Americans!

This gene apparently does its dirty work by slowing the body's use of food intake. But the difference between persons with and without the gene was all of thirty-six calories a day—basically the equivalent of a piece of hard candy, a dollop of mayonnaise, or four minutes on a treadmill. If you are unfortunate enough to have two copies of the gene, you have an extra eighty calories a day to deal with, meaning two pieces of hard candy or eight minutes on a treadmill.[22]

This also applies to the results of a study you may have heard about in which obese black women were found to burn about ninety calories fewer a day than a comparison group of white women. Ninety calories hardly means a destiny of obesity. Indeed, the comparison white women who burned those extra ninety calories a day were on average slightly fatter and had higher BMIs than the black women![23]

In short, even if you are that very rare individual who has both copies of the gene, you are hardly condemned to a life of obesity, much less gross obesity. It can't possibly account for your weighing 250 pounds, much less the 300, 350, 400, or more pounds many Americans these days weigh. It means a tiny bit of sacrifice or extra work beyond that of your neighbor who has no copies of the gene.

"There are genetic differences, but they aren't things that can't be overcome by eating right and getting exercise," says G. Ken Goodrick of the Baylor College of Medicine in Houston. "A lot of my patients say they're exercising regularly and eating very little and I look them square in the face and tell them they're violating the law of physics."[24] "Genes don't cause obesity. They make people more susceptible to obesity, says William Dietz, M.D., of the New England Medical Center. "That means the process by which the gene operates can be modified, to either make people overweight or to be controlled in a way that people don't become overweight."[25] And says Rockefeller University's Jules Hirsch, M.D., "No matter what genes you have, if you don't eat the food, you're not going to get fat."[26]

THE NATIVE EXPERIENCE

An obesity hormone "does not account in my mind for the remarkable increase in obesity that has occurred even in this decade," said Theodore van Itallie, M.D., an obesity researcher at Columbia University's College of Physicians and Surgeons in New York. Nor, he added, "does it account for the fact that people moving from one country to another will change their weights."[27] Which brings us to some fascinating research showing that as native peoples move into a Western culture their weight has a tendency to absolutely explode—and thereby explode the myth that obesity is all in one's genes.

Consider the sad case of the Pima Indians in the American Southwest. At least one group of Pima living on a reservation has a rate of diabetes almost twenty times higher than a comparison group of whites.[28] Because they have such a terrible obesity problem, the Pima Indians have been subjected to a terrific amount of studies to determine if their problem is genetic. Some scientists have speculated that the Pima may suffer from a genetic defect. But this was not borne out in two studies that actually measured Pima metabolism. One study comparing Pima adults with white adults in fact found the Pimas had a faster metabolism per pound of fat-free mass,[29] while another of children found that they had the same metabolism as comparison white kids.[30] In yet a third study, National Institutes of Health researcher Eric Ravussin did find a difference of seventy calories burned a day between fatter and less fat Indians.[31] Over time one can see how that seventy calories could make a difference. But again, one can see how easily a little more exercise or a bit less eating could counteract it.

Indeed, what researchers have found is that compared even to American whites, the Pima are a sedentary people. One comparison between Pima and white children found that across the board, Pima boys and girls engaged in less sports, less physical playing, and more TV watching than white boys and girls.[32] In any event, once again we see that even if genes are a problem they are not destiny. One study comparing active Pimas to more sedentary ones found that the more active ones were also leaner.[33]

Another fascinating study compared Pima in Arizona living it up the American way with those in Mexico who still live to a great extent as they have for centuries. The results were startling. The Mexican Pima women averaged only 132 pounds, while their Arizona counterparts squeezed the scales at 198. Mexican Pima men weighed 153 pounds compared to 199 for the Pima males in Arizona. Part of the difference is that the Mexican Pima were shorter on average, but comparing by BMI we see again the huge difference. Mexican Pima women averaged a BMI of 25.1 and Mexican Pima men 24.8; for the Arizona ones it was 35.5 and 30.8, respectively. In short, the Mexican Pima are at worst borderline overweight, while Arizona Pima men are obese and the Arizona Pima women are terribly obese.[34] It wasn't genes that condemned the Arizona Pima to obesity; it was nationalities—which country they happened to live in. The Pima are proof of a point I've tried to make throughout this book: The very act of living in the United States puts you at great risk for obesity.

Another ethnic group that has aroused great interest are the Samoans. Western Samoa is part of the Samoan group of islands, located approximately midway between Australia and Hawaii. It comprises the two large islands of Upolu and Savai'i, plus some smaller islands. Apia, on the island of Upolu, is the main town and center of government. The majority of Western Samoans are full-blooded Polynesians thought to have originated in Southeast Asia some 3,500 to 4,000 years ago.

Early European explorers of the Pacific Ocean were impressed by the large and muscular physiques of the island inhabitants, particularly in Polynesia and Micronesia. In 1996 there was an exhibit at the Metropolitan Museum in New York displaying photographs of Samoans between 1875 and 1925. The men and women shown were as lean as the cast members of *Baywatch*, albeit lacking the rippled abdomens, silicone implants, and collagen-injected "bee-stung" lips.[35]

Now that has all changed. In Apia, many work in sedentary jobs and the diet includes a high proportion of imported foods. In rural areas, subsistence agriculture and fishing remain important sources of food but differences between rural and urban areas have diminished markedly as increased cash incomes and improved transportation have made imported foods more available in rural areas. As their lifestyle has changed, so has the Samoans' weight—and incredibly so. At least as early as 1978, it was clear that something was terribly wrong in Western Samoa, that the inhabitants were suffering extraordinary rates of obesity and Type II diabetes. But since then the problem has grown dramatically worse. Between 1978 and 1991 in the rural area of Tuasivi, obesity increased by almost 300 percent among the males and it more than doubled among the women. And in Apia in 1991, over 58 percent of the males and an amazing 78 percent of the females were obese. In the thirty-five to forty-four age category, just shy of 90 percent of all the women were obese.[36]

Prior to this period, when the Western Samoans were relatively thin, it was found that when they left their traditional culture for modern ones they became dramatically fatter. Data collected in 1979 showed Western Samoan females averaging slightly above 130 pounds when in Western Samoa, while those who were in the American-controlled part of the islands weighed in at about 170 pounds. Those in the United States proper but still in a relatively native population—that is, those residing in Hawaii—weighed a few pounds more. Finally, those on the continental United States, who were completely submerged in American culture, were the fattest.[37]

In his book *Radical Chic and Mau-Mauing the Flak Catchers*, Tom Wolfe describes the Samoans as seen in San Francisco: "You get the feeling the football players come from a whole other species of human, they're so big. Well, that will give you some idea of the Samoans, because they're bigger. . . . They start out at about 300 pounds and from there they just get *wider*."[38] Actually, that's a bit of an exaggeration. The California Samoans studied weighed about 185 pounds on average, or more than 40 percent more than the Samoans back in Western Samoa. Concluded the researchers, "the California Samoan population may be the world's heaviest."[39] A separate study found that Samoan women in Hawaii were three times more likely to be overweight than those in Western Samoa.[40]

The Japanese have had a similar experience. Like the Samoans, the closer the Japanese get to the continental United States, the fatter they become. To choose just one age range to illustrate, among those forty-five to forty-nine, less than 4 percent of the men living in Japan were obese when the study was done. But among those living in Hawaii it was 12 percent and among those in California it was about 14 percent. Why were the Japanese living in

America so much fatter? No secret; they ate more. They were probably considerably less active, too, but the study didn't measure activity.[41]

African-Americans have also been compared with Africans in Nigeria. The American blacks were about a fourth heavier than their counterparts in the Old World.[42]

One set of researchers at the University of Hawaii came up with a terrific idea. They took 20 natives and placed them on a "pre-Western-contact Hawaiian diet" for 21 days. The food consisted of such things as taro (a starchy root, similar to a white potato), sweet potatoes, yams, breadfruit, taro leaves, fruit, seaweed, fish, and chicken. All foods were served either raw or steamed in a way to imitate ancient styles of cooking. The diet turned out to have a very low fat content (7 percent) and a very high fiber content. The results were simply amazing. Despite being told they could eat all the traditional foods they wished (except a limit was placed on the fish and chicken), average daily caloric intake decreased from 2,594 calories a day (actually probably more, according to the researchers) on the Western diet to only 1,569 a day on the native diet. They also lost on average more than 17 pounds, and they saw their cholesterol levels and blood pressure drop as well. This almost incredible amount of weight loss was possible only because the men were so terribly obese to begin with.[43]

These studies on native peoples teach us an invaluable lesson. Genes may count for something, but the overwhelming factors in obesity are culture and individual behavior. The first explains why Americans are so much fatter than people in other countries, the second explains why some Americans are so much fatter than other Americans. Obesity gene research is certainly interesting and may eventually lead to help for some individuals. So far though, it's had nothing but a pernicious effect, allowing people to blame something other than their own behavior. "But people don't want to hear that," says John Foreyt of Baylor College. "They don't want to hear it's all themselves to blame."[44]

What if we applied the obesity "gene defense" to something else, say intelligence? There's ample evidence that intelligence has a genetic component. But what would the appropriate response for a teacher be if a student approached her with his test marked "D" and explained that he had determined that he was genetically intellectually disadvantaged and therefore a "D" was the best he could do. Any good teacher would say, "Well, Johnny, if that's true I guess it just means you'll have to study a bit harder than some of the other boys and girls, but I will expect the same results from you I expect from them." To do any less is to guarantee that Johnny turns in nothing but "D" tests for the rest of his life.

That's the sort of defeatism that some in the media and the fat acceptance movement are fostering. It must be resisted. The bottom line on genes is this: If you are blessed, you have an obligation to not push your luck and overcome your predisposition by becoming fat anyway. If you are cursed, you have an obligation to resist that curse even while you wait for the first anti-obesity gene therapies. There is no excuse for self-defeatism, much less throwing your lot in with the fat acceptance movement and working to spread your self-defeatism to the American population as a whole.

THE SETPOINT MYTH

No one dietary myth prompts more satisfaction and—paradoxically—more despair than that of the "setpoint." If you've thrown in the towel and joined the fat acceptance movement, setpoint theory tells you you've made a proper decision. On the other hand, if you're overweight and still hope to slim down, the mere utterance of setpoint can send you into spasms of anguish. It seems so unfair. But, it's not just unfair; it's untrue.

The setpoint, as is generally understood, means that your body has somehow decided that it wants to be a certain weight and, depending on whom you ask, changing that weight is anywhere from terribly difficult to utterly impossible.

In discussing how she and other fat activists are attempting to alter the way obesity is perceived, Carrie Hemenway says, "We share a common language. 'I've reached my setpoint,' I tell a friend. The word 'setpoint' is ours."[45] Indeed it is. Evidence that the setpoint theory has trickled down to the masses and is being used as a license for gluttony was a letter in 1996 to the editor of *The New York Times Magazine*. "Study after study has shown that our bodies naturally gravitate toward a set weight, and that diets don't work," wrote Emily Harrison of New York. "When are Americans going to go back to just enjoying themselves and their food?"[46] Another letter stated, "The body has a certain setpoint and will fight like crazy to stay there. . . . Let's accept ourselves as we are. Whether a person weighs 110, 160, 250, or 350. . . ."[47] Naturally, someone had to also go and write a book called *The Setpoint Diet.*[48]

Before looking at the science, let's just apply a little common sense here. We know that Americans are getting fatter by the year, that in 1994 they weighed on average eleven to twelve pounds more than in 1977–78.[49] Are we to believe that our bodies are engaging in some sort of national conspiracy to raise everybody's setpoint? Is this a plot for an Oliver Stone movie? For *The X-Files?* ("Next week on *The X-Files*: Are UFO's raising our setpoints?")

In reality, all the setpoint means is that your body tends to want to be where it is now. If you've been 110 for some time, your body wants to be 110. If you've been 350 for some time, your body wants to be 350. This is a basic rule of physics, that things will tend, at least in the short run, to stay the way they are. That's why my apartment tends to stay so messy. (On the other hand, when it is clean it seems to get messy awfully fast. Let's not take that analogy too far.) But to say that something tends to stay the way it is hardly means it's unchangeable.

THE ROCKEFELLER STUDY

The mother of all setpoint studies, conducted at Rockefeller University in New York, was reported in a March 1995 issue of *New England Journal of Medicine.* The article led to such news reports as *The New York Times*'s, "Metabolism Found to Adjust to a Body's Natural Weight."[50] Many of the stories told people trying to lose weight to pretty much just hang it up. "Think You'll Ever Be Slim Again? Fat Chance!" was the title columnist Joan Beck used when taking on the subject.[51] One newspaper told readers, "Even the Best Dieters May Be Doomed; Study Bolsters Setpoint Theory,"[52] while another headline read, "Dieting Won't Be of Much Help to the Obese; Body Weight Not Voluntary, Authors of New Study Say."[53]

Actually, the study skewered a couple of myths the fat acceptance people propagate. One is that "yo-yo" dieting permanently slows the metabolism. Once the subjects regained their weight, their metabolisms were right back where they started. The study also showed once again that obese people do not have unusually slow metabolisms.[54] Somehow neither of these findings made their way into any of the fat acceptance literature that discussed the study.

Instead, what interested most people was the study's finding of a metabolism reduction that came about when people ate less, and a metabolism increase that happened when people ate more. Specifically, the study found that a "10 percent increase or decrease in the usual weight was accompanied by a 16 percent increase or 15 percent decrease, respectively" in resting metabolic rate.[55]

To understand this, you have to understand that metabolisms go up with more eating and down with less eating for two reasons. The first is simply that as you lose fat you usually also lose a certain amount of the muscle that was needed to support the weight of that fat. The less muscle you have, the lower your metabolic rate, because less muscle means less need for energy. Another way of looking at it is that your lighter body now needs less energy to get around just as a light little Honda uses less gasoline to travel the same distance as a big heavy Cadillac. But that's not what the Rockefeller study was talking about. It was talking about the other aspect of metabolism. That's the tendency of your body to either conserve energy when you reduce caloric intake because it thinks a famine might be setting in, or conversely its tendency to burn off extra calories when you overeat.

I never hesitate to criticize the media when it's deserved. But here the media could hardly be blamed for characterizing the study as they did because all three of the doctors who conducted it, especially the chief one, Rudolph Leibel, M.D., gave it the same spin. On a television news segment with the pessimistic title "Why You Can't Lose Weight by Dieting," Leibel said people can't help being fat "anymore than Michael Jordan can help his height."[56] He told a news magazine, "To claim that obesity is a problem under voluntary control is comparable to blaming somebody for their skin color or their height or their hair color."[57]

This coverage caused a lot of hearts to sink. "When I had to go to class that night," said fitness and weight-loss guru Richard Simmons, "there were 300 women waving [an] article in their hands like a *Citizen Kane* segment in his movie. They were scared. It took some of their motivation away."[58]

New Age guru Deepak Chopra, M.D., author of the perfectly silly book *Perfect Weight*,[59] gave the idea the worst—and dumbest— spin when he told a news show that eating less actually *packs on* the fat. ". . . The major misconception people have is that if you cut down the amount of calories you're going to lose weight," he said. "What happens is, when you drastically reduce your caloric intake, is that your body perceives a famine coming on and it actually slows down its metabolism and the more you cut down, the slower the metabolism gets and the more you gain weight. So, losing weight and optimizing your weight is not dependent on cutting down your food intake."[60] No obesity doctor anywhere that I've ever heard of, including the three from Rockefeller, ever claimed that calorie reduction actually makes you *fatter*. The most they've said is that your body shows resistance against attempts to become thinner.

But let's leave behind Chopra's foolishness and consider Leibel's assertion, again applying a little common sense. In the last ten years, Michael Jordan has neither gained nor lost height. But in that same decade, tens of millions of Americans have either gained or lost large amounts of weight and maintained that loss or gain.

Let's look at a specific individual, say, Sally Smith, president of NAAFA. Smith reportedly weighs 350 pounds. But she wasn't born that way. She got that way through persistence. Month after month, year after year, she ate more than she burned off in energy. Setpoint be damned, she worked her way up to 150, then 200, then 250, then 300, finally arriving at 350. Now she says that setpoints are virtually impossible to defeat even as she's living, breathing proof that they cannot only be defeated but utterly put to shame. If the Sally Smiths of the world can work their way up the obesity ladder with setpoints tugging at their heels, they can work their way down, as well.

The way some writers have tried to deal with such embarrassing facts is to say that the setpoint can be moved. Thus Glenn Gaesser writes in his fat-acceptance tome, *Big Fat Lies*, that "a lot of people's setpoints will keep them from ever satisfying the insurance industry and government weight recommendations,"[61] but just two pages later he tells us that "in fact the setpoint can itself change. . . ." Wait a second here. A moving setpoint is not one of those cute oxymorons we're always hearing, like jumbo shrimp, military intelligence, and journalistic integrity. Yet all the time, you hear people promising a magic formula to "change your setpoint." The very cover of the aforementioned book, *The Setpoint Diet*, says, "Finally, lose ALL the weight you need to and keep it off forever by lowering your setpoint."[62] You can buy and eat jumbo shrimp, but if a setpoint is a setpoint, then by golly it's a *set* point. Otherwise it loses all its meaning.

In any case, Leibel seems to be proposing (and most of the fat acceptance people adopting) what we would call not simply a setpoint but a "ratchet-wrench setpoint." It can go up but not back down. But nothing in his study supports that. Remember, in fact, that it showed that subjects' metabolisms sped up to compensate for extra calories just as they slowed down to compensate for fewer ones. In other words, the whole time Sally Smith was eating more and more, her metabolism was racing faster and faster to try to burn off some of those extra calories. Yet she defeated all that in her climb to 350 pounds.

The Rockefeller authors would also have you think that metabolic change is permanent. Said one, Jules Hirsch, M.D., "the person who lost . . . body weight is forever different in respect of needing calories."[63] Similarly, another Michael Rosenbaum, M.D., claims there's "no evidence that maintaining the new weight for an extended length of time changes your setpoint."[64]

But other obesity researchers disagree. "That was the major criticism of the Rockefeller study," says their colleague, Steven Heymsfield, M.D., of the adjoining St. Luke's–Roosevelt Hospital. "The real question is what happens after a year or so that you've been at that weight. It by no means indicates that reduced obese [formerly obese people] have a permanently lower metabolic rate." He adds that while the Rockefeller researchers have done very provocative work and good work in other areas as well, "I think they're very polarized in their views and that a vast majority of scientists have different views on obesity. They're definitely out on a limb."[65]

Again, let's consult our old friend Common Sense and pick on poor Sally Smith just one last time. At one time she was 150, but now tilts the scales at 350. So isn't her metabolism working desperately to pull her back down to her 150-pound weight? No, because it's now settled in comfortably at the 350 level. She worked her way up to that and held it long enough for her metabolism to adjust.

Metabolism adjustment has been evident in numerous studies that Leibel, Hirsch, and Rosenbaum conveniently ignored. (Their own study was too short to allow such a determination.) For example, in an experiment lasting almost a year, University of Pennsylvania School of Medicine researchers put two sets of obese women on diets. One group ate 1,200 calories a day. The other also ate 1,200 calories a day, except for two weeks when they consumed only 420 calories per day. Ultimately, both sets of women lost the same amount of weight. During the first five weeks of the experiment, both groups also showed steep declines in metabolic rates. But by the end of the study those rates had risen to within 10 percent of their original levels. That missing 10 percent simply reflected the reduced size of the women's bodies (Remember my heavy-car-versus-light-car analogy?), not the slowdown in metabolism that is part of the body's antifamine defense mechanism.[66]

Metabolisms do readjust. It's just a matter of waiting it out. The length of that wait varies from person to person and perhaps depends on other factors, such as how quickly the weight was lost. The point is that you need to give yourself time. Your metabolism will catch up to you. This is one reason it's wise for the extremely obese to lose weight in stages. Drop part of your weight, give yourself at least a few months for your metabolism to start to rise back up, then lose some more weight. Repeat as necessary.

Yes, to maintain your new, slimmer body you will always have to eat less (or exercise more), simply because you'll be sustaining less weight. (Don't force me to invoke that heavy car–light car analogy again.) But no, you won't be stuck permanently with a metabolism that is trying to defend you from famine, trying desperately to push you back to your old poundage. And just as permanent weight gain has obviously been attained by many Americans, so can permanent weight loss.

The setpoint theory has its place, but its place is alongside goblins, fairies, dragons, honest high-ranking politicians, and other creatures of mythology.

THE "IT'S A MYTH THAT FAT PEOPLE EAT
MORE THAN THIN PEOPLE" MYTH

The debate over whether fat people eat more than thin ones is truly historic. In his classic book, *The Life of Samuel Johnson*, biographer James Boswell (1740–95) recalls a conversation between himself and the famed philosopher regarding an extremely corpulent fellow. Johnson (1709–1804), who himself is rather fat, tells Boswell, "He eats too much, Sir." Replies Boswell, "I don't know, Sir; you will see one man fat, who eats moderately, and another lean, who eats a great deal." Replies his mentor: "Nay, Sir, whatever may be the quantity that a man eats, it is plain that if he is too fat, he has eaten more than he should have done. One man may have a digestion that consumes food better than common; but it is certain that solidity is increased by putting something to it."

Today we hear it repeatedly—and not just from fat people—that scientific research has proven that fat people eat no more than thin ones.

- Covert Bailey, in his megaseller *The New Fit or Fat*, has one chapter titled, "Fat People Eat Less Than Skinny People."[67]
- Joel Gurin, now editorial director of *Consumer Reports* magazine, wrote in the June 1989 *Psychology Today* of recent studies showing "absolutely no connection between calorie intake and body weight."[68]
- Diane Epstein and Kathleen Thompson, in their fat acceptance book *Feeding on Dreams*, put in a sidebar, "A study of three thousand people that was reported in the *British Medical Journal* revealed that the fattest subjects ate the least and the thinnest ate the most."[69]
- Dale Atrens tells us in his book, *Don't Diet*, that "Fat people are no more likely to overeat than are lean people, yet fat people are widely assumed to be gluttons."[70] He adds that, "To further indicate just how baseless a prejudice the notion of the fat glutton is, most of the available data (inadequate as they are) show that fat people eat less than thin people!"[71]
- Dawn Atkins, writing in a NAAFA publication, states: "The myth that a person who is fat eats more or differently has

not been proven by studies. In fact, at least twenty studies have tried to show that fat people either eat great quantities, or less nutritionally sound food than thinner people. . . . Only one study found a higher consumption by fat participants."[72]

Here's what all these people *didn't* tell you. Yes, there are numerous studies indicating that the obese don't eat more than the lean, but these simply take the subjects' word for it. They're based on recall.[73] But what if that recall is wrong? In fact, study after study has shown just that.

The best-known of these studies questioning eating recall was done at the Obesity Research Center at St. Luke's–Roosevelt Hospital in New York and appeared in the *New England Journal of Medicine* in 1992. It evaluated a group of nine women and one man who claimed that their metabolisms were defective, causing them to be obese even though they said they were eating 1,200 calories or fewer a day. Some of them were taking thyroid medicine, in the belief that a thyroid malfunction was causing their metabolisms to be slow. The study compared these ten to a group of eighty people who didn't claim to have such a defect. Like earlier researchers who found consistently that obese people ate less, these researchers asked the subjects to recall how many calories they had eaten. But in addition, this study actually *measured* the caloric intake using a technique called "doubly labeled water."

Put simply, the doubly labeled water technique involves subjects drinking water containing two nonradioactive atomic isotopes. It doesn't taste like Dom Pérignon, but it's quite harmless. The subjects then give urine samples each day for analysis. The technique shows how much energy is used; the more burned up, the more carbon dioxide is produced and the faster one of the isotopes disappears from the body relative to the other.

Using this, the researchers compared the number of calories the ten obese people said they ate versus the calories the double water technique showed they actually did consume. They found the subjects had *understated* how much they'd *eaten* by one half. Moreover, they had *overstated* how much they had *exercised* by the same amount. Using a different system to measure metabolic rate, the researchers found that the obese people burned calories at the same rate as the control group who had not claimed to have slow metabolisms.[74]

"These people positioned themselves, in a sense, as being different from other people who are obese, in that they ate very little and they couldn't lose weight," said one of the researchers, Steven Heymsfield. "And we found, in a sense, that they were not different than other obese people in terms of their metabolism. What distinguished them was the fact that they severely underreported what they were eating."[75]

Did these people intentionally lie to the researchers? Apparently they were lying to themselves. Indeed, the St. Luke's–Roosevelt doctors reported that the obese people "were distressed when they were given their study results."[76]

In explaining such underreporting, one obese patient told CNN News, "I mean, you don't want to tell about the chocolate cake in the middle of the night, mostly because you want to forget."[77] Rosemary Green in *Diary of a Fat Housewife* said that when she was trying to fight her obesity through keeping a food log she would often sneak food in the middle of the night, reasoning that it was too late to go on the previous day's log but too early to go on the next day's.[78] "Whatever I ate during those 'magic' hours has no caloric effect on me," she wrote in her diary. (Of course, at some level she knew better.) Obese comedienne Beth Donahue reports playing a mind game in which "the faster you drink the [chocolate] syrup, the fewer calories you ingest. If I can just gulp it down quick enough, there's no way it will register on the log-in system that catalogues what goes down in my mouth every day." She adds, "We've all told ourselves that one!"[79]

Fat activists howled when the St. Luke's–Roosevelt study came out, insisting, as one put it, "the conclusion of this one study is contradicted by many studies showing that, on average, obese people do not eat more than thin people."[80] What they ignored (or possibly didn't know) was that this was just the latest in a litany of such findings. Indeed, to my knowledge, every single study ever done that has actually measured food intake, as opposed to taking a person's word for it, has found the same thing.

A report in the April 1996 *American Journal of Clinical Nutrition* states, "These results indicate that energy intake derived from food records is an imprecise measure that substantially underestimates energy intake."[81] This confirmed a previous one in the October 14, 1995, *British Medical Journal* that found, "In agreement with other studies, a direct relationship was seen between obesity and dietary underreporting of energy and protein."[82]

Studies showing systematic underreporting by the obese go back for decades, so there's no excuse for fat activists or diet book authors to be ignorant of them. One from 1978 found obese persons underestimated their intake by 800 calories a day, "suggesting that estimates of energy intake by overweight individuals are at least moderately uncertain and may often be quite unreliable,"[83] while a 1982 study used direct observation to report that obese patients understated their calories by about half.[84]

FAT PEOPLE HAVE *HIGHER* METABOLISMS

Most studies actually indicate that obese people have higher metabolic rates than lean ones. Let me just shoot a few of the titles past you: "High Levels of Energy Expenditure in Obese Women," "Elevated Metabolic Rates in Obesity," "A Positive Correlation Between Energy Intake and Body Mass Index in a Population of 1,312 Overweight Subjects."[85] Notes yet another, "The finding of elevated energy expenditure in overweight subjects is so consistent, regardless of the method used, that any survey that fails to note an increase in the mean caloric intake of a group of overweight subjects should be considered unrepresentative of their usual nutrient intake."[86]

Now actually, per pound of muscle, obese people have the same metabolic rate as thin ones. But in order to support their excess fat, obese people have to grow more muscle. The more muscle you have, the higher your metabolic rate. So no, pound for pound of muscle, fat people don't have faster metabolisms. But overall they do have faster ones, because of that extra muscle supporting the extra fat. This means that if 350-pound Sally eats a fried chicken leg and 125-pound Betty eats an identical leg, Sally is actually going to burn off more of those calories and convert less to fat than Betty.

Is there anybody out there who can truthfully claim that his or her fat is from a slow metabolism? "I think it's an urban legend," Heymsfield told me. "I've never found anybody with a very low metabolism like people often think they have. We have people who come here and they say, 'Oh my metabolism is so slow,' but when we measure we find that 99 percent of the population is within a range of plus or minus 10 or 15 percent. The notion that they could be 25 percent below normal is ridiculous unless they have a disease like hypothyroidism."[87]

It is true that even a metabolism that's 10 percent lower than average will lead to some weight gain, but Heymsfield puts it in the range of perhaps ten or fifteen pounds more than the person otherwise would be. "When we get people who say they eat 800 calories a day we find that their resting metabolic rate alone is 1,000 or more a day," says Heymsfield. "These people [who can maintain obesity with 800 calories daily] really just don't exist."

Well, then, what about hypothyroidism? "Hypothyroidism can slow the metabolic rate," says Heymsfield. "I don't know the frequency in population exactly but it could be as high as one in a hundred." Nonetheless, he says doctors often prescribe thyroid medicine to fat people just to get them out of the office. Still, some people really do have a thyroid deficiency and "There does seem to be a small weight gain in the twenty- to twenty-five-pound range," he says.[88] But obesity is just one of the symptoms. If you don't have the others, such as hair loss, dry skin, and intolerance to cold, there's probably nothing wrong with your thyroid.

If there's no evidence that fatter people have slower metabolic rates, then how about those people we all seem to know who are terribly thin yet claim to eat like hogs and always seem to be eating around you? I've known them, too. But when I interview them I find they don't eat nearly as much as they think they do, or that they expend tremendous amounts of energy. I had one skinny roommate who each night for dinner ate half a chicken and half a cake, albeit unfrosted. But his job was delivering pizzas and he jogged daily. Further, the pizzas he delivered were so crummy I had no illusions that he was eating on the job. In another case a friend told me he felt his thinness must be for the most part genetic. But under pressure (I threatened to shoot his dog), he readily confessed that he exercises regularly both by walking and by lifting weights and has a diet that is almost as tightly controlled as that of a rat eating premeasured portions of chow.

When I asked Heymsfield if it were possible that some people have considerably higher than average metabolisms, he said probably not. Still, he conceded that there's almost no medical literature on the subject "since these people haven't complained."[89] Makes sense, doesn't it?

With such a mass of medical evidence—and simple common sense—telling us one thing, why do so many people cling to the myth of the undereating or "metabolically impaired" obese person? Pretending there's no relationship between intake and obesity serves any number of disparate agendas. It allows the fat acceptance people to pretend they're not gluttons and even claim victim status. It allows people selling exercise as a magic solution to claim that since fat people don't differ in caloric intake, only exercise can make a difference. It allows the "fat-free" hawkers, be they writers of books or sellers of dessert cakes, to claim that since fat people don't differ in caloric intake, the only difference must be the fat content of the food. In a nutshell, saying that obesity is caused by *something* other than overeating allows the sky to be the limit on what that something is—and every shyster in the world is going to have his or her own magic formula.

THE UNDOUBTING DOCTORS

Yet doctors have also added to the misinformation. "It would . . . seem that some nutritionists and physicians are engaged in a sort of denial as they continue to dwell on 'metabolic factors' and ignore the inaccuracies of dietary histories, while paying so little attention to the psychodynamics of obesity,"[90] observed Gilbert B. Forbes, M.D., in the October 1993 *Nutrition Reviews*.

Indeed, in an editorial accompanying the St. Luke's–Roosevelt study in the *New England Journal of Medicine*, Elliot Danforth Jr., M.D., and Ethan A. H. Sims, M.D., were absolutely bristling. Clearly they did not want to believe that fat people are responsible for being fat, but just as clearly they could not refute the data. "It would be unfortunate," they wrote, "if the results of the study were misinterpreted by others, including the lay press, as proving that obesity is simply the result of gluttony and sloth and that obese people fool themselves and others about their eating and physical activity."[91] In fact, that is the only logical interpretation.

Back when I wrote my first book, on the subject of AIDS and how it is transmitted, an epidemiologist with the New York City Department of Health explained to me why so many doctors willingly accepted that their clients had gotten the disease from a prostitute when the evidence indicated they probably got it from a homosexual lover or intravenous drugs. Doctors, he told me, hate to believe that their patients would deceive them. It's "the old clinician's perspective: 'that my patients wouldn't dare lie to me,' " he said. "Doctors aren't in the business of determining if patients are lying or not."[92]

Doctors who treat the obese fall into two categories: Those who believe patients who claim to maintain 300 pounds of weight on a chicken drumstick and a piece of lettuce a day, and those who don't believe them. One doctor told me about one of his patients who, while grossly obese, claimed she ate like the proverbial bird— nothing but low-fat vegetables. But when he applied his stethoscope to listen to her heartbeat, he heard an alarming crunching sound. Turns out he stumbled onto the potato chip cache under her blouse.

It's understandable that doctors would not want to think their patients are deceiving them, but if it hurts their pride to admit it, that's too bad. "Change starts with recognizing and taking responsibility for existing behavior," noted a letter to the editor of the *New England Journal of Medicine* challenging Danforth and Sims. "Researchers and clinicians might assist patients in this process, rather than abetting them in their denial."[93]

A lot of people are going to hate me for what I've done here. I've taken away their excuses about abnormal thyroids and slow metabolisms. I've shown them in no uncertain terms that they're fat because they eat too much and exercise too little, and that if they think otherwise they've been dishonest with themselves. But I hope at least some of them will realize the favor I've tried to do them. I've tried to immunize them against their own excuses. George Mann, M.D., in an editorial in the *New England Journal of Medicine*, put it strongly, saying, "There is an old and treasured notion that obesity is caused by a metabolic defect, whether acquired or inherited, and this makes obesity a kind of act of God. It removes all blame and postpones successful management. . . ."[94] No reader who has paid attention to this chapter will continue with such a belief and postpone successful management. If people know that losing weight means taking in fewer calories and burning off more, and that there's no avoiding that equation, some of them will do just that. They'll make no more efforts at hiding behind their thyroids or their genes. They'll do what it takes and they'll lose weight.

Further, Samuel Johnson was right. Even if you did have a slow metabolism, if you are fat it is evidence that for *your* body you are overeating or underexercising. It's possible that somebody else out there eats as much or more than you do but is nonetheless slimmer. But that is not your concern. Your concern is your own body.

If you read the introduction to this book, you'll recall my saying how my own research led to my weight loss. None of that research was more important to that accomplishment than what I learned for this chapter. For I, too, blamed what I was sure was a slow metabolism. And who knows? Maybe my metabolism *is* a bit on the slow side. I've certainly got things coded on my genes courtesy of Mom and Dad that I wish I hadn't received, like allergies. Maybe I've got one of those nasty old obesity genes, too. But when I learned what I've told you here, I realized that it wasn't my metabolism literally weighing me down, but my habits. As soon as I started losing my excuses I started losing weight.

WHY "FAT ACCEPTANCE" IS UNACCEPTABLE

In more ways than the obvious, the "fat is beautiful" and "fat acceptance" movement is growing. Claiming legitimacy by medical research, obesity activists are demanding not just to have the same rights as thinner Americans but that obesity also be completely accepted socially. They are attempting to popularize the term "fatphobic." Because a phobia is by definition a mental illness, fatphobic means that anyone who believes there's something wrong with being obese, even grossly obese, has a mental disease. Groups like the aforementioned National Association for the Advancement of Fat Acceptance (NAAFA) hold workshops around the country to convince obese people that they should be proud of their appearance.

These people are generally not just a bit on the heavy side.

NAAFA doesn't collect measurements of its membership, but it did produce a telling survey when it polled members on whether they felt they've been discriminated against. Male respondents classified as "moderately fat" averaged 209 pounds while women averaging 186 pounds were so labeled. To earn a classification of just plain "fat," men had to weigh a whopping average 315 pounds and women 289.[95] These are people who, in a less polite age, were considered grotesquely, horribly, obscenely fat.

NAAFA members periodically go to regional and national meetings where they give each other psychological support, tossing around expressions like "We have more bounce for the ounce, and more cushion for the pushin'."[96] The fat acceptance movement has its own lapel ribbon, light blue in color. Among NAAFA's recommended activist activities for groups on International No-Diet Day are public protest rallies, picketing diet or weight-loss surgery establishments, boycotting foods from companies with diet product lines (good luck finding a food company that doesn't have one), closing down public scales, publicly destroying bathroom scales, and "get[ting] a large garbage can or dumpster and throw[ing] away symbols of fat oppression: diet soda, foods, and products; calorie counters; food scales; etc."[97]

In October 1994, Ithaca, New York, celebrated its second annual "size acceptance month" dedicated to "body weight liberation." Marking the event was a "speak out" celebration of weight diversity, workshops at nearby Cornell University, and a downtown event where the public was invited to bring scales and "other oppressive dieting paraphernalia" to be destroyed with sledgehammers on the city common. Organizers reported the measure has already been copied by St. Paul, Minnesota.[98] Some fat acceptance advocates have even gone so far as to suggest bombing weight-loss clinics.[99]

The fat activists seem to take great comfort in the growing American waistline, seeing it as both a confirmation and a matter of safety in numbers. In his NAAFA newsletter essay on finding clothes for obese men, Harry Gossett writes, "The good news is that today there are more big men in the United States."[100]

Likewise, NPR commentator Daniel Pinkwater says smugly, "Fat people are on the march—and our numbers are expanding, our ranks are swelling." He concludes, "A fat day is dawning, America. Remember, you heard it here first."[101]

But there's no safety in numbers for the extremely obese fat activists. That's because no matter how fat the country gets, there will always be a subpopulation that's far fatter than the others. Future members of NAAFA will be that subpopulation. When we're all 100 pounds overweight, society will still likely discriminate against those who are 200 pounds overweight.

FAT ACCEPTANCE MYTHOLOGY

Although the Tobacco Institute is famous for its repeated denials of the hazards of cigarette smoking in the face of overwhelming evidence, its people appear mere amateurs compared to the fat activists in their effort to deny the hazards of obesity. Pinkwater claims that being fat is no more pathological than being left-handed or having green eyes. Obesity, he says, "was classified as a disease [simply] by virtue of being a deviation from the norm," along with "something that could be profitably treated."[102]

When asked if being overweight is unhealthy, NAAFA spokesperson Frances White replied, "Now, would you say that no thin person has high blood pressure, no thin person is prone to heart disease? I don't think so."[103] By that logic, cigarette smoking isn't unhealthy, because nonsmokers get lung cancer and heart disease, too.

Chef Paul Prudhomme, famous for his numerous books and TV appearances touting his Cajun cooking recipes, isn't a fat activist, but his capacity for denial is representative of the ilk. In explaining why his dieting *goal* was 350 pounds, though he's just five feet nine inches tall, Prudhomme said, "I think everyone in the world is different. To say everyone has the same weight needs is like saying everyone should eat the same foods."[104] In other words, he's asserting that his "natural weight," as fat activists put it, is around 350 pounds. Prudhomme, in case you've never seen him on TV or in person, gets around on a motorized scooter because, as he admits, his tremendous weight puts too much of a burden on his knees.[105]

Some fat activists admit that overweight people seem to have special health problems, but blame it not on the fat per se but on efforts to get rid of it. Terry Nicholleti Garrison in her book, *Fed*

Up!: A Woman's Guide to Freedom from the Diet/Weight Prison (co-authored with David Levitsky, M.D.), says that "it may be repeated dieting rather than obesity itself which accounts for the greater incidence of hypertension in the obese."[106] Others have even gone so far as to blame society's intolerance for fat people's health problems.

At a London obesity conference I attended, British researcher John Garrow dismissed this as nonsense. "There is this interesting view that people die younger from being fat because they're being treated beastily," he said. But he pointed out that the Pima Indians in Arizona have no social stigma against obesity, "yet they have a terrible diabetes rate. Stigma is certainly not the cause of their liability."[107]

Dale M. Atrens's 1988 book *Don't Diet* (underwritten, interestingly, with the "largest life sciences grant ever made by the Australian government")[108] is a dream come true for any fat person who's given up on losing weight. All one need do is read the cover (and probably that's all a lot of people did do) to see there's absolutely no harm in being overweight and even if there were, you might as well relax and enjoy it because there's not a damned thing you can do about it. In what is perhaps the longest book subtitle in history, Atrens informs us: "The Rationale for Dieting Is Wrong. Diets Don't Work. Exercise Does Not Cause Weight Loss. New Research Proves: Fatness Is Not Due to Overeating. Fatness Is Not Due to Underexercise. Fat Does Not Cause Cancer. Fat Does Not Cause Early Heart Disease. Fat Does Not Cause Early Death." Actually, there's more but you get the picture. To be sure, Atrens's book was published back in 1988, long before some of the most damning evidence about the health risks of obesity were proven in medical studies. But already by 1988 there was enough research to indicate Atrens was wrong on every count.

The irony is that even Atrens admits that extreme obesity is life threatening and virtually all fat activists are extremely obese.[109] That's why the fat acceptance movement hasn't embraced him. Because they entail the very heaviest of the heavy, they cannot accept his compromise position—that only extreme obesity is harmful. Fat is harmless in any amount, they insist. Even 300 pounds? Yes. Even 500 pounds? Yes, damn it! Don't confuse us with the fat facts; our minds are made up.

The "Fatlash" Books

Just as the same diet schemes keep appearing under different book titles, so do books that pooh-pooh obesity. So it was that in 1996, eight years after Atrens's book, Glenn Gaesser came out with his *Big Fat Lies*, with three of the six endorsements on the back coming from members of NAAFA (Pat Lyons, Charles Van Dyke, and William J. Fabrey). One endorsement, from the group's chairman of the board, Charles Van Dyke, gushes: "Finally, truth and justice for the fat person. People will vary, and cannot all fit some insurance chart."[110] It would take three insurance charts laid end to end to fit Charles; he weighs 600 pounds.[111] Gaesser's work came out just before another fat acceptance book, Richard Klein's *Eat Fat*,[112] and half a year before yet another, Laura Fraser's *Losing It*.[113] But it has potential to do much more damage because the Klein and Fraser books come across as written by fat people trying to justify their conditions rather than change them. Klein's book, as one can guess from the title, is also only meant to be taken with limited seriousness. But Gaesser is thin! He also writes in a much more scholarly (meaning less-fun-to-read) fashion.

In the introduction, Gaesser claims, "There is a large and ever-growing body of scientific evidence, most of it still confined to professional journals, showing that fat may not be so bad, and in fact thin may not be so good."[114] Yes, just what people with large and ever-growing bodies want to hear. Later in the introduction he says, "This book was written with the hope of discrediting the myths that obesity is a 'killer disease,' that weight loss is good, that thinner is necessarily healthier, and that the height-weight tables measure something meaningful."[115] True to form, he spends the first part of the book twisting various studies and picking and choosing from others to make his points.

But a curious thing happens later on as he presents information that undoes what came before. He informs us, for example, of a Duke University study of 600 obese men and women who completed a low-calorie, low-fat diet and exercise program lasting at least four weeks. They all lost weight, yet all were still obese.[116] He then notes that their cholesterol levels, their blood pressure, and the amount of fat in their bloodstreams all fell. The point, he says, is *"It is possible to greatly improve or even 'cure' diabetes and other serious health problems while still remaining markedly overweight* [emphasis his]."[117]

Now wait here. This is a guy who told us that saying that "weight loss is good [and] that thinner is necessarily healthier" are "myths." He has a whole chapter disparaging diets with a title that could hardly be stronger: "Diet and Die."[118] Now he's citing a program of *diet* and exercise in which weight loss correlated to improved health indicators as somehow supporting his thesis.

Also toward the end of the book Gaesser admits that fat under the belly appears to be responsible for "such killers as heart disease, cancer, and diabetes, for example."[119] Well, anyone who's extremely fat carries a large amount of fat above the belt—or above the hips if they're too big to wear a belt. Charles Van Dyke's abdominal fat alone probably weighs more than I do. Ultimately, the "bad" type of fat becomes almost every fat person's concern.

Apparently the fat acceptance people who endorsed *Big Fat Lies* didn't read much past the introduction. I sure hope the people who buy the book do, lest they become Big Fat Corpses.

AIDERS AND ABETTORS

In terms of sheer numbers, the fat acceptance movement is quite small. But their numbers are multiplied manifold by a media that's largely sympathetic. Thus, when any major obesity study comes out you're likely to see a news program featuring a doctor as one guest and a NAAFA member as the other. The media don't feel any compunction to counter NASA scientists with members of the Flat Earth Society. You don't see Holocaust historians balanced with anti-Semites who insist the Holocaust was a hoax. But the media stand ever ready and willing to give equal time to fat acceptance people.

In 1995 *GQ* magazine decried what it called on its cover "America's War Against Fatties." The article inside documents the troubles of the aforementioned 600-pound Charles "Charlie" Van Dyke. The writer, Mike Sager, is clearly impressed that Charlie hasn't gained any weight in fourteen years. "How many 44-year-old men can say that?" he asks.[120]

How about that "war"? Well, "one prospective employer turned

Charlie down because the company's drafting tables were lined up too close together," while another "firm that did hire him instructed him not to sit on the new sofa in the waiting room." They didn't want their couch broken? Such bigotry! Then there was the petroleum company that was going to hire him until they found out they didn't have a fireproof suit large enough for him. Sager concludes by rattling off all the obesity myths such as the setpoint, concluding "it is not Charlie's fault that he is fat. He was born that way." Pity poor Charlie's mom, giving birth to a 600-pound baby.[121]

Similarly, a 1994 *Working Woman* article by fat acceptance advocate Laura Fraser stated, "Recent research . . . shows that discipline has very little to do with obesity. The vast majority of studies have shown that, on average, obese people eat no more than average-size people; their bodies are simply predisposed to burn food at a different rate."[122] As I write this, the British edition of *Vogue* has announced it's planning a "nonwaif issue," saying, "We want round and lovely roly-poly women. . . . So, stand up, fat girls of the world—it's time to make your mark."[123]

As an answer to the prayers of the fat acceptance people, several movies extolling the virtues of the horizontally challenged appeared or began production in 1995. (As a *USA Today* review put it in its headline, "Hollywood Is Falling for Hefty Heroes."[124]) Of one, *Heavyweights*,[125] which takes place at a summer camp for overweight boys, the writer-director said, "This movie isn't about losing weight; it's about empowering kids." In another movie, heartthrob Chris O'Donnell is the campus hunk at a Dublin college who "falls for a chubby co-ed over her slim, more conventionally beautiful pals."[126]

Canada has even gone so far as to use tax dollars to fund fat acceptance propaganda films. One, paid for by the National Film Board of Canada, is a documentary called *Fat Chance: The Big Prejudice.* In it a 400-pound man tries to lose half his weight but eventually discovers the fat acceptance movement and in the closing proclaims, "A lot of people were wrong: doctors, the media, the press. Now I feel that the chains are off, and I'm walking with freedom." A NAAFA reviewer called it "very important to the size acceptance movement, especially when we're trying to 'open the eyes' of the general public."[127]

"I believe that theater, film, and TV presentations with size acceptance themes are proving to be a supremely important way of combating size discrimination where it starts: in the minds of the people," wrote a columnist for *Radiance* magazine.[128]

Fat activists are also infiltrating the medical community. Among the movement's successes has been the infiltration of Kaiser Permanente, the world's largest health maintenance organization (HMO). The NAAFA newsletter of March—April 1995 boasted that fat activist Pat Lyons, a registered nurse, is a regional health education consultant for Kaiser Permanente of Northern California. (Lyons was listed as the first endorser of Glenn Gaesser's book, and was identified with Kaiser.) In this role she "has been instrumental in spearheading an effort to shift the weight/health paradigm at Kaiser," which "introduces the ideas of self-acceptance and size acceptance with an emphasis on both strategies to empower individuals as well as activities to effect social change." The newsletter tied Lyons's activities to Kaiser's holding "a teleconference with more than 800 physicians in order to educate them about counseling patients about weight and health. As a result, most physicians reported that their knowledge about fatness increased and that they would incorporate the new information in their recommendations for patients."[129]

The Obesity Backlash Backlash

The two groups of people most sympathetic to fat acceptance are those who have always been thin despite eating what they want (and perhaps feel a bit guilty about it) and those who are themselves extremely fat. The persons least sympathetic are those who have been fat themselves but no longer are. Their own experiences demolish the fat acceptance excuses. One such person is Ken Hecht, a TV producer and writer in Los Angeles, who wrote a column for *Newsweek*'s "My Turn." A permanent loser of 128 pounds, Hecht said that fat people "love to wallow in failure and believe that, in the end, they really have no control over their weight." But, he says,

> The fact is we have more control over what we put into our mouths than over almost any other aspect of our lives. Face it, Chubbo, when

was the last time you were force-fed? I know my tone may seem cold, harsh and lacking in understanding. But reality often comes in a cold, harsh package. And I understand the devastation to the quality of one's life caused by these feelings of hopelessness and self-loathing. What I also understand is that excuses and the never-ending search for magic bullets keep the overweight stuck where they are: miserable and low on self-esteem.

So forget excuses and magic bullets. When you blouse your waist or put on dark colors, don't tell yourself you don't look so bad. You do. . . . I've lost and kept off 128 pounds. I did it and so can you, fatties.[130]

Susan Estrich, campaign manager to Democratic presidential candidate Michael Dukakis and one of the nation's most prominent feminists, wrote in her *USA Today* weekly column, "Fat is no longer a feminist issue. It's a question of health and personal responsibility." She continued:

It's harder for some of us than for others, but the obesity gene is no more an excuse for gorging on fatty fast food than poverty is for committing crimes. We can't control our genes, but we can control what we eat and how much we exercise.

I know how hard it is to lose weight. If there's a fat gene, I've probably got it. In the last two years, after a lifetime of diet failure, I've gone from a size 12 to a size 4. And I'm not oppressed by male notions of beauty, thank you very much. I'm just happier. And healthier. It's worth it. It's the feminist thing to do.[131]

There's probably nobody less sympathetic to the fat acceptance movement than Rosemary Green. Her heartbreaking diary documenting repeated failures to lose some of her 250-plus pounds of weight is the subject of her book, *The Diary of a Fat Housewife*. Green pulls no punches and takes no prisoners. For example, she scores touchy-feely advice columnist "Dear Abby" for having "quipped the all-time unthinking skinny-person remark" to an obese letter writer, namely, "I applaud you for accepting yourself as you are." Writes Green, "Obesity is a disease, a sickness, Abby. It is physically detrimental, possibly fatal. Yet the *mental and emotional* consequences are even more serious, more damaging. Would you applaud the diabetic who refuses to take insulin, or the hearing-impaired man who refuses to wear a hearing aid? Would you applaud the alcoholic who refuses to quit drinking because he 'likes himself the way he is'? Then why do you applaud this very sick, obese person who gives up on a cure for her sickness?"[132]

Green's book is filled with shame at her condition, which she repeatedly admits is entirely self-inflicted. But fat activists say she has it all wrong. Fat is something to be proud of, they say. "At workshops around the country, women are touting a new reason for pride," said a CNN reporter.[133] But those workshops are going to have to do some heavy work, because indications are that most fat people desperately do not want to be fat. One survey asked formerly severely obese people if they would rather be obese again or suffer some other form of disability. Usually when you ask disabled people a question like that, they chose their own disability, the study noted, preferring the devil they know to the one they don't. But obesity turns this on its head. The forty-seven survey respondents, down to the last person, said rather than be fat again they would become deaf, dyslexic, diabetic, or have heart disease. More than 90 percent said they would rather suffer an amputation and almost 90 percent said they would rather be legally blind. When asked to choose between being normal weight or severely obese multimillionaires, all the patients said they would prefer to be of normal weight.[134] So much for fat pride. You can be fat and happy, but very few people are happy about being fat.

THE THIN DISCRIMINATORS

What the fat activists want more than anything else is to be seen as victims. Society is out to get them because of something over which they have no control. They're mad as hell and they're not going to take it anymore.

In his 1995 book *A Nation of Victims*, Charles Sykes chronicles legal complaints filed by the obese in the name of fat acceptance. There was, for example, the Chicago man who complained to the Minority Rights Division of the U.S. Attorney General's Office that McDonald's was violating federal equal-protection laws because their restaurants' seats are not large enough for *his* seat.[135] Commenting on the complaint, *Chicago Tribune* columnist Mike Royko noted that despite the man's attempt to equate his status with that of blacks and other minorities, he "was not born with a sixty-inch waist and an enormous butt. After a certain age, he created himself and his butt. They are his responsibility. And even the most liberal of liberals would have to agree that [this man's] sixty-inch waist and awesome butt should not be the responsibility of the United States of America."[136] In any event, it certainly didn't appear to occur to the man that if he ate in McDonald's a little less often he might be able to fit when he did.

Another case Sykes documents is the 640-pound contractor in Baltimore who attempts to cash in on his truly exceptional status to qualify as a minority under the city's plan setting aside a certain percentage of work for members of minority groups—this even though he was unable to visit construction sites because he falls through wooden stairs.[137]

One might think that if there's one business that has a right and a duty to maintain weight standards it's the military. But Minnesota resident Nyleen Mullaly felt otherwise. She sued the Army National Guard for violating her rights by saying she should weigh no more than 155, when she tips the scales at 220. Mullaly says she's protected by law, though, because she's handicapped. Her handicap? She overeats.[138]

But is discrimination against fat people as widespread as we are to believe? In purely social terms, it's true, people are far less likely to choose fat mates than thin ones. But (so far at least) the government has stayed out of this area. In terms of areas the government does regulate, studies indicate that fat people aren't nearly as bad off as the activists would like us to believe. Thus, although it's common to hear that discrimination against fat people leads to substantial earnings losses, a 1989 review of the data found that overweight persons earn as much as lean ones when health differences are taken into account.[139] It hardly seems fair to blame employers for paying less money to people who spend more time in bed because of obesity-related illnesses.

To the extent that there is discrimination against fat people, it may be provoked by their own actions. In a Vermont study, obese and non-obese women conversed on the phone. Judges, who did not know the weight of the women, listened to audiotape recordings of the conversations. They rated the obese women as less likable, less physically attractive, and with inferior social skills.[140] Professors John Foreyt and G. Ken Goodrick of Baylor College, in the book *Living Without Dieting*, speculated that these women probably subtly communicated their lower self-esteem in their manner of speech.[141]

There is at least one area in which fat people are clearly discriminated against. Although they repeatedly tell us that "fat is beautiful," to look at the models in the fat activists' own publications is to be struck by a certain realization. No matter how many issues of *BBW/Big Beautiful Women* I pored over, I never found a model who appeared to weigh more than 250 pounds. Most seemed to hover in the 170-to-200-pound range. Apparently fat is beautiful only so long as there isn't too much of it.

It is built into us to favor healthier-looking specimens. This isn't some sort of manufactured prejudice, like racism. Rather it is biologically decreed that animals should favor healthier-looking animals, the better to maintain the species. Men have favored the classic "hourglass" or "Coke-bottle shape," long before there were Coke bottles. This has held true, even though the overall width of the hourglass has waxed and waned through history. Artist Peter Paul Rubens' models were certainly fat compared to today's models, but they still had that basic hourglass shape. The bell shape of NAAFA members has never been in vogue. *Newsweek* magazine, in a cover story on the concept of beauty, noted the work of Devendra Singh, a University of Texas psychologist. "He has surveyed men of various backgrounds, nationalities and ages," it noted. "And whether the judges are eight-year-olds or eighty-five-year-olds, their runaway favorite is a figure of average weight," whose waist circumference is 70 percent of that of her hips.

Providing biological evidence for why this would be, Dutch researchers have found that even a slight increase in waist size relative to hip size can signal reproductive problems. Thus they found that among 500 women who were attempting to become pregnant, those whose waist measurements were 80 percent of their hip measurements were a third less likely to conceive than women whose waists were only 70 percent of their hip measurements. If their waist measurements were 90 percent of their hip measurements, their fertility dropped by another third.[142] In the modern age, many traditional biological signs of attractiveness—such as height in a male—have become archaic. But a woman's weight does matter.

At some points in history, Rubenesque women may have been desirable, but this was only because it meant they had a lifestyle that could pay for a combination of food and labor-saving servants. Given a choice between an overweight woman or someone so thin and frail as to be likely to die in childbirth, it might have made sense to choose the fat woman. Obviously things have changed. Now anyone in our culture can afford enough food and little enough manual labor to sustain obesity; indeed, the poorest Americans are among the fattest. Today obesity signals health problems, ranging from premature death to simply not being able to climb stairs.

The fat activists aren't just at war with society, but with biology itself. What they have to accept is that society as a whole doesn't accept their attitudes toward sloth and gluttony. By insisting that we don't force our values on them, they are forcing their values on us.

They are also trying to remove a tool that society has long successfully used to prevent excess stigma. There's strong evidence that one reason black women are so much fatter than black men or white women is that their culture simply considers their obesity to be acceptable.[143] A study of weight loss and maintenance among middle-aged men put it scientifically but bluntly: "Perceived well-being at baseline was inversely related to weight loss."[144] The better the men felt about being fat, the less likely they were to lose weight. The worse they felt about being fat, the more likely they were to lose weight.

Social pressure also explains why at Indian Rocks Beach on Florida's Gulf Coast potbellies and fat thighs prevail, even among the young people, while at Manhattan Beach in Southern California the order of the day is washboard waists and slender hips. It explains why young homosexual men are thinner than their heterosexual counterparts. No doubt it also plays a role in why Americans are so much heavier than Europeans. As one British newspaper put it, "No one needs to feel fat in America. No matter how thunderous the thighs or elephantine the gut, or how the elastic waistband strains on your XXL stretch sweatpants, or your neck flows over the collar of your 'I Love Beer' T-shirt, there will always be someone fatter. Much, much fatter."[145]

THE "CRAB-BUCKET" SYNDROME

In his book *The End of Racism*, Dinesh D'Souza documents the self-defeatism that characterizes the attitudes in many black schools. "Getting ignorant" is considered a virtue. Black students who earn honors are labeled "nerd," "sell-out," and "whitey." Teachers at such schools refer to the "crab-bucket" syndrome: when some crabs try to crawl out of the bucket, the rest pull them back down.[146]

The fat acceptance advocates are the counterparts of the ignorance acceptance advocates; they, too, try to pull their fellow "crabs" who don't want to be fat back into the bucket. "Stay right here," they say. "It's the natural place for you." A 1995 fat acceptance book carries the title *Self-Esteem Comes in All Sizes*, with the subtitle, "How to Be Happy and Healthy at Your Natural Weight."[147] Laura Eljaiek, program director of NAAFA, claims, "Fat is a natural state for most women," and that "We feel people should accept their weight without shame or denial."[148]

But the term "natural weight" has no meaning scientifically or medically; rather, it's just a term of convenience invented by the fat acceptance movement. Cancer is perfectly natural. It was completely natural when diseases like smallpox and polio ravaged the land, killing, crippling, and scarring millions. If your actions make you fat, it is natural that you will suffer all sorts of medical problems as a result. If your actions make you thin, it is natural that you will not suffer those illnesses, or at least not to the same degree.

Even if you feel your obesity isn't "natural," there's not a damned thing you can do about it, say the activists. "Most fat people have no more chance of getting thin than short people have of growing taller,"[149] claims NAAFA's Sally Smith. "All too often we're told, 'Get some control, and you won't have that problem,' " she says. "Fatness is a very complex characteristic, but it's not a matter of control."[150] Weight-loss "treatment always fails," avers NPR's Daniel Pinkwater, thereby stating that anybody who claims to have lost significant weight and kept it off, including the present author, is a liar.[151] But Pinkwater has grasped an important concept. To admit that *anybody* has been able to lose weight and keep it off is to give away the store. Likewise, to say that something is impossible is to keep others from even trying—and thereby discovering that weight loss is possible. The fat acceptance message is simple: Don't even try.

While many thin or slightly overweight people may laugh at the antics of the fat acceptance movement, many fat ones take their nonsense quite seriously—and pay the price. Writing in a recent issue of *Good Housekeeping,* Karen Wilson related that "All my life I've been overweight. . . . I just liked to eat." She added:

> For years I read *BBW/Big Beautiful Woman* magazine and was comforted by its message that big is beautiful. I read newsletters from [NAAFA]. And on a TV talk show that I saw, a woman who was so big that she needed a wheelchair to get around insisted that fat was fine. All this pro-fat talk gave me the excuse I needed to stay heavy. Before I knew it, my weight exceeded 300 pounds.[152]

But then she was diagnosed with endometrial cancer and had to undergo surgery and radiation therapy. "During the weeks of radiation treatment that followed," she wrote, "I read everything I could get my hands on" and learned that "obesity is recognized as a major risk in endometrial cancer."[153]

Wilson has now gotten her weight down to 220 pounds and says, "I have an important message for every woman who, like me, has let excess pounds pile up. I don't want women to be casual about big weight gains or misled by pro-fat propaganda. I want them to know they can take control and avoid the life-threatening dangers of obesity."[154]

Some years ago I had a dear friend named Mike Virella who washed dishes at the restaurant where I bussed tables. He was one of the smartest and nicest people I ever met. He was also one of the fattest. He died of a heart attack at the age of twenty-nine. Today I watch the same fat acceptance groups that preached to him preach to the other Mike Virellas of the world that there's nothing they can do about their weight, nothing literally but eating, drinking, and being merry. Until that one day, early in life, when it all comes to a stop.

"How do you feel about fat people?" Rosemary Green asked me. "I mean, how do you really feel about them?"

The answer I gave her off the cuff is still the one I would give. "I feel empathy for those who are somewhat overweight or slightly obese," I said, "because I've been there." For people who are extremely overweight, like she was, "I can only feel sympathy," I said, "because I don't know what it's like to suffer from that." But for those who go around preaching to other such souls that there is nothing that can be done about their state, that nature has mandated that they weigh 300 or 350 pounds, that all diet and exercise regimens are doomed to failure, "For them," I said, "I have nothing but the utmost contempt."

Author Jean Garton has said, "the human mind is never more resourceful than when it is involved in self-justification."[155] The fat acceptance people have been very resourceful. But make no mistake about them. Some may be very nice as individuals, but they are doing very bad things to our society and especially to those struggling with weight problems. They have turned what had been two of the Seven Deadly Sins—sloth and gluttony—into both a right and a badge of honor, complete with light blue ribbon to signify it. That's a sin in and of itself.

6 The Profiteers

The American dieter surely hath no greater enemy than the American diet book. Like modern-day Ponce de Leóns, tens of millions of Americans scour the landscape looking for the miraculous fountain. Each time they plunk down the $22.95, they think they may have found it. Each author is like Lucy holding the football for Charlie Brown. She swears that this time she won't pull it away. Like poor little Charlie Brown, the dieter finds herself sore and bedazzled. But Charlie Brown knows Lucy is to blame for his failure, while the dieter tends to blame herself. After all, the book sold a million copies. It must have helped a lot of people, why not her? Of course, that's just what the other million purchasers are telling themselves. Which is why after more than thirty years of best-selling diet books, Americans are fatter than ever and yet diet books continue to be best-sellers. In fact, sales figures for diet books, videos, and audio cassettes are projected to jump from about $600 million in 1996 to over $1 billion by the end of the century.[1] While nobody knows exactly how many diet books have been written, one on-line bookstore, *Amazon.com*, claims to have access to almost 2,000 different diet book titles.[2]

"It's one crazy diet after another," says Yale obesity expert Kelly Brownell. "They all have a brief flurry in the market. They're all condemned by health professionals either because they're dangerous or because there's no data to support them. And then another comes along, and people say, 'Oh, maybe this is the real one.'" He adds, "When I get calls about the latest diet fad, I imagine a trick birthday candle that keeps lighting up and we have to keep blowing it out."[3]

Diet gurus and their books must be seen in the overall context of quackery, both now and through the ages. Quacks have no doubt always been with us. What do you want to bet that mastodon and woolly mammoth foreskins were once ground up and sold as aphrodisiacs? Even from ancient times, men sought a cure for being follically impaired—you know, back when it was called baldness.

It's important to realize that even the smartest people can fall victim to quacks. An eighteenth-century quack convinced Britain's longest-serving prime minister, Sir Robert Walpole (1676–1745), to drink a solution of one part soap and three parts limewater daily in order to prevent the formation of kidney stones. At the time of his death, apparently hastened by this "treatment," it was calculated he had consumed at least 180 pounds of soap and 1,200 gallons of limewater. An autopsy revealed that nonetheless he had three stones in his bladder.[4]

The point, gentle reader, is that you shouldn't feel like a total idiot if you have fallen for the scams of one of the diet gurus. You are a mutton chop in a den of hungry lions. Quackery is their job; that's why they're good at it. Your job is to be a teacher, housewife, secretary, businessperson, or whatever—not to spend your free hours in medical libraries and calling nutritional experts. That's my job.

There have always been counter-quacks, but they've always fought an uphill struggle to win over people's minds. In part that's because wishful thinking is a powerful enemy. In part it's because magazines and newspapers have always greatly profited from "quackvertising,"[5] while book publishers reap the big bucks by producing quack books. Indeed, one publisher turned down the proposal for this book saying, in so many words, that diet books have brought in so much money for them that they dare not publish a book that may make people stop buying diet books.

In America a decade ago, quackery was estimated to be a $10-billion industry, with an unknown amount of that devoted to various instruments, potions, pills, schemes, videos, and books claiming to help you easily lose weight while lying around like a slug and eating like a sow.[6] Unfortunately, one side effect of the rapid progress of science in recent decades is that it's actually encouraging quackery. Consider that at one time staples of the quack were cures for baldness, for wrinkles, and for cancer. Now we actually do have medicines that treat baldness, creams that diminish wrinkles, and we've made tremendous progress against some types of cancer. Thus, the pump is primed for the shyster who claims miracle formulas to deal with these and other problems, including obesity. It's so easy now for a scam artist to get away with saying that his findings are on the cutting edge of science—so cutting edge that you've never even read about it in the newspapers. Selling snake oil has never been easier, and we may well be in the golden age of quackery.

You've seen the magazine and newspaper ads for instant results for any number of problems, real or perceived—too little hair, too much hair, too much weight, too little weight. On a single page of Continental Airlines in-flight magazine I found ads for seven highly dubious products. Two were for cheaply, painlessly banishing wrinkles, one for permanently removing hair without electrolysis, and the remainder were for weight loss. My favorite was for the Lipo Slim Briefs with "thousands of thermo-active micropore cells [that] produce a gentle massage that destroys deep fat particles and liquid molecules which are the cause of excess fat." But a close runner-up was the Elysee Electro Exercise System, four pads that when fastened to your body "send tiny modulated electrical impulses" to make "your muscles contract and expand as they would in a strenuous physical workout."[7] I couldn't really tell what the third miracle weight-loss product was and the fourth was an abdomen exerciser promising abdominal muscles that would put Granny's washboard to shame.[8]

If you don't want to invest $79.95 for a device, how about only $3.95 for a magazine promising the same results? During a single trip to a bookstore I found the following titles on the covers of magazines aimed at women: "Weight-Loss Motivators," "Swim Yourself Thin," "Lose Ten, Fifteen, Twenty Pounds or More," "Get Lean Now," "Pedal Your Butt Off!," "Abs, Butt, and Thigh Blaster," "The New Millennium Diet," "Six Quick Tricks to Lose Pounds in Just

Days," "An Easy Diet for Women Who Can't Lose Weight," "Twenty-five Guilt-Free Snacks," "Seven-Day Plan to Go Longer, Feel Better, and Burn More Calories," "Eat Up and Drop Five Pounds in Five Days," "Drop Nine Pounds in One Week," "Be Tubby No More," "Forty Painless Ways to Trim the Fat," "Make Your Body Burn Fat Faster," "Take Three Inches Off Your Hips in Thirty Days," "Drop a Size with 'Somersize,'" "Eat Pizza, Shed Pounds," "Slim Down, Power Up," "Winning at Weight Loss," "Resize Your Thighs," "Drop Those Hard-to-Lose Ten Pounds," "The Cabbage Soup Diet," "Craving Zingers," "Fifty Ways to Be Fat Free by Fall," "Lose Those Last Ten Pounds," and "The Amazing Fat-Melting Diet."

Dear reader, in how many ways must I state the obvious, that these things don't work? Okay, here's one way. Go to your friendly neighborhood bookstore right now—yes, right now; the burning pot on the stove can wait. Look at the covers of those women's and fitness magazines. You'll see those same titles all over again. But the articles didn't help anyone when they first appeared and they won't help anyone now.

The ultimate quack weight-loss device is the diet book. For those of you who aspire to write a weight-loss best-seller, here's the formula:

- Be fat.
- Lose weight.
- Pretend that having lost the fat you are now an expert in the area.
- Come up with a gimmick that distinguishes your book slightly from previous diet books.
- Intersperse a bunch of anecdotes from formerly fat people cured by your formula. Slap a slew of recipes or a fat counter guide onto the back so your 15,000-word article now has the heft of at least a 75,000-word book.
- Keep the weight off long enough for the book tour and the appearances on the *Good Morning America* and *Today* shows.
- And—most important—don't forget to offer your readers something for nothing.

Whatever you do, don't tell people they have to eat less than they want to. In fact, if you want a really successful book, tell them that what they believe to be their vices are actually good for them and that if they indulge even more, they'll weigh less. This something-for-nothing promise is often in the titles themselves, like *How to Become Naturally Thin by Eating More*, the best-selling *Eat More, Weigh Less*, and the subtitle of Cliff Sheat and Maggie Greenwood-Robinson's best-selling *Lean Bodies*, which is *The Revolutionary New Approach to Losing Bodyfat by Increasing Calories*. One cover strains so far to convince the reader to do nothing uncomfortable that it carries the contradictory title of *Fight Fat and Win: How to Eat a Low-Fat Diet Without Changing Your Lifestyle*.[9] Presumably if your lifestyle already included a low-fat diet, you wouldn't have any use for this book, but never mind.

Books promising the equivalent of divine intervention are nothing new. Martin Schiff, M.D., had one such book back in 1974 with *Dr. Schiff's Miracle Weight-Loss Guide*.[10] Now we have Adele Puhn's 1996 best-seller, *The Five-Day Miracle Diet*.[11] Interestingly, just before Puhn's book came out, another one appeared called *The Miracle Diet: Fourteen Days to New Vigor and Health*.[12] It went nowhere. After all, who wants to wait an extra nine days for a miracle? (It's too late now, but I should have immediately published a book called *The Four-Day Miracle Diet* and taken away all Puhn's business.)

Other books don't have a something-for-nothing promise in their titles, but it certainly appears in their pages or otherwise on their covers. Susan Powter in *Stop the Insanity!* says on the cover that the key to being skinny is to "eat, breathe, move," albeit in the right ways.[13] What could be finer than breathing off pounds? Richard and Rachael Heller in their best-selling *Carbohydrate Addict's Diet* tell readers they can eat absolutely anything they want so long as they eat almost all their carbohydrates at the evening meal. And, oh yes, the evening meal absolutely must be consumed within an hour.[14] Tough rules!

Barry Sears and Bill Lawren's *The Zone* says right on the back: "You can burn more fat watching TV than by exercising."[15] Could that be why they've sold over 400,000 books?[16] Between *The Zone* and *Lean Bodies* it appears we'd be a nation of beanpoles if we just watched TV twelve hours a day and ate potato chips the entire time. And then, of course, there's *How Sex Can Keep You Slim*,[17] which says . . . well, you get the point.

In the "give 'em what they want to hear" world of diet books, nothing is too ludicrous. How about a book saying you can lose weight through eating chocolate? It's been done. Twice. Nineteen-ninety-five saw the publication of *The Chocolate Lovers' Diet* and Debra Waterhouse's *Why Women Need Chocolate*,[18] which is a strange thing to say about something that most of the world's population wasn't exposed to until the seventeenth century. (Imagine the appeal to a sun-worshiper that the answer to premature wrinkling is to get a deeper tan or telling a child that large amounts of candy will prevent cavities.) The only problem, of course, is these diets don't work. Yet it is a common theme in diet books that the reader, no matter how obese, is already pretty much doing everything correctly. He or she just needs to tweak his or her habits a bit.

Probably the ultimate in diet books catering to wishful thinking is Debbie Johnson's 1994 *How to Think Yourself Thin.* It's going to be hard for anyone to top that. In it Johnson provides such valuable advice as: "The subconscious is an extremely powerful a vehicle [*sic*] within us which can easily control the body's weight."[19] Right, if it's so darned easy, how come so many of us are so darned fat? The book is accompanied by such illustrations as a woman eating a thick wedge of layer cake telling herself, "Everything I eat turns to energy."[20] So many people bought Johnson's line—and her book—that in 1996 it was picked up and republished by a major New York publishing house, Hyperion.[21] These are the same folks who brought us *Why Women Need Chocolate.* They ought to package the two together with an accompanying advertisement that a woman can lose weight very quickly if she thinks thin thoughts while popping Hershey bars and truffles.

I was studying the weight-loss books in a store recently when something struck me. Why is it that so many have pictures of the authors on the cover? There they are, smiling at you: Cliff Sheats, Susan Powter, Dean Ornish, Art Ulene, Covert Bailey, Adele Puhn, Richard and Rachael Heller. Debra Waterhouse's *Outsmarting the Female Fat Cell* (hardback edition) has photos of her on both the front *and* back. What's going on here?

First, the picture shows that the author is slim. It conveys the message, "I'm thin and so can you be if you read this book." But more than that, we tend to put more trust in people we can see. And diet-book authors need all the trust they can get because it's usually all they have to offer. Almost none of their books contain notes, for example. One diet book I found contained a huge bibliography, but upon inspection it became obvious that this was the old high school trick of slapping a thick bibliography onto a text to make it look heavily researched when actually the bibliography has nothing to do with what's written. Occasionally a weight-loss book will refer to a couple of medical journal articles, yet I have identified well over one thousand important articles on obesity from 1985 to the present, with thousands more of lesser importance. Building a thesis or a book around just a couple of these is simply nonsense.

Likewise, "miracle" weight-loss books are virtually devoid of endorsements by experts in the weight-loss field. When an editor at HarperCollins told *Publisher's Weekly* "endorsements matter," she should have explained how HarperCollins sold more than 400,000 copies of *The Zone* without having any. For that matter neither did *Stop the Insanity!*, *Fit for Life*, *Dr. Atkins' Diet Revolution*, the *Complete Scarsdale Medical Diet*, *The Carbohydrate Addict's Diet*, or *The Rotation Diet*—each a mega-seller—carry any endorsements. The number one best-seller, *The T-Factor Diet*, did carry a whopping seven endorsements.[22] The endorsers' names were A.S., A.K., J.I., J.B., R.V., M.S., and V.K.

People with good medical reputations do not risk them by endorsing dumb books, but dumb books with good sales pitches will outsell smart books with good endorsements every day of the week.

I want this chapter to serve as an inoculation of sorts against diet quacks and especially the book industry. I want to vaccinate you against hype so that never again will you get that urge to spend good money and high hopes on parasites who feed off your dreams.

A HISTORY OF DIET SNAKE OIL SALES

The first diet guru was William Banting, who actually got his diet from the British ear surgeon William Harvey. Banting lost weight on it and later published the diet as *Banting's Letter on Corpulence.* Since Banting's background wasn't in health, but rather he was an undertaker, this established the precedent that diet gurus need know nothing about nutrition or physiology.

The first heavily marketed diet plan was that of Romanian-born gynecologist Herman Taller, M.D. The title of his 1961 book *Calories Don't Count*[23] introduced into popular parlance a phrase that continues to wreak havoc to this very day. Naturally, it was one many dieters wanted to hear and so 2 million of them rushed out to buy it. Taller agreed with most diet book authors today that "all calories are not the same." But whereas today the diet gurus say it's the fat calories that will do you in, Taller blamed the carbohydrate ones. He divided all foods into two groups—the first "good," regardless of caloric content, the second "bad," again regardless of calories. He then warned the reader that while "You do not have to count calories," you should not "eat *any* of the foods that are not permitted [emphasis originial]." The following list of impermissible foods included essentially all carbohydrates and refined sugars. He then went on to encourage readers to consume unsaturated fats (those that are not hard at room temperature, like cooking oil). "When you eat large quantities of unsaturated fats," he explained, "you set in motion a happy cycle. You *stimulate* body production of certain hormones which work to release fats stored around the body. You *limit* the production of insulin, a substance which seems to prevent the release of stored fat. And you change the character of your fat. The hard, tough fat, difficult for the body to utilize, softens."[24] All nonsense, you say? Sure, but Taller sold 2 million books.

As it happens, Taller got into a bit of trouble for his lack of ethics. He had mentioned a particular mail-order company as a source for safflower oil capsules. Turns out he owned an interest in the company, which netted him a good chunk of additional change but also conviction on twelve counts of mail fraud, conspiracy, and mislabeling. Alas, his suspended sentence and fine of $7,000 probably equaled the royalties of a few days' sales.[25]

Such a successful formula was sure to inspire imitators, and indeed many of them were successful as well. They included the *Air Force Diet Book* (neither developed by nor endorsed by the Air Force); *The Drinking Man's Diet*; Irwin Stillman's *The Doctor's Quick Weight-Loss Diet*[26] and its companion volume, *Doctor's Inches-Off Diet*; and *Dr. Atkins' Diet Revolution.*[27] All offered readers essentially the same high-protein, low-carbohydrate diets that were first popularized more than a century ago by our coffin-making friend, William Banting.

Dr. Irwin Stillman's *Doctor's Quick Weight-Loss Diet* said, for example, "The usual basic restriction at its strongest may be summed up in one sentence: don't touch carbohydrates, sugar, salt, fruits, cereals, bread, rice, potatoes, and alcohol." Another such list included bran, whole wheat bread, cereals, grapes, pasta, oatmeal, potatoes, and yams.[28] This book may have been the inspiration for the scene in Woody Allen's *Sleeper* in which the hero wakes up after a century of sleep to find out that scientists have determined that fudge is good for you.[29]

Psychiatrist Richard Mackarness, in a 1962 book called *Eat Fat and Grow Slim*, actually urged readers to gorge themselves on fat. "Eggs, fish, meat are the stand-bys," he wrote. "You can eat as much as you like of these, preferably sauteed in butter or cooking oils or deep fried in fat, BUT WITH NO FLOUR, BATTER, OR BREAD CRUMBS [emphasis original]."[30]

By 1985, the pendulum had swung in the other direction. That year, *The New York Times*'s health columnist produced a book titled *Jane Brody's Good Food Book: Living the High-Carbohydrate Way*.[31] It was that rarest of gems, a book aimed (in part, at least) at dieters that was nonetheless factual. More bizarre yet, it actually spent nine weeks on *The New York Times* best-seller list. No doubt this was in great part due to Brody's deserved reputation as one of the nation's top health reporters.

But as they say about that old suit or dress of yours hanging in the closet, hold on to it long enough and it will come back in style. Now the low-carbohydrate books are back with a vengeance, leapfrogging over each other to the top of the best-seller lists.

High-protein, low-carbohydrate diets work in the short run for several reasons. First, they greatly restrict your choices. Most Americans get half their calories from carbohydrates. Give people menus that greatly reduce their access to that half and they will be hard pressed to make up the calories from fat and protein. In essence, then, you're probably also restricting their calorie intake. Restricting calorie intake does result in weight loss.

Another way they work is that they temporarily suppress the appetite by creating something called "ketosis." Deprived of carbohydrates, the body burns off some fat but also considerable muscle, producing ketones that must be extracted through the kidneys. Some ketones are exhaled during respiration, giving you what one weight-loss expert calls "rotten-apple breath."[32] Between the loss of muscle and the water loss from the kidneys excreting the ketones, and the appetite-suppressing effect of ketosis, weight loss comes quickly but little of the weight is actually from fat. In any event, soon the body rebels against this unhealthy regimen. It adjusts to the ketosis, the hunger returns, and the weight loss stops.[33] But by then the dieter has already told ten friends about how great the book is and they've bought it themselves. They then tell ten friends about the book before it fails them, and the cycle continues like one of those weird chain-letter schemes. In this way, a diet-book author can sell a million copies by word of mouth without actually making a single person slim, much less helping her stay that way.

In the meantime, other diet fads have come and gone. One that was dormant for awhile was the one-food or food-group diet. A couple of examples are Joel Herskowitz's 1987 *Popcorn Plus Diet* and Judy Moscovitz's 1986 *Rice Diet Report*.[34] (Neither of these carried endorsements, though *The Rice Diet Report* had a fetching photo of the author on the back.) Another is Judy Mazel's million-selling 1981 book *The Beverly Hills Diet*, which restricted the dieter to exotic fruits such as mangoes and papayas for days at a time. Such a diet would require the average woman to eat about eight pounds of mangoes a day to supply her normal energy requirement. It's hardly surprising that it worked until such inevitable time as the dieter got sick to death of eating exclusively from a menu that looked like it belonged on Carmen Miranda's head. "It's a terrible book," wrote Philip White, director of the American Medical Association's department of foods and nutrition. "Its effort at medical or scientific backing comes directly from the nineteenth century. There is very little in the book in the way of explanation of nutrition, biology or digestion that is in fact the truth."[35] He could have said that about most diet books. In any case, Mazel was back in 1996 with *The New Beverly Hills Diet*.[36] She has no doubt calculated that everyone will forget that her book didn't work fifteen years earlier, remembering only that lots of people bought it.

When it comes to diet plans, there's no such thing as something that's too outlandish, though some schemes are just too simple to be made into books. One was the water diet, which prescribed a certain number of glasses a day to "wash away" fat. Sorry, but fat doesn't "wash away." The water diet might work only in that you spend practically half your waking hours drinking and the other half urinating, leaving little time for other activities, including eating. Maybe I'll write a book called *The Prune Juice Diet*, which will have a similar effect. No, better yet, *The Four-Day Miracle Prune Juice Diet*.

Food combining is a fad that is still with us. It says that foods eaten in different combinations can somehow fool the body into absorbing fewer calories than the individual foods contain. The king of these fads is Harvey and Marilyn Diamond's *Fit for Life*, the paperback edition of which claims it's "America's All-Time No. One Health and Diet Book" with "Over 3 million copies in print."[37] In it the authors propose that it does not so much matter what you eat, but when you eat it and in what combination foods are consumed. Their plan includes recommendations such as not eating anything but fruit before noon, and never eating protein at the same time as carbohydrates. (And while you're at it, don't have sex during the full moon, else you conceive a child who becomes a werewolf.) The Diamonds offer nothing but anecdotal evidence to support their claims. "It would be difficult to choose the most ridiculous diet book ever written," write Stephen Barrett and the editors of *Consumer Reports* in their book *Health Schemes, Scams, and Frauds*, "but surely *Fit for Life* . . . would be right up there."[38] William Jarvis, president of the National Council Against Health Fraud, clearly agreed, saying "*Fit for Life* seems unprecedented in the amount of misinformation contained." He added, "Its only socially redeeming feature is that its popularity may alert American educators to their failure to impart the most fundamental knowledge about health and nutrition to the students entrusted to their care."[39]

C. Wayne Callaway, M.D., a Washington, D.C., physician, in his book *The Callaway Diet*, relates that when he met the Diamonds in a television debate, "They seemed to view me as one of the most despicable creatures known to man: a medical expert." Callaway asks, "But where are the Diamonds now? . . . How many of your friends are marveling about the way *Fit for Life* has given them great results?" I'll tell you where the Diamonds are, Dr. Callaway. They're probably sunning themselves on their yacht, which ought to be called the S.S. *Sucker*, in loving memory of all those folks who bought their book.

For every diet there may be some successful adherents. If somebody swears up and down that they lost weight and kept it off with *Dr. Quack's Gummi Bear Diet*, who am I to argue? But there are no magical formulas with weight loss. If they're offering you something that sounds too good to be true, it is.

Let's look at some of the biggest of the recent diet gurus and see how they do just that.

STUART BERGER'S BALONEY

The late Stuart Berger, M.D., authored three best-sellers: *The Southampton Diet, Forever Young: Twenty Years Younger in Twenty Weeks*,[40] and *The Immune Power Diet*, his biggest seller. He also operated a clinic that catered to many celebrity clients, including the perpetually tanned George Hamilton, singer Roberta Flack, and former New York Congresswoman (and wearer of funny hats) Bella Abzug. *The Immune Power Diet* essentially blamed obesity on food allergies. It also tied such allergies to various other problems, including loss of vitality; contracting colds, flu, and other infections; insomnia; vague aches and pains; stress; and loss of memory and concentration.[41] Perhaps most reprehensible, Berger claimed his diet could forestall the development of AIDS in HIV-positive persons.[42] This was all the more vicious considering that Berger was himself a homosexual.

As with other diet gurus, much of Berger's credibility was based on his own weight loss. He claimed a reduction from 420 to 208 pounds, which was fairly slender considering he was six foot seven. Much of the rest of his credibility came from his having graduated Harvard Medical School. But as the then dean of the Harvard School of Public Health later pointed out, "Berger did not take one single course in nutrition and took no research on the psychology of dieting while he was here." He added, "I am embarrassed and offended that he used the good name of Harvard for his sales pitches."[43]

Claiming he was using "dispatches from the frontiers of medicine and microbiology,"[44] Berger nonetheless cited no published studies. Like any good diet guru, he completely ignored the role of caloric consumption, instead blaming food allergies for stimulating the immune system to cause excess accumulation of fat. He claimed, "Recent research has just begun to show us that each of us has allergies to certain foods,"[45] and that body fat is caused by these allergies.[46] Actually, only about 2 percent of adults and 5 to 10 percent of children have food allergies,[47] but no matter. Only by eliminating these, said Berger, can you begin eating normally. As an alternative to telling you to get tested for these allergies, he fills most of his book—as do most diet-book authors—with recipes. What's unique about them, he says, is that they don't allow you to become exposed to any one food more than once in a four-day cycle. This prevents them from challenging the immune system.[48]

At a glance, one can tell why his diet might work. It's simply low-calorie. You'll lose weight on it not because of anything to do with the immune system but because the calories it provides are almost surely lower than the number you're already consuming. As such, it carries the benefits—and drawbacks—of any low-calorie diet. The main drawback with most of these diets, and Berger's, is that you can't stick to them.

Interestingly, the con man was himself shammed out of more than $2.5 million. Most of it he gave to a man to invest in high-paying but unfortunately non-existent Australian bonds. Then he gave the same man $75,000 for a down payment on 2 million British condoms that were to be traded to Russia for frozen chickens and in turn sold to Saudi Arabia for a $3 million profit.[49]

Unbeknownst to his clients and readers, Berger was a total glutton. Zabar's, his favorite New York delicatessen, shipped over a daily order of quail eggs, sides of smoked salmon, several buckets of cream cheese and pickled herring, and dozens of bagels and roasted chickens. But while he fooled millions of Americans, there was somebody he couldn't deceive: that fellow who wears a hooded black robe and carries a scythe. In 1994 Berger died at age forty of a heart attack; he weighed 365 pounds.

SUSAN POWTER'S INSANE MESSAGE

A lot of people don't trust diet gurus or the diet industry anymore. Susan Powter knows that and has turned it to her advantage. In her best-selling book *Stop the Insanity!* she opens up her life to her readers, telling them of her abusive ex-husband (sarcastically dubbed "Prince Charming"), and even of her days as a topless dancer. Every salesman knows he must build a bond with his target, but nobody knows it more or does it better than Powter. At every turn she urges listeners or readers to treat everyone else as a liar; only she holds the truth. "You don't have the problem," says Powter in her book. "The diet and fitness industries have the problem. They have been lying to you, ripping you off, and setting you up for failure. You and I are not the failures, they are."[50] Elsewhere in the book she refers to nutritionists as "arrogant, egomaniac[s]."[51]

All of which is to say that Powter, who didn't finish high school, can't even pretend to have a background in nutrition or health or anything that could possibly apply to what she writes about. Smartly, she turns her weakness into her strength. "I'm not a dietician, not a doctor. I'm a housewife with no degree who figured it out," she says. "*Stop the Insanity!* is about how I broke the system."[52]

Powter's huckster career began when, as a Texas aerobics instructor, she was discovered by public relations men Richard and Gerald Frankel, who went to her class and were impressed by her boisterous style. They took that style and her tight, aerobicized body and built it into an incredible moneymaking machine for Powter and their firm. Within two years of its first airing, her *Stop the Insanity!* infomercial, where she stomps around and screams at viewers and urges them to buy her video, had already taken in a reported gross of more than $100 million.[53] Her *Stop the Insanity!* book at this writing has sold an additional half million copies and has been followed up with several more books. She also had a short-lived national talk show and a short-lived nationally syndicated newspaper column that despite being sent out by the prestigious New York Times Syndicate never seemed to show up anywhere but the *Fresno Bee.*

For all the talk about being different from everyone else, Powter sells the same low-fat mythology that has dominated the diet-book market for several years now. Still, absolutely none of the low-fat diet gurus are more adamant that calories from carbohydrates and protein somehow magically slip through your digestive system. "It's not food that makes you fat," she writes in *Stop the Insanity!* "It's fat.

I promise," she exhorts her readers.[54] "Your body does not manufacture fat, it comes from the end of your fork."[55]

So does that mean that if I avoid fat I can make an absolute pig of myself? That I can eat two dozen fat-free Fig Newtons, a pound of hard candy, and chase it with a half gallon of Classic Coke? Yes indeedy! "Eat as much as you want" is one of the only two rules she lays down.[56] Tough rules!

When Powter says calories don't count, she really means it. Referring readers to a chart, Powter says, "You can have 1 cookie or 20 cups of rice."[57] Her reasoning is that they both contain the same amount of fat and therefore are equivalent. But her own chart shows the cookie has only 78 calories while all that rice packs 3,242 calories—about twice the calories one of Powter's female readers should be consuming in a day. At a seminar she gives, she tells her excited audience that for the amount of fat in a hamburger they could swim in (and eat) a bathtub of noodles or consume 452 cups of grain. "You can eat truckloads of grain."[58]

Powter herself claims to take in some 3,500 to 5,000 calories a day.[59] But the math shows that if this is true she must work out like an absolute dog. First, let's average that off to 4,250 calories. She appears to be about average in height, meaning she can sustain herself on perhaps 1,600 to 1,800 calories. That leaves at least 2,425 calories unaccounted for, which would take over four hours of aerobic dance to work off. It's doubtful that Powter could have the busy schedule she claims[60] (part of her effort to endear herself to readers is to keep emphasizing all the things she does as a mother) and still have four hours a day for exercise. But in any case, what she offers is not a regimen for the masses. Only the idle rich, persons whose jobs depend on it, or would-be Olympic athletes have time for such diversions.

The bottom line is you cannot follow Powter's dietary advice and be thin. "Susan Powter is making women's lives a misery by promoting a bizarre eating pattern," says Tom Sanders, M.D., of Kings College, London, adding, "This obsession with eradicating fat entirely from our diet is no more than modern voodoo."[61]

In January 1995, Powter filed for personal bankruptcy, citing legal fees in tussles with her partners in the Susan Powter Corporation. In typical Powter fashion, she says the filing was "all about women saying, 'Excuse me! Excuse me! You don't own me. You have to treat me like a human being.' " In actuality, it was about her efforts to get out of the deal she had negotiated with the Frankels, which looked great when she was a nobody aerobics instructor yelling at thirty students at a time, but having been made into a media megastar it no longer looked so good.[62]

Later that year, Powter announced that she was launching her own line of health and fitness centers at former Nutri/System locations around the country. The relationship later fell through, and both sides sued each other for millions of dollars. Responding to the suggestion that she had sold out to the very diet industry she had blasted, Powter said, "It's not even worth acknowledging." But the centers used exercise, counseling, and prepackaged foods just as the Nutri/System clubs did. Indeed, her backing was from the Nutri/System L.P. holding company.[63] So don't acknowledge it, Ms. Powter. But if it walks like a duck and talks like a duck, it's generally considered a duck. Susan Powter sold out.

CLIFF SHEATS'S SHAM

With so many diet-book authors already promising that calories don't count, it takes something special to stand out in the crowd. Cliff Sheats and his co-author Maggie Greenwood-Robinson found that something special. They revealed that eating *extra* calories actually makes you thin. Indeed, they worked this into the 1992 book's title: *Lean Bodies: The Revolutionary New Approach to Losing Bodyfat by Increasing Calories.* To reassure the incredulous, the book also says at the top of the paperback edition: "It's true. It's a proven fact! The secret to losing weight is eating more!"[64] The paperback also declares the book to have been a national bestseller, which of course it was. How could a book telling you to eat more calories and lose weight fail to become a best-seller?

So just how much food do you have to stuff down your craw before you just watch those pounds melt away? "On our new Lean Bodies program, you can and will lose body fat by increasing calories to 1,800, 2,500, even 3,600 calories a day—all while you get leaner and fitter than you have ever been in your life," swear the authors.[65] Gee, does that mean that if I can somehow force down, say, 5,000 calories I'll be so thin that I'll be hospitalized for anorexia?

But wait, Sheats and Greenwood-Robinson aren't through yet. They also tell you just what you want to hear about exercise: it's really been overrated.[66] Yeah! Throw away that treadmill and put the walking shoes to pasture! So long as I can stand to wolf down 3,600 calories a day, I'll be a lean, mean fighting machine!

It's true that by eating more you can increase your metabolism, specifically that part of the metabolism called "dietary thermogenesis." But the increase in metabolism will not be enough to match the intake in energy consumed, no matter how few calories are contained in the food you're eating. It hardly makes sense to eat an additional 200 calories to burn an additional 20. But that's exactly what Sheats advocates.

To put to lie Sheats's claim, let's go to the country of Cameroon in Africa to observe a rather bizarre ritual of one tribe in which during a process called *Guru Walla* young men are absolutely stuffed to the gills over a period of two months. It's probably rather fun at first, and would be especially so if chocolate were made available, but it's not. In any case, the young men just eat and eat as if they were at a perpetual Las Vegas smorgasbord. The researchers found that the men's metabolisms accelerated tremendously to try to handle all that food, increasing almost 50 percent. Nonetheless, despite this the young men gained on average more than thirty-seven pounds. If Cliff Sheats were right these men would have been scarecrows by now. Incidentally, the fat content of these men's food was only 15 percent of calories, less than half the rate for Americans and Western Europeans.[67]

Other studies closer to home, including those at Cambridge University in the United Kingdom, the University of Colorado in Denver, and elsewhere [68] all show the same thing: eat a lot, weigh a lot; eat less, weigh less. A study by the U.S. Department of Agriculture found that 85 to 90 percent of excess food consumed was stored on the body, and mainly as fat.[69]

In case you're wondering, there is also no such thing as foods that cause you to lose weight, to borrow the title of a very irresponsible book by Neal Barnard, M.D., the founder of the Physicians Committee for Responsible Medicine.[70] The book's subtitle is *The Negative Calorie Effect*, and again, there's no such thing. All foods have calories; most excess calories convert to fat. There's also no such thing as a "fat-burning food," despite such book titles as Judy Jameson's *Fat-Burning Foods and Other Weight-Loss Secrets.*[71]

But who cares about scientific studies when you pack your book with testimonials from people who all have last names containing only one letter. Joe O. "eats about 3,500 calories a day, has lost more than 50 pounds, and is down to 20 percent body fat," write Sheats and Greenwood-Robinson.[72] Robbie W. dropped from 30 percent body fat to 24 percent and lost 20 pounds by increasing caloric intake to 2,500 calories a day and says, "I feel wonderful."[73]

Testimonials from people whose names consist of initials are almost always a sign of a scam artist at work. If you see a weight-loss book filled with them, throw it down and run screaming from the bookstore. Well, don't throw it. And don't scream. And don't run. But you get the idea. And don't buy Sheats and Greenwood-Robinson's 1995 follow-up nonsense, *Lean Bodies, Total Fitness,* which again promises on the cover that you can eat "increased calories."[74]

THE HELLERS' HORRIBLE SCIENCE

"So It May Be True After All; Eating Pasta Makes You Fat." Thus ran the bombshell title of a 1995 front-page *New York Times* story by food reporter Molly O'Neill. It contained much useful information on how Americans were still getting fat despite low-fat diets because they were simply eating too many carbohydrates. But O'Neill went astray when she tried to tie this into a theory of "insulin resistance." Indeed, where she really went astray was in relying on the expertise of Richard Heller, who had just published a new book with his wife called *Healthy for Life.*[75] She quoted Heller saying, "The majority of overweight people are insulin resistant. Carbohydrates are the worst thing they can eat because it causes them to overproduce insulin, which stimulates appetites, encourages the production of body fat and, over the long term, has serious health implications."[76]

The O'Neill article prompted a firestorm. "This is such a disservice; it's so unfair," Bonnie Liebman, nutritionist with the Center for Science in the Public Interest, told *USA Today.*[77] The paper did an analysis of one day of the Hellers' diet and found it added up to more than 4,000 calories, of which 49 percent were from fat and 19 percent from saturated fat, widely considered the worst kind.[78]

Meanwhile, *The Harvard Health Letter* countered *The New York Times* with a lead story, "Pasta Is Not Poison," which said that Italians called the article "an anti-spaghetti conspiracy." One Italian nutritionist said it reminded him of a news story published in a reputable French paper that said drinking Coca-Cola makes women give birth to daughters. (How silly! Everybody knows it's Pepsi that makes women give birth to daughters.)[79]

Gerald Reaven, M.D., professor of medicine at Stanford University Medical School, aptly summarized the O'Neill article when he said it "mixed up apples and oranges." The story, Raven said, "was probably supposed to be about how Americans are eating lower fat diets but aren't losing weight. [But] insulin resistance is a different issue. While some overweight people subsequently become insulin resistant, the two are sometimes totally unrelated." Agreeing was George Blackburn, M.D., associate professor of surgery at Harvard and director of nutrition services at Boston's Beth Israel Deaconess Medical Center, who told the *Health Letter*: "If the two are related it's that insulin resistance is sometimes the consequence of obesity, not the cause of it."[80]

Further, says Reaven, "You're no more likely than anyone else to gain weight if you're insulin resistant. You are, however, more likely to suffer potentially dangerous side effects." Like anyone else, insulin resistant people only gain weight if they eat too much and exercise too little.[81]

Who are the Hellers who cracked open this hornet's nest, anyway?

Richard is a psychologist while Rachael is a pathologist. Together they run a clinic in New York called the Carbohydrate Addict's Center, where they claim a success rate of more than 80 percent.[82]

The Hellers don't go as far as *The Zone* in claiming that "Eating fat does not make you fat."[83] But like *The Zone*, they definitely finger carbohydrates as the bad guys. They explain that, "When a carbohydrate addict eats carbohydrates, his or her body releases too much of the 'hunger hormone,' insulin, into the bloodstream. Rather than telling the brain the hunger has been satisfied," they write, excess insulin "causes the carbohydrate addict to desire more food after eating." This they say, causes more cravings for foods high in carbohydrates.[84]

Actually, as I described in chapter four, there's some controversy over whether this really happens even with pure sugar. But if it does, it's much less a problem with complex carbohydrates such as the potatoes the Hellers repeatedly rail against. That's because the fiber and other ingredients in complex carbohydrate foods slow the intake of the sugar, allowing the pancreas to more carefully adjust its output of insulin. What the Hellers should be saying is simply "eat less sugar." But you don't sell a whole lot of books that way.

Among the most evil of the Hellers' vegetables, those which should only be eaten once a day (at the "Reward Meal") are beets, broccoli, carrots, kidney beans, legumes, peas, and of course potatoes. They *hate* potatoes. Good thing they didn't live in Ireland 150 years ago.[85]

Though they do not say that obesity is always caused by carbohydrate addiction, the Hellers claim, "Our test results proved that more than 75 percent of those who came to us were carbohydrate addicts."[86] Elsewhere they say that "Evidence indicates that there is an 85 percent incidence of carbohydrate addiction in overweight Americans." What that evidence is, they never say.[87]

In addition to blaming carbohydrates, the Hellers emphasize food combining. Indeed, allegedly what makes their book superior to the previous Demon Carbohydrate books like Taller's and Stillman's is that the Hellers say you can actually eat all the carbohydrates you want so long as you do it all at once.

The solution to breaking "carbohydrate addiction" is somewhat similar to Stuart Berger's solution for beating "fattening" food allergies. In Berger's case, he said you break the cycle by never having the same food until four days have gone by. In the Hellers' case you do it by loading all your high-carbohydrate foods into a single meal, called the "Reward Meal." "Once a day at your Reward Meal, you can eat any food you desire (allowing for any dietary limitations imposed by your physician)," they write. "*All* foods are allowed at the Reward Meal, and quantities are *not* limited." They explain that "Having been fooled by two consecutive Low-Carbohydrate Meals, the body will release far less insulin than if you had been eating carbohydrates at every meal."[88] But there is a catch to this wonderful plan. They say, "you may eat whatever you desire, in whatever quantity you wish, but you have to complete that meal *within one hour.*"[89]

Yes, that's it. That's the only catch. Considering that a generation of Americans raised on fast food can wolf down a whole meal in five minutes, that's like telling a child he can have a chocolate bar only if he finishes his ice cream. I'm waiting for somebody to offer me a free Ferrari, but only so long as I also accept a free Porsche convertible as well.

A Few Good Books

None of this is to say that all books relating to weight loss prior to this one are bad. At my editor's suggestion (actually I *had* kind of thought of it first), I list some books that provide useful information and may inspire you. I don't necessarily endorse everything in them. Further, the list is surely incomplete, since I don't claim to have read every weight-loss book ever written—though I have read far too many.

- *Living Without Dieting* by John P. Foreyt and G. Ken Goodrick[90]
- *Jane Brody's Good Food Book* by (yes) Jane Brody[91]
- *Habits Not Diets* by James M. Ferguson[92]
- *Lean and Mean* by Morton H. Shaevitz[93]
- *The Callaway Diet* by C. Wayne Callaway, M.D. (don't worry, it's not really a diet)[94]
- *Diary of a Fat Housewife* by Rosemary Green[95]
- *Thin for Life* by Anne M. Fletcher[96]
- *Intuitive Eating* by Evelyn Tribole and Elyse Resch[97]
- *Weight Loss Through Persistence* by Daniel S. Kirschenbaum[98]

These books do not promise miracles. They do not say that you can eat like a sow and lay around in a mud puddle all day and still be thin. A couple of the books do put the authors' pictures on the cover but, hey, nobody's perfect. A few even made the best-seller lists, *despite* their accuracy and honesty.

Sometimes nice books do finish first, though in the weight-loss industry, 'tis a rare book indeed. Rest assured, the quack books will always dominate the heap. C. J. S. Thompson concludes his book, *The Quacks of Old London*, with: "If any one is bold enough to assert that he has a remedy which cures certain diseases and reiterates it often enough and loudly enough [Susan Powter?!], he is sure to get a following of believers among whom will be found persons of ability and position. This is confirmed again and again in the history of quackery."[99] At one time, in Austria, Germany, and Russia, quackery was a crime punishable by death.[100] That seems a bit extreme today—even for Miss Powter. The best way to punish these people is to simply remove their audiences and their incomes. That starts with you.

THE DEVIOUS DIET INDUSTRY

The late celebrated nutritionist Jean Mayer once said, "Overweight, like offshore oil, is a natural resource that adds to the GNP." In 1995 some 7.5 million Americans spent $1.78 billion at commercial weight-loss centers, according to Marketdata Enterprises, Inc., of Tampa, Florida, which tracks the diet industry. About 90 percent of their clients are women, though in recent years weight-loss centers have been making more efforts to attract men.

But as popular as they are with customers, many of these centers are far less so with nutritionists, doctors, and consumer activist groups. "We're getting fatter and fatter," says John Foreyt, director of the Nutrition Research Clinic at the Baylor College of Medicine and co-author of a 1994 Institute of Medicine study critical of the centers. "We're losing the war as the industry is booming."[101] He could have added that the industry is booming because we're losing the war.

Programs are divided into three major categories: medically supervised liquid diets, powdered-formula products that can be purchased over the counter at stores, and commercial weight-loss centers without medical supervision.

At one time, diet drinks (such as Slim-Fast, Ultra-Slim-Fast, Dyna Trim, and Nestlé's Sweet Success) were all the rage. By 1990 they were a $1.3-billion business, and hawked by numerous former fatties, ranging from L.A. Dodgers manager Tommy Lasorda to former New York Mayor Ed Koch to TV personality Willard Scott. But Scott and Lasorda became fat again (I haven't seen Koch lately to judge) and diet drink sales have plummeted—44 percent just between 1991 and 1992. Why? Probably because everyone else was having Willard Scott's and Tommy Lasorda's experience. Lasorda even had a heart attack and had to retire from baseball. The very concept of these drinks strikes me as silly. Instead of a hearty meal, you have a drink that, while it does have some fiber in it, really isn't all that much more filling than a glass of water. Why have a glass of Slim-Fast when you can have three apples instead? Even a hamburger (the old-fashioned, pre–Quarter Pounder size) has barely more calories, and it's a lot more satisfying.

As for the commercial weight-loss services, among the major ones are: Weight Watchers International, Inc.; Jenny Craig; Optifast; Medifast; Health Management Resources (HMR); Physicians Weight Loss, the Diet Center, Inc.; United Weight Control Corporation; Nutri/System, Inc.; Herbal Life; Dick Gregory's Bahamian Diet; and Slim Time Weight Loss Center.

The following is a summary of the largest programs:[102]

- Weight Watchers International, the oldest and largest commercial diet program, has been in business for 35 years and has more than 600,000 members. Its revenue in 1995 was about $1.35 billion. Clients pay a registration fee of $14 to $17 (at this writing), plus weekly meeting fees of $10 to $14. Purchase of food products is optional and some are available at supermarkets. The company changes its program as the science appears to dictate, with one of its more recent programs being "Fat and Fiber," emphasizing fruits, vegetables, and whole grains.
- Jenny Craig, the second-largest program, has some 600 centers. Its 1995 revenues were about $400 million. Clients pay enrollment fees of $99 to $279, depending on which program is chosen. Purchase of Jenny Craig food is mandatory and the average cost of meals is about $70 per week. This cost, however, drops as dieters begin substituting their own meals. Clients meet individually with a consultant each week. The company's maintenance program for participants is free with the premium enrollment fee. The company has also recently begun emphasizing exercise and has developed a series of motivational videos and audiotapes.

- Nutri/System, Inc., also has about 600 centers nationally, with 1995 revenues between $200 and $250 million. Enrollment costs $99 to $399, depending on the program. Purchase of their food is mandatory and the cost is about $49 per week. Clients receive a health assessment and a customized diet plan. More recently, it has made itself into something of a prescription mill for the weight-loss drug combination phentermine/fenfluramine and the drug dexfenfluramine.

- Physicians Weight Loss and Diet Center Worldwide came under the same ownership in 1995. At that time, Physicians was down to 89 centers from 500 in 1989. Diet Center Worldwide had about 600 stores, way down from about 2,300 in 1988. Revenues in 1995 were a little more than $100 million. The name implies supervision by doctors knowledgeable about weight loss, yet according to the firm's marketing and advertising director, the only nutrition and obesity training many company doctors receive comes from the company itself. Two of the programs are not physician-supervised at all.

The basic allegations against the commercial centers are many: They lure customers in who shouldn't really be there; they understate their prices; they refuse to verify their alleged results, and ultimately those results are poor.

PUSHY PEDDLERS

Clearly some weight-loss centers are all too eager to accept clients. One gets the idea that many would eagerly sign up Popeye's emaciated girlfriend, Olive Oyl. During an investigation, the New York City Department of Consumer Affairs sent people to such centers to see if they would be accepted. The Slim Time Weight Loss Center told one city employee he needed to lose 18 pounds, though according to the Consumer Affairs report he was just a little high on the weight chart and was extremely muscular. In another case a male staffer who stood at five feet eleven inches and weighed a mere 142 pounds visited the Diet Center, claiming he had gained weight and couldn't fit into his clothes. Instead of pointing out that he was actually two pounds below the bottom of the range in the 1983 Metropolitan Life Table, the sales representative told him he could lose eight pounds in two weeks. The representative told the Department of Consumer Affairs staffer to ignore the chart because "your clothes let you know what's right." On the other hand, an Optifast Center and Medifast program turned down these men, saying they didn't need to lose weight.[103]

Diane Epstein and Kathleen Thompson, in their book *Feeding on Dreams*, document many instances of such abuse. They quote a former Jenny Craig counselor commenting on one of her clients: "I was shocked. I looked at the client's chart before she started the program. She was five, two and weighed 108 pounds. The computer said her weight range was 104 to 114, so they sold her a program to lose four pounds. Imagine! There is something wrong with that woman and it's not her weight."[104]

Leila Farzan, an attorney with the Center for Science in the Public Interest (CSPI) in Washington, D.C., says that when she showed up at weight-loss centers they tried to enroll her even though "I'm normal weight." Says Farzan, "They're preying on a vulnerable population. People assume if they [salespeople] wear white lab coats they know what they're talking about. Obviously these people didn't know what they were talking about."[105] Or they did and didn't care.

This isn't to say that some people, like models, might not want to be extraordinarily thin and wish to use a commercial program. But in this case, it should be the client trying to convince the sales representative, not the other way around.

When *Consumer Reports* asked in 1993 if readers experienced strong pressure to join or stay in the program, 34 percent of the survey respondents said yes of Nutri/System and 31 percent of Jenny Craig. Only 12 percent said so of Weight Watchers and 11 percent of Medifast.[106]

Another way programs suck in clients is through physician referrals. One doctor testified before Congress that an income prospectus circulated by Medifast, Inc., boasted that doctors could make potential earnings of up to $15,000 a year from a quota of just fifteen patients on the Medifast plan.[107]

HIDDEN COSTS

We all know the expression "you get what you pay for." Often enough, it's true. As a frequent traveler, for the longest time I went through piece after piece of cheap luggage. Handles snapped off, zippers broke, and one piece, notwithstanding its five-year warranty, broke the first time I picked it up after it was packed. Finally I shelled out for some quality luggage and countless trips later it's still with me.

The commercial diet industry, however, turns the axiom on its head. Rarely do customers get the results they hope for and rarely do they pay what they think they will.

The main way these programs stick you is through food sales. This is most especially the case with Jenny Craig, which makes fully 90 percent of its profits from its food, according to Marketdata. Nutri/System gets about 75 to 80 percent of its money from food, while with Weight Watchers it's around 65 to 70 percent.[108]

As comedienne Beth Donahue puts it, "Jenny's ads say you can 'Sign up now for just six cents a pound.' What they don't tell you is that you should cash in all your 401K savings if you want to be able to afford Jenny's 'cuisine.' "[109]

That's a bit extreme perhaps, but the point is valid. Said one Nutri/System client, "Lose your first ten pounds free. Sounds good. I had about seventeen pounds to lose according to the computer. Even though the first ten pounds came off in less than four weeks, that was still $360 worth of food. Hardly free. I had to purchase a program for the other seven pounds. They never came off, but it still cost me another $360 to struggle for four more weeks, plus a $99 Guaranteed Program fee." Concluded the woman, "Eight hundred dollars is a lot of money for a free program."[110] The average client spends about $600 for a four-month period in a typical commercial program, according to Marketdata.[111]

The companies assert that their prepackaged meals help dieters learn portion control, freeing them from the need to weigh or measure food. Well, maybe. But at some point the training wheels have to come off. Measuring food shouldn't be an exact process any more than counting calories should. Learning to eat properly comprises two things: the type of food and the amount of food. The proper amount of food varies from person to person and day to day. It's a matter of satisfying your hunger and nothing more. As difficult as it is for many of us in our culture to differentiate true biological hunger from simple appetite, certainly Jenny Craig doesn't know what your hunger level is.

Still, if prepackaged breakfasts, lunches, dinners, and snacks teach Americans that the portions they're used to being served in restaurants are obscenely huge, then perhaps they serve a temporary purpose. But if that's the case, there are plenty of choices of such prepackaged foods in the stores and you can bet they're cheaper than what the diet centers are hawking. "We did comparison shopping and Jenny Craig offers a container of tomato soup for $2.20 and we bought it at a store for 50 cents and got twice as much," says CSPI's Leila Farzan. "They have 6.5-ounce frozen lasagna for $4.79 and Stouffer's Lean Cuisine was $1.46 for the same serving and it had half the fat and fewer calories."[112]

If a diet program insists you buy only their food, I'd suggest you insist on taking your business elsewhere. That means telling Jenny to take a jump and saying nix to Nutri/System. But it will also require some willpower at Weight Watchers. While dieticians praise Weight Watchers for not pushing its own brands too forcefully in its classes, *Fortune* magazine has observed, "the message gets across anyway. Handouts at lectures often include coupons, and staying on the complex diet can require such tedious calculations that many dieters just stock up on Weight Watchers food instead."[113] Remember that Weight Watchers is owned by a food company, Heinz, and that company makes the Weight Watchers food. It's all a very cozy relationship.

But being pressured to buy food is one thing and having no choice another. Indeed, when *Consumer Reports* asked if the programs "have higher costs than you were led to believe," 47 percent said yes of both Jenny Craig and Nutri/System. Only 7 percent said yes of Weight Watchers, while 17 percent said yes about the liquid-fast program HMR.[114]

SUCCESS RATES—OR LACK THEREOF

In May 1996, CSPI filed a forty-nine-page petition with the Federal Trade Commission (FTC) demanding that certain commercial weight-loss centers be required to disclose their full costs and dieters' prospects of success. CSPI was particularly critical of the promotions and practices of Physicians Weight Loss Center, Nutri/System, and Jenny Craig. It was much less critical of Weight Watchers. In a statement, Weight Watchers said it agreed that "industry-wide standards should be developed," though it did not explicitly endorse the specifics of the CSPI petition.[115] CSPI was joined in its action by such groups as the American Society of Bariatric Physicians, the Association of Schools of Public Health, the Association of State and Territorial Public Health Nutrition Directors, and various consumer groups.[116]

One specific complaint of CSPI was that "Advertisements continue to include testimonials from celebrities and others who claim to have lost significant amounts of weight even if such weight losses are not typical or cannot be maintained. Such ads need only disclose in small print that weight loss may vary among individuals." Another was that "ads continue to tout the price of enrollment, but fail to disclose the cost of other mandatory fees. The FTC merely requires that such ads disclose in small print that some mandatory fees are not included in the advertised price." Thus, it said, such ads "are filled with nearly illegible 'mice type' that most people do not notice or cannot read."[117] This is all the more outrageous when you consider how few mice have the ability to read.

What CSPI was actually asking for was *further* FTC action. On numerous occasions the agency has pursued diet programs for false advertising and had forced changes. For example, in March 1993, the agency released the results of a full-scale investigation of the state of the diet industry. One outcome was that it signed what one official called an "out-of-court agreement" with thirteen diet programs to change their advertising claims, claims that implied "long-term weight loss" and "cure." So far, though, the two biggest, Jenny Craig and Weight Watchers, have refused to give in and are battling it out with the FTC in court.

I really hate to agree with bureaucrats, but the FTC was clearly right on this one. The diet industry has played fast and loose with its "evidence." For example, Jenny Craig published results of a survey in the journal *Addictive Behaviors*, which found that 82 percent of clients who reached their goals remained within 10 percent of those weights a year later. But the study was based on surveys mailed to clients, of which only half responded. "You have to assume the other half gained weight," says Wayne Callaway. Or at least a lot of them. More importantly, the study did not address how many people who began the program reached their goal.[118]

Weight Watchers in 1993 claimed that of 1,200 lifetime members 53 percent maintained their goal weight for two years and 37 percent maintained it for five years or more. But Baylor's Foreyt is unimpressed. "The proof of the pudding is always in the publication of the data and a peer-reviewed scientific journal. So it's very important for all organizations, including Weight Watchers, to submit their data to journals and to publish it,"[119] he says. To date, Weight Watchers has not done so.

Other companies have made outright false claims. In 1991, Stanford University, along with Jenny Craig and Weight Watchers, filed suit against Nutri/System, charging the company with false advertising. The ads in question cited a study published in *Healthline* magazine, edited by a psychologist at Stanford University, ranking Nutri/System as number one among well-known weight-loss programs. Stanford officials said the ads, which carried the Stanford seal, misled readers into thinking the study was based on research sanctioned by the school though it had no official connection either with the study or with *Heathline*. The suit said Nutri/System paid *Healthline* $25,000 for the article.[120] (Unfortunately, ads made to appear as articles are actually quite common in some health and women's magazines.) In 1990, Nutri/System advertised that it met American Heart Association guidelines, three years after it had asked permission to make such a claim and was turned down. That time it backed down with just the threat of a suit.[121]

Appearing on the CNN show *Sonya Live* in 1994, a representative from Nutri/System essentially admitted the organization had a sad record of helping people keep weight off, saying "the weight management programs of the eighties do not have long-term success rates. They do, though, I think, have laid [*sic*] the foundation for a new generation of programs that you will see come into existence in the nineties. . . ." Specifically asked for "the numbers" on successful weight loss, he simply avoided the question.[122] In other words, as of 1994, Nutri/System was not having much success in slimming its clients.

Of course, you can always make up "the numbers." When *Vogue* magazine writer Laura Fraser went to a Jenny Craig clinic in 1994 posing as a prospective client, the sales representative told her that their success rate was "much better than any other weight-loss program. It's 96 percent."[123] Meanwhile, "Medifast estimates that 30 percent to 50 percent of its dieters keep the weight off after a year while HMR [Heath Management Resources] claims a 60 percent maintenance rate after two years," the *American Medical News* reported in 1990.[124] They forgot to add that pigs really can fly and that white alligators plague the sewer system of New York City. A year later, the FTC made them back down on their claims.[125]

As of this writing, only one diet center has published what could be considered reliable data. And what it shows is not encouraging. In a peer-reviewed study of 4,026 obese patients who went on the Optifast program, one fourth dropped out within the first three weeks, and of the majority of dieters who achieved significant weight loss, only 5 to 10 percent maintained their reduced weights after eighteen months.[126] Other than this, says Foreyt, "There's no good long-term data on any of these programs other than testimonials and certain individuals' before-and-after photos."[127]

Facing this data dearth, *Consumer Reports* did its own survey in 1993. "On average, our respondents reported that they stayed on the programs for about half a year and lost 10 to 20 percent of their starting weight," said the magazine. "But the average dieter gained back almost half of that weight just six months after ending the program, and more than two thirds of it after two years." It also found that "None of the top five diet programs were better than others in helping people lose weight during the program or keep it off six months later. As a group, people on the three liquid-fast programs did lose weight more rapidly than those on regular diet programs—but they gained it back at roughly the same rate."[128]

CONSUMER REPORTS' SURVEY:
RATINGS OF THE WEIGHT-LOSS PROGRAMS

Diet Programs	Satisfaction with Weight Lost	Satisfaction with Maintenance	Percent of Weight Lost End of Program	Six Months After
Weight Watchers	74%	54%	8%	5%
Jenny Craig	65%	35%	11%	6%
Physicians Weight Loss Center	65%	37%	12%	7%
Diet Center	68%	38%	10%	6%
Nutri/System	63%	34%	11%	7%
Liquid-Fast Programs				
Health Management Resources	82%	43%	20%	15%
Optifast	73%	24%	20%	12%
Medifast	65%	23%	15%	8%

Source: *Consumer Reports*, June 1993.[129]

There's a caveat to this chart. To just look at the results of the liquid-fast programs, they appear more successful both in overall weight loss and at the six-month follow-up. In fact, this is just the nature of the beast. Liquid-fast programs clearly cause the greatest, quickest weight loss. The question is: Does it stay off? The aforementioned Optifast study indicates few of their clients keep it off. The 15 percent or 12 percent weight loss the chart shows at the six-month mark will probably have practically disappeared by the twelve-month or eighteen-month follow-up. Of course, this is likely to have happened also with those in the solid-food diet programs, too.

"Despite all this," said *Consumer Reports*, "a significant minority of our respondents—about a quarter of them—did get some apparent benefit from their weight-loss regimen. Two years after finishing their program, they had kept off most of the weight they had lost."[130]

Some professionals also hold out hope for those looking to commercial programs. "Many people who come to see me for help have gone through every single one of the commercial diet programs first," says Elizabeth Ward, a registered dietician and spokeswoman for the American Dietetic Association. "However, I don't want to bash those programs because it really does depend on the person and his or her ability to think long term and make changes in habits."[131] Chairwoman Marion Nestle of the New York University Department of Nutrition says of the commercial programs, "They all work for some people and if that's what it takes, it's all to the good. If people think they have to spend money at some place, that's fine. But unless they exercise more and eat less, they're not going to lose weight, no matter what the gimmick."[132]

As far as which program to choose, well, *Consumer Reports* threw in its lot with Weight Watchers. "Since no diet program was especially effective," it said, "anyone who wants to play the commercial-diet game should choose a program on the basis of cost, comfort, and common sense. By those criteria, Weight Watchers was our readers' clear favorite. It costs less than the others, emphasizes healthful dietary habits, encourages relatively slow weight loss, and generally appears to provide the most satisfying, supportive experience." Said the magazine, "Compared with customers of the typical diet program, Weight Watchers customers experienced less sales pressure, had fewer problems with the diet, felt less hungry, and were less often surprised by unexpectedly high costs."[133]

Other consumer advocates and medical authorities with whom I've spoken seem to agree. I attended one Weight Watchers meeting perhaps ten years ago. I learned some practical things and thought their program made sense, though it depressed the hell out of me to hear this huge lady in the back row talk about eating twenty ice cream sandwiches in a single sitting.

In any case, I never went back, and I rather agree with the twenty-six-year-old woman who had been a client in three different programs. "I don't know that diet programs are worth the money, because I've learned from being in several there really aren't any secrets," she said.[134]

If it's just emotional support you're looking for, there are a couple of very inexpensive organizations around. One is called Take Off Pounds Sensibly (TOPS) and another is Overeaters

Anonymous (OA), patterned after Alcoholics Anonymous. (There's a book about Overeaters Anonymous that, fittingly enough, was anonymously written.[135]) They won't give you diet plans (which you may see either as a plus or a minus) and they won't foist food upon you. But what they will do is put you in the company of other people who have the same problem you do. Depending on your outlook, you may find that encouraging or depressing.

But the commercial centers remain an option. For all their misrepresentations and raising of false hopes, commercial weight-loss centers really want to help their clients lose weight and keep it off. It's nonsense to believe, as some writers have alleged, that these programs conspire to keep their patients' weight yo-yoing in order to keep them on a permanent basis. "We couldn't stay in business if it weren't for the repeats," Diane Epstein and Kathleen Thomson quote one diet program counselor saying ominously in their book *Feeding on Dreams*.[136] But with about 80 million Americans obese and three fourths of Americans overweight, as the old miner put it: There's gold in them there hills! Nothing would extract that gold (in the form of new clients) better than having real, demonstrable success with current clients. That's real incentive to successfully treat as many clients as possible. Hey, it's like Michael Douglas's slimy Gordon Gekko character said in the movie *Wall Street*: "Greed works."[137]

7 Diets Don't Work —

Except When

They Do

If there is one expression that has absolutely taken the weight-loss industry by storm in recent years it is: "Diets don't work." Actually, that's not strong enough. How about: "DIETS DON'T WORK!" There, much better. It has been the title of countless magazine articles and book chapters and even a best-selling book.[1] Depending on how you define "diet," the phrase may be true. But unfortunately it's an expression that has launched a thousand myths, many of them self-serving. In general, it has been broadened to mean that you can't lose weight and keep it off by restricting your caloric intake. And the medical science indicates that's just not true. Moderate calorie restriction done correctly can remove and keep off excess weight.

In 1958 the University of Pennsylvania's Albert Stunkard summarized in just two sentences the results of the previous thirty years' efforts to control obesity through diet: "Most obese persons will not stay in treatment for obesity. Of those who stay in treatment most will not lose weight, and of those who do lose weight, most will regain it."[2] We can see by that statement that progress has been made in the clinical treatment of obesity. Now research trials of moderate caloric restriction combined with behavior modification indicate that 80 percent of patients will remain in treatment for twenty weeks and that about half will achieve a weight loss of twenty pounds or more.[3] It is only on point number three, the part about regaining, that we're still lacking.

Time and again we're told that official government figures say as many as 95 percent of all dieters fail. It happens this is partly true; it just doesn't mean a whole lot.

THE "95 PERCENT" FALLACY

In 1992 a panel of obesity experts from around the country was convened by the National Institutes of Health (NIH). That panel made headlines when it suggested that 90 to 95 percent of dieters regain all or most of their poundage within five years.[4] No doubt many an overweight person, upon hearing this, just threw in the towel and headed for the refrigerator. Such defeatism is a travesty, because the 90 to 95 percent figure is far gloomier than the facts merit.

The most glaring problem is the source of the data. Kelly Brownell, M.D., a Yale obesity researcher, says the failure rate may look higher than it is is because it is based on the "hard-core" overweight, people with the most pounds to lose who have failed many times over. Because they've had so much trouble with their weight, they may be drawn to university-based research studies. Conversely, people who are successful—particularly those who lose weight on their own—tend not to wind up in the research studies from which the statistics come. "What we don't have, and what we need," Brownell says, "are statistics from the average group of people who go on diets on their own. I think people are doing a lot better than we think."[5] Xavier Pi-Sunyer, M.D., of St. Luke's–Roosevelt Hospital in New York City estimates the actual relapse rate for dieters is closer to 85 percent[6] while the aforementioned 1993 survey by *Consumer Reports* puts it at around 75 percent.[7]

A paper in the 1993 *Journal of the American Dietetic Association* agreed with Brownell's theory, noting that "several studies have indicated higher long-term success rates for individuals who lost weight without the assistance of formal programs."[8] One such person is the present author. I took off lots of weight and kept it off. But I'll never make it into any government weight-loss database. And you can imagine how irritating it is to hear that what you've done is not do-able. It would be like Sir Edmund Hillary, having reached the top of Mt. Everest, hearing years later that the world's tallest peak has yet to be conquered. In fact, the vast majority of dieters—95 percent of men and 87 percent of women, according to one 1993 survey in the *Annals of Internal Medicine*—do exactly what I did and design their own weight-loss programs. They do not take part in organized plans.[9] The ones who end up in the monitored programs tend to be the ones who couldn't make it on their own. Once in such a program, they'll likely fail again.[10]

There's also a definitional problem with statements like "95 percent of diets fail" because dieting is not an all-or-nothing proposition. Consider a review of numerous diet programs that found a mere 3 percent kept off their lost weight entirely. Just 3 percent! But these researchers realized that keeping weight off is not an all-or-nothing proposition and noted that 18.5 percent maintained at least half their losses for at least four years, while 34 percent kept off at least a quarter of their loss. For an obese person, keeping off a quarter of one's excess weight can still bring substantial health benefits.[11]

Let's face it though: One way or the other most people who lose weight do probably eventually regain much or all of it, and that's not a good thing. But then, that is hardly unusual for a chronic illness, which is what obesity is. Relapse rates for drug, alcohol, and smoking treatment programs are reported to be in the range of 50 to 90 percent.[12] Funny, I can't remember the last time I heard anyone say there's no point in trying to quit drugs, drinking, or smoking because most people who try fail, especially in their first efforts. There are no equivalent groups to the National Association for the Advancement of Fat Acceptance (NAAFA) for drug abusers, drunks, or smokers who claim that just because something's difficult to do it shouldn't even be attempted.

Instead of bemoaning the high recidivism rate of weight loss, we need to look at why it happens to try to prevent it.

The "Yo-Yo" Myth

The first step in this direction is get rid of the notion that even trying to lose weight is harmful. But what about this concept of yo-yo dieting? The alleged terrors of the yo-yo—losing and gaining weight repeatedly—are threefold. First, it is supposed to damage your health. Second, it is supposed to make it more difficult to lose weight when you try again. Third, it is supposed to end up making you fatter than when you started to diet.

Shysters have eagerly embraced the yo-yo theory. "Every time you diet and then go off it, it becomes harder for you to lose weight the next time you diet," says diet guru Cliff Sheats in *Lean Bodies: The Revolutionary New Approach to Losing Bodyfat by Increasing Calories*.[13] "With each [new] diet you have less of what it takes to lose weight and more of what it takes to gain weight,"[14] says Debra Waterhouse in *Outsmarting the Female Fat Cell.*

Naturally, fat activists love the yo-yo. "Physically, a series of diets makes you fatter. If, after the first few diets, you only go back to your original weight, don't be fooled," claim Diane Epstein and Kathleen Thompson in *Feeding on Dreams.* "Today's number on the scale is not the whole picture. You *are* becoming fatter. Each time you put the weight back on you are adding fat cells. And they never go away."[15]

In fact, says St. Luke's–Roosevelt Hospital's Pi-Sunyer, "There is no convincing data for the claim that yo-yoing makes you fatter but it has somehow gotten into the media in a large way, so people have gotten confused about whether they are actually harming themselves by trying to lose weight."[16]

Here's why the yo-yo doomsayers are wrong. As discussed earlier in this book, it's true that when you lose weight your metabolism drops, for two reasons. One, you lose some muscle. Most of this muscle was infrastructure needed to carry around your fat, so when you lose the fat the muscle goes, too. Two, your metabolism also dips in order to conserve energy because the body sees a drop in calories as a threat of famine. But when you regain the fat, the muscle comes back to support it. And when the body no longer perceives a famine threat, that part of the metabolism rebounds as well. Hence, at the end of the yo-yo cycle, while all your fat may be back, at least all of your metabolism is, too.

There's plenty of medical literature showing this. The conclusion reached by one set of authors writing in the January 1996 *International Journal of Eating Disorders* was, "Results of this study do not support claims that weight cycling reduces [resting energy expenditure] in obese patients" who had lost and regained an average of forty-one pounds. "Consistent with several other recent studies, our findings also failed to show that weight cycling increased the deposition of fat in the upper body or the ratio of fat to lean tissue."[17] In other words, the women regained their fat in the same places they had lost it, and they lost no muscle tissue during the cycle.[18]

How about the allegation that yo-yoing damages your health? Glenn Gaesser's *Big Fat Lies* has a chapter titled "Diet and Die," with a subheading, "The Weight-Loss Paradox: Yo-Yoing to Death."[19] The point is made, is it not? Analyses of some large epidemiological databases have linked body weight fluctuation to excess deaths from all causes and especially heart disease. But the aforementioned *International Journal of Obesity* study also looked at this data and again concluded there's nothing to fear. It noted, among other things, that "None of the studies was originally designed to address the health hazards of weight fluctuations. Consequently, important information is missing," including information on why the people lost weight.[20] For example, we know that weight loss usually precedes death by cancer, AIDS, and numerous other diseases. The database picks up the cancer or AIDS patient because of the weight loss but doesn't factor in the disease. All the database analysis really shows is that weight was lost. So if you look at the data without thinking about what went into it, you can erroneously conclude that weight loss is a killer.

A study that came out after the *International Journal of Obesity* review looked at the specific issue of weight cycling and heart disease. In it, University of Pittsburgh researchers found that those who lost and regained twenty pounds or more over a thirty-month period had no greater risk of heart disease than others who maintained their original weights.[21] "Concern about weight cycling shouldn't keep overweight people from trying to lose weight," says chief author Rena R. Wing, M.D.[22] Likewise, the National Task Force on the Prevention and Treatment of Obesity, set up by the NIH, did its own review of medical literature between 1966 and 1994. "There is no convincing evidence," the task force concluded, "that weight cycling in humans has adverse effects on body composition, energy expenditure, risk factors for cardiovascular disease, or the effectiveness of future efforts at weight loss."[23]

GET THIN SLOWLY

Still, if weight cycling isn't harmful, certainly it's better to stay down once you're down. And apparently one "secret" to doing this is to go down slowly.

Wayne Callaway, M.D., notes that marketing studies conducted by one weight-loss organization found that, when dieting, most women expect to lose between two and three pounds a week and most men expect between three and five pounds a week. If the expectation is unmet, dieters will discontinue the program by the third week. Not for nothing do you hear slogans like Slim-Fast's "Give us a week and we'll take off the weight."

"To remain financially successful, commercial operations try to meet this expectation, even when they know that most of the early weight loss is from water and that a water retention cycle will eventually follow," says Callaway. "Virtually all the experts—from the Surgeon General to well-respected popular health and nutrition writers such as Jane Brody . . . agree that diets designed to meet these expectations always fail over the long term."[24]

"Rapid water loss is the $33-billion diet gimmick," says Callaway. "It looks good on your bathroom scale and it raises your hopes. But the initial water-weight loss is completely meaningless in terms of your ultimate goal. You are not losing fat; you are not getting leaner. It's only a trick, a gimmick, the temporary side effect of not eating enough carbohydrates to supply your brain. . . ."[25]

Remember that virtually any diet can cause you to lose weight; the real problem is keeping it off. With that in mind, choose a regimen that emphasizes not speed but permanency. While one often hears that no more than two pounds a week should be lost, it appears even this is too much for most people who are not extremely obese. (Obviously, the fatter you are, the less of an overall percentage of your fat two pounds is. So with some people, two or even three pounds might be OK.)

George Blackburn, M.D., chief of surgical nutrition at Beth Israel Deaconess Medical Center in Boston, is considered one of the nation's foremost authorities on weight loss. He suggests you begin by aiming to lose no more than 10 percent of body weight at the rate of no more than a pound a week. Only after maintaining that loss for six months and receiving permission from your physician, he says, should you attempt to take off another 10 percent.[26] In my case, after I began writing this book I initially lost 14 percent of my weight, which struck me as a good goal since it brought me to the weight that I was at when I joined the army at age eighteen. So I went a bit overboard, perhaps, but not by too much. In any case, it brought me down to a good, healthy weight. Then I went conservative and held that weight not for six months but for a whole year before trying to drop more. Then I said, "Congratulations, you did it. Now it's time to try to reach your ultimate goal, which is to be not only healthily slim but downright athletic." I'm not advising that for all my readers. But this was what I wanted for myself and I did it.

The main reason to aim for slow weight loss is because you are seeking to permanently change your eating habits. The calorie deficit you create should be close to what will be your permanent calorie level and certainly no lower than 1,200 to 1,300 calories. The further you go below this, the more likely you are to suffer from hunger—and nothing defeats a weight-loss regimen more quickly than hunger.

Paradoxically, for a while an extremely low energy diet of, say, 600 calories a day, stops hunger after a few days.[27] You may feel tired and listless but your hunger will leave you. Yet the calorie deficit is so deep that when the time comes to move to a maintenance stage, you will have to make drastic changes. That's the point at which the appetite-suppressing effect of a very low-calorie diet abates and leaves you ravenously hungry.[28]

Another big advantage of slighter reductions in calories is that evidence indicates you may lose somewhat less muscle this way than with sharper calorie restrictions.[29] In what is probably a best-case scenario, researchers at the University of Pennsylvania put one set of obese subjects on a very low-calorie diet consisting of 500 calories a day and other set on a low-calorie diet of 1,000 to 1,200 calories daily. While those on the very low-calorie diets saw their resting energy expenditures drop by more than 17 percent within a few weeks, their counterparts saw only a 2 percent drop, all of which could be accounted for by their lost weight.[30]

Very low-calorie diets may be necessary for those few cases where people need to lose a lot of weight quickly because of serious health problems, such as the need for surgery. Other than this, I believe they have little going for them—though all too many doctors continue to recommend them to patients. Studies comparing the two types of weight-loss regimens have found that you definitely get more bang for the buck with less caloric restriction. That is, you lose more fat off your body per calories reduced with milder restriction. Consider severe energy restriction as a jackhammer while lesser restriction is more like a hammer and chisel. You can break up rock more quickly with the jackhammer but more to your liking with the delicate instruments.

CONSTANT CRAVINGS

"To lose weight, you've got to control your appetite." So goes the sales pitch for an over-the-counter drug that has mild appetite-suppressing properties. Let me put a different spin on the phrase, though. To lose weight (and keep it off) you've got to find out what your appetite is. Our society has come so far from the time when food was seen primarily as sustenance that, for many of us, the idea of food as a source of energy needed to survive—as opposed to being a source of recreation—is utterly foreign. In short, we have lost our ability to distinguish appetite from hunger. All "I'm hungry" necessarily means today is "I feel like eating." And for many of us, eating whenever we get the urge to have something nice in our mouths is the road to obesity.

As facile as it sounds, one of the most important tools in weight control is to eat primarily only when hungry. But we have largely forgotten how to do that. "We tend to use the food on our plate instead of the way our stomach feels as the standard for how much we should eat," says Jane Hurley, senior nutritionist at the Center for Science in the Public Interest.[31] Our society has so thoroughly disconnected eating from hunger that detecting true hunger is something we must relearn.

Registered dieticians Evelyn Tribole and Elyse Resch, in their book *Intuitive Eating: A Recovery Book for the Chronic Dieter*, urge us to chuck calorie counting and instead listen to our hunger. It is rather bizarre that they should feel it necessary to list symptoms of what hunger feels like, but in the America of the 1990s for many of us it *is* necessary. Their listed hunger symptoms are:

- Mild gurgling or gnawing in the stomach
- Growling noises (from your stomach, not your dog)
- Light-headedness
- Difficulty concentrating
- Uncomfortable stomach pain
- Irritability
- Feeling faint
- Headache[32]

If you don't have any of the above feelings and yet you're reaching into the refrigerator, you should stop at least long enough to ask yourself why. And if your answer resembles that of the mountain climber—"because it's there"—you need to think again about eating that food. This isn't to say all recreational eating is bad. Sometimes when a piece of creamy cheesecake or a thick, rich brownie screams, "Eat me," you've got to answer the call of nature and at least eat part of it, lest you spend the next two weeks wishing you had. But if you're overweight and you're doing a lot of purely recreational eating, don't wonder that the two might be connected.

In his 1996 book *The Garden of Eating*, Jeremy Iggers talks of being "mindful" of what you're eating. "At the risk of reducing the ancient wisdom of the Orient to just another weight-loss gimmick," he says, "when you eat mindfully, pausing to take note of the flavor and the texture of the food, and of the sensations on the tongue, you're likely to eat more slowly, and to eat less." He adds that "this same conscious eating may also make us more exacting about what we eat: The difference between flavorless, cottony white bread and whole-grain bread becomes dramatic."[33]

Tribole and Resch write:

> One of our clients aptly suggested that *Intuitive Eating* is about *waiting* and learning to be patient. She finds herself *waiting* to eat until she is hungry. Then she describes *waiting* during a time-out in the midst of her meal to see if she is full. When she is experiencing a difficult feeling that she used to cover up with overeating, she now sits with the feeling and *waits* it out until she feels better. And in the bigger picture, she is *waiting* for her eating to normalize so that her body will return to its natural healthy weight. She says that

this process has taught her to be more patient than she has ever been in her life. She has decided that patience is golden, that what she has learned about herself as she patiently *waits* is more valuable than all the pounds she has lost (and of course, regained) and all the money she has spent on her failed diet.[34]

This very much describes my own experience. Getting down to my proper weight meant gaining control. Being overweight was both the problem and a symptom of the problem.

It has long been believed that emotions can lead to overeating, and indeed whole books have been written on the subject. While it would be wrong to blame emotions for the national obesity problem, in recent years there has emerged evidence indicating that on a personal level emotional eating can lead to overweight.[35] One study, for example, found that "A significantly increased probability [of overeating] was observed when subjects checked [on a list] 'tired,' 'bored,' and 'irritable,' while checking 'hungry' was associated with a significantly lower probability of overeating." Likewise, impulsive eating was associated with being "tired, depressed, bored, stressed, irritable, and nervous. A lower probability of impulsive eating was associated with hungry and happy." The study concluded that "eating behavior is at least partially under situational control, partly under cognitive control, and easily disregulated by emotions."[36]

"Two thirds of all obese persons may be carbohydrate cravers who eat not for hunger but to combat tension, anxiety, mental fatigue, and depression," estimate John P. Foreyt and G. Ken Goodrick, of Baylor College.[37] Dean Ornish quotes one of his patients saying, "When something's eating me, I eat. When I'm lonely, which is much of the time, I eat. And then I eat some more. I keep trying to fill up the void with food, but the feelings of emptiness keep coming back. I use food to stuff my emotions, to keep the sadness from coming in."[38]

Many of us can sympathize with this, myself included. When I was working in Washington, D.C., and didn't have a girlfriend to spend Friday nights with, I would ritualistically spend the night with two rented videos, a pizza that was so crummy as to be indistinguishable from the cardboard box holding it, and ten Reese's peanut butter cups. That's enough calories to choke a small elephant. I thought about writing to the Hershey company and insisting they send me a free pass to the Hershey amusement park as a reward for my patronage.

But as least I was able to hold this binge to one night a week. Many of us engage in such rituals nightly. After that, I moved from Washington and found a girlfriend, but I still had an eating problem. As you've probably figured out by now, I'm a writer. And a writer's life is a lonely one. This is especially true when you work out of your home and only have a dumb rabbit to keep you company. I have often wished I were in a "people" job like bartending or at least photographing models for swimsuit magazines. I was a waiter in law school and thoroughly enjoyed the job because I met so many neat people and could play the role of both server and entertainer. But writing is my job and there's no helping that. And while during the day I spend much of my time bantering on the phone with people I'm interviewing or who are interviewing me, at night it gets mighty lonely. For the longest time I used food to keep me company. No more of that ten-candy-bar nonsense, but food nonetheless.

One day in the early stages of writing this book, I realized that food should not be your friend. Food is sustenance and sometimes it's entertainment. But never, never make it your friend. People should be your friends, pets should be your friends, books should be your friends.

Now I carefully monitor not only what I'm eating but *why*. Hunger is always a justifiable motive. Entertainment may well be, in very small doses. But if it's just for comfort, forget it. My comfort is in knowing that I control food, not the other way around.

The problem with making food your friend is it can so quickly become your enemy. And that's why it's no mystery at all that Americans have developed a love-hate relationship with food. It makes perfect sense that a country that invests so much value in food is going to be an overweight country and that, realizing that overweight is bad, will loathe that food. It makes perfect sense that even as we get fatter by the year, tremendous numbers of us claim to be on diets—diets we can't possibly stick with because we have invested so much value in food. It makes perfect sense that the fattest Western nation on earth would also have the most eating disorders.

As hard as it is to detect when you should begin eating because you're physiologically hungry, it may be that much tougher to detect when you should stop. The best way of dealing with this is to eat slowly and let your body do its work in sending a signal to the satiety center of the brain. Aside from this, you need to keep a mental record of what it takes to really satisfy yourself. (Unfortunately, this will vary from food to food, so you won't accomplish this in just a couple of days.) Start with breakfast, which tends to be the most fixed meal of the day. If you normally eat two eggs and two strips of bacon for breakfast, try eating just one of each. If you're still hungry twenty minutes or so later, the next time you have breakfast add back one egg or one strip of bacon, or maybe just part of an egg or a piece of bacon. Actually the best thing of all would be to exchange these foods entirely for a high-fiber cereal breakfast, but the idea is the same. And just because you're eating a high-fiber cereal breakfast doesn't mean you can eat all of that you want either. Again, experiment to see what your body is really demanding.

FAT IS NOT A FEMINIST ISSUE

While discussing the connection between emotions and excess eating, some may think of the smash best-seller *Fat Is a Feminist Issue*.[39] Written by psychologist Susie Orbach, now known as therapist to Princess Diana, it was summarized by the author as saying, "Fat . . . is an individual (conscious or unconscious) rebellion against an imprisoning social role."[40] In the book itself, subtitled *The Anti-Diet Guide to Permanent Weight Loss*, she writes, "Fat is a social disease, and fat is a feminist issue. Fat is not about lack of self-control or lack of willpower. Fat is about protection, sex, nurturance, strength, boundaries, mothering, substance, assertion, and rage. It is a response to the inequality of the sexes."[41] Women become fat, says Orbach, because they think, "If I get bigger like a man then maybe I'll get taken [as] seriously as a man."[42]

No talk of excess calories or energy surpluses here. Instead, everything can be explained and treated by psychotherapy, which by amazing coincidence is Orbach's profession. Some feminists leapt to their feet and applauded Orbach's assertions, with Susan

Faludi demanding that it "be read by every American woman."[43] That would indeed be unfortunate. Orbach's books (she penned a sequel, with the inspired title *Fat Is a Feminist Issue II*[44]) may provide useful insights on the state of women's rights, and certainly there must be some women with eating disorders who fall into categories Orbach describes. But Orbach's thesis cannot explain why there are just about as many obese American men as women. It cannot explain why European women—less liberated than American women by most standards—are much thinner than their American counterparts, nor why female obesity has been growing in the United States at the same time women have been making great gains in job opportunities, pay, "reproductive rights," and virtually every area considered important by feminists.

In fact, the National Academy of Science's Institute of Medicine has expressly rejected Orbach's kind of thinking. "For many years," it stated, "obesity was considered a disorder with pronounced psychological underpinnings. The obese were considered to overeat in response to negative feelings such as insecurity, sadness, and frustration, or more particularly because of their inability to establish positive interpersonal relationships. More recently, this traditional view has changed dramatically on the basis of new research findings."[45]

Whatever solutions Orbach provides, she provides no answer to female obesity. Instead, she just joins the long list of other writers who steal attention away from real causes, victimizing both women and men. Women, as well as men, deserve scientific answers about their weight problems, not psychobabble.

DON'T SKIP, DON'T BINGE

Just as you should make eating when not hungry a rare event, you should always make sure that when you are hungry you do eat. You've heard the advice about not skipping meals. Take it. Studies show that, as one stated, "meal patterning is important in that skipping meals was associated with increased probabilities of uncontrolled behaviors at subsequent eating episodes."[46] In nontechnical terms: "If you totally try to deny a craving, it just makes it worse. You're just going to want it more and more and more, and then by the time you allow yourself to have it, you may go way overboard," says registered dietician Chris Rosenbloom.[47]

The medical term for "pigging out" is a binge. Bingers fall into two categories: those who follow the binge by vomiting, called bulimics, and those who leave the food in their bellies. Bulimia can lead to the wearing away of tooth enamel, chronic heartburn, and choking. Being a binger who doesn't purge leads to weight gain. From 20 to 40 percent of obese patients report significant problems with binge eating.[48]

So (with rare exceptions), eat only when hungry and with *no* exceptions *always* eat when you're hungry. To violate either of these rules is to risk obesity. Presently we will look at former fat people to see how they keep their weight *off*. But here's a glance at current extremely fat people to see how they keep their weight *on*.

A 1992 study of severely obese patients to see how they maintained their weights found that they ate vast amounts of food. The women averaged 3,260 calories a day and the men 4,475 calories. More than that, though, it found that "hunger did not appear to be the usual initiator of food consumptions and feelings of fullness and/or discomfort did not usually result in the cessation of eating." It also observed a high amont of bingeing, including fourteen ounces of chocolate chip cookies, an entire cake or Danish ring, six servings of meat loaf with gravy, or a pound of bacon.[49]

It's possible to be fat without bingeing, and it's possible to binge without being fat. But the two are closely related. Avoid bingeing at all costs.

LET ME COUNT THE CALORIES ... OR MAYBE NOT

As I noted, Tribole and Resch advocate chucking calorie counting altogether in favor of what they call "intuitive eating." There are no medical studies on this of which I'm aware, probably because they would be so hard to conduct. But I have sympathy with their position. The only European country in which people routinely attempt to count calories as we do in the United States is the United Kingdom, and even in the UK there is nowhere near the obsession we have here.

"I don't think anybody can accurately count calories," says Marion Nestle. "That's in part because we're so bad at estimating portion sizes, despite the FDA-mandated labels," she says.[50] Most of us ignore the portion size part of the label, anyway. A National Consumers League survey found that while 52 percent of people check the fat content on food labels, only 1 percent make sure the serving size on the label is what they actually eat.[51]

Also, sometimes the labels are wrong. When Nestle and fellow New York University researcher Lisa Young weighed a number of randomly selected single-serving packages of cookies, muffins, and brownies, they found that virtually all weighed more than they said they did, providing as much as 100 to 175 more calories per package more than they claimed.[52] CNN did an analysis of a product sold in the New York area called a "Skinny Roll," which claimed to have one gram of fat but proved to have twenty-one. Rather than the 125 calories claimed, it had 438. When confronted, the manufacturer—a company called Genesis Two—said it was no longer selling the Skinny Roll, then changed its story to say it had a new Skinny Roll with new labels. But a lab analysis found it still had three times the fat and calories claimed.[53]

Even when labels are accurate, "Most people don't have a clue as to what's in the food they're eating," says Nestle. "Even a trained nutritionist can't estimate [very accurately]. What you can do is see that something has a lot of calories, but precise numbers aren't very helpful."[54] The best advice for us as a nation, it seems, is to eat the right foods, eat when hungry, get a decent amount of exercise, and the rest should fall into place. Follow this plan and if you're overweight, the weight should start to come off. Otherwise, you can try to shoot for that 1,200-to-1,300-calorie range I talked about earlier. Still, exact numbers are not only impossible to calculate but fairly unimportant.

While on the subject of calories, many people have asked me about the importance of those from alcoholic drinks. Alcohol plays a major role in the dietary intake of some Americans. One study estimated that among the drinking-age population in the United States it contributes about 160 calories a day. While heavy drinkers may use alcohol in the place of food, for most of us it appears these calories are additional to food.[55] (At least one study, though, has found that alcohol did decrease the consumption of candy and sugar for women.[56]) Since alcohol adds to calories, it would seem to also add to waistlines and this has been borne out.[57] This only applies to moderate drinking, though. It has long been thought that very heavy drinkers are exceptionally thin. There was even a successful book back in the early 1960s called *The Drinking Man's Diet*. Such a diet does appear to work, but only if you drink enough to damage your liver.[58] There are much better ways to lose weight than walking around in a stupor all day long and turning your liver into a pâté.

DO SHEEP HAVE THE RIGHT IDEA?

Another issue worth debate (yet rarely debated) concerns eating the traditional "three squares" versus recent admonitions to "graze," taking in the same amount of food but through more meals. The common wisdom these days clearly favors grazing. But though many of us have been fleeced by diet quacks, we are not sheep.

The apparent advantage of grazing is that you can more closely time your eating with your hunger, although people who stick to regular mealtimes often find their hunger matching the mealtime. The problem with grazing is psychological. For one thing, it can turn into what's called "reverse deprivation mentality." Instead of completely giving up on "bad" foods, you will eat a small amount— a Twinkie here, an Oreo there. But then guilt keeps you from having a decent meal at the appointed time, leaving you truly hungry and ready to go back to nibbling. This sets up a cycle in which you are never really satisfied but always eating.

One drawback is that many Americans are always looking to eat more than they should. The math says that 2,000 calories divided by six is still 2,000 calories. But for too many of us, I think the reality is that 2,000 calories divided by six ends up amounting to more like 2,500 calories. It's a lot easier keeping track of what you're eating and why when you do it less frequently.

Another drawback of grazing is that it tends to favor snack food over food that takes longer to prepare. At a recent Food Marketing Institute meeting in Chicago, a speaker from a consumer survey group predicted that with grazing taking over as a dominant eating style, snack foods would soon become the number one grocery category.[59] If she's right, we're all in a lot of trouble. Clearly snack-food consumption is already on the rise for some reason. It rose steadily from 17.5 pounds per person in 1987 to 21.7 pounds in 1994, before dropping slightly in 1995.[60]

Abandoning fixed mealtimes in favor of letting the whole family just graze from the refrigerator and freezer can have consequences far beyond dietary ones. Indeed, a 1996 survey found that the more often teenagers ate dinner with their parents, the less likely they were to use illicit drugs than those who didn't.[61]

On the other hand, overly large meals are also clearly bad. Why? Because they stretch your stomach and make you more likely to eat a large meal the next time around. (Don't confuse this with the old belief that fat people necessarily have larger stomach capacities as a result of being fat. True, from the outside their stomachs are larger, but that's because of fat layered on top of the abdominal muscles and below them, not necessarily because the stomach itself is larger.) But what recent research from St. Luke's–Roosevelt Hospital in New York has shown is that consistent eating of large meals does actually stretch the stomach. And the larger the stomach, the more food it takes to sate the person possessing that stomach.[62] It becomes a vicious cycle. The more you eat in one sitting, the likelier you are to eat more at the next sitting. This is not a call for skipping meals. "Many overweight people skip breakfast and have a very small lunch," says the chief author of the study, Allan Geliebter. "That's probably not enough time to shrink stomach capacity. And by the time their dinnertime rolls around, they're ravenously hungry and devour huge volumes of food. Night after night following this eating routine might eventually increase stomach capacity."[63]

The good news is that Geliebter says, "If I had to guess, I'd say the process of altering stomach capacity begins in a few days,"[64] meaning that within a few days of not eating stomach-stretching meals, your desire for them should begin to abate.

Meanwhile, another way of keeping your stomach from feeling empty is to make it feel smaller from the outside. Geliebter's research shows that form-fitting clothes or a tight belt might discourage you from overeating.[65] (You've perhaps heard the expression "belt soup.") Thus, the habit so many obese Americans have of wearing shorts or sweatpants with elastic bands (what have been called "eating clothes") might be helping them maintain that obesity. Psychologically, I also think it probably helps to wear tight clothes if you're someone who has to watch your weight. Like a rubber band around the wrist, it serves as a constant reminder.

Where does this leave us in the grazing debate? Again, you have to use your own brain instead of letting a diet guru do your thinking for you. If you think that you will use grazing as an excuse to overeat (and if you don't know for sure, keep a log of your eating), stick to three meals and a snack. If, conversely, you can divide three meals into five or six and be literally dividing and not adding, and if you think this makes you more satisfied, then go for it. But bear in mind that throughout most of American history, back when we were much thinner, we maintained that weight on three squares a day. Not three big, fat meals with bagels the size of Frisbees and steaks that make the dinner table creak and groan under their weight, but three meals comprising moderate portions. It worked for Grandpa and Grandma and it will work for us as well.

VARIETY IS THE SPICE OF OVEREATING

When it comes to the question of why people are fat, you'll see books blaming practically everything under the sun. But there's one culprit you'll never see labeled as such in any diet book. In fact, the recipes in most diet books (and most diet books fill their pages with recipes) actually contribute to this problem. It's called variety.

Yes, a certain amount of variety is both good and necessary to get all the vitamins and minerals you need. But variety has also clearly contributed to the American obesity problem.

I first realized the importance of variety in obesity from observing my rabbits. Rabbits eat an enormous amount of food by human standards—yes, even Americans—and compared to cats and dogs, as well. In essence, they're furry little poop machines, so efficient at consuming massive quantities that they sometimes eat and defecate at the same time. Yet if I fill the food tray high enough with their pellets, even they will be sated. That is, until I give them a treat—a piece of lettuce, an apple core, and, yes, carrots. (They are wholly insensitive to the fact they're perpetuating a stereotype.) Suddenly these previously sated creatures are ravenous.

Variety sparks appetite, and not just for rabbits. Rats increase their eating when offered tasty high-fat[66] or high-carbohydrate foods.[67] University of Pennsylvania researcher Barbara Rolls has demonstrated that variety caused rats offered chow plus three different cafeteria foods to gain more weight than those offered only one cafeteria food plus chow.[68]

Rabbits and rats, but humans? You bet. "During the course of a meal the pleasantness of those foods not eaten remains relatively unchanged," observes Rolls. "We have called this form of satiety 'sensory specific satiety.' " The result is that "more is eaten of a varied meal than a monotonous one."[69]

Americans today are bombarded with a vast number of different food choices. Rockefeller University obesity researcher Jules Hirsch, M.D., estimates that there are about 50,000 foodstuffs available to Americans today, compared with perhaps just 500 a century ago.[70] Supermarkets now carry twelve times as many different products as they did in 1961, an average of 30,000 items in a single store.[71] But even that doesn't tell the whole story. As a middle-class American I can afford virtually every one of those 50,000 foodstuffs, even if I couldn't afford much of some of them. Yet a century ago a family might actually eat fewer than a dozen foods on a regular basis. Until the great famine beginning in 1846, many Irish subsisted almost entirely on just potatoes and buttermilk with an occasional turnip. And surely you haven't forgotten that rhyme you learned as a child: "Pease porridge hot, pease porridge cold,/Pease porridge in the pot, nine days old."

Try eating pease (peas) porridge, hot or cold, for nine straight days and see how much weight you'll lose. In fact, this is the key to those bizarre diets that emphasized just jelly beans or grapefruit or popcorn.

If you're watching your weight, try to watch your variety. Discard the diet books that offer you a different menu for every day of the month. Pick a small number of foods with low calorie density (that give you the full spectrum of vitamins and minerals you need) and primarily stick with them. Save extraordinary items for extraordinary occasions, such as eating out. And console yourself that if nothing else, at least you aren't eating pease porridge for the ninth day in a row.

How Do the Winners Keep It Off?

At one time the science of weight loss was devoted almost entirely to inducing the loss itself. Researchers generally didn't even conduct follow-ups to see if the weight remained off. Only in more recent years, as scientists and the public began to realize that most people don't keep the weight off for very long, has preventing relapses even begun to be studied, much less treated. But scientists are now conducting experiments and engaging in observation to see what truly works to keep the pounds off once they've been lost.

The largest ongoing observation program is the National Weight Control Registry, maintained by the University of Pittsburgh School of Medicine and the University of Colorado School of Health Sciences at Denver. The program tracks persons who have lost thirty pounds or more and have kept the weight off at least a year. As of the end of 1995 it had 831 people, ages nineteen to eighty-one. "There are two beliefs out there," says Pittsburgh's Rena Wing, M.D., who along with Denver's James Hill, M.D., administers the registry. "One is that almost nobody succeeds at weight loss. The other is that for the few people who do, success requires such an extreme sacrifice that they basically do nothing but count calories and exercise all day. We see no reason to believe either is true."[72]

Among the preliminary findings of the registry:

- 94 percent of successful losers increased their physical activity level, with walking the most common activity
- 98 percent decreased their food intake
- 57 percent got professional help, including doctors, registered dietitians, Weight Watchers, and others
- 92 percent are continuing to exercise to maintain weight loss
- 98 percent are still watching their diets

"We have to debunk the myth that there are no successful losers," says Wing. "There's no magic to why people lose and keep it off. They just keep exercising and watching what they eat."[73] Says Hill, "It's not that, gee, these people have figured out what to do. Nearly everyone knows what's required: take in fewer calories than you burn. It's that they've figured out *how* to do it."[74]

One "trick," if you will, for maintaining weight loss seems to be weighing yourself regularly or wearing tight clothes and getting right back "on the wagon" if your weight or girth starts to go up. "Reversing small weight gains immediately, as they occur, is the single most important skill that patients fail to learn in conventional weight-loss programs," says Thomas Wadden, M.D., director of Syracuse University's Center for Health and Behavior.[75] Anne Fletcher, for her insightful book *Thin for Life*, rounded up 160 "masters at weight control, all of whom have managed to keep off at least twenty pounds for a minimum of three years."[76] She says the vast majority of these people stopped gaining before they put on more than five pounds, while most others allow themselves no more than ten pounds.

One 1990 study of women who were able to keep lost weight off and women who weren't drew a contrast so important and fascinating that I reprint much of the study conclusion verbatim, along with the chart that accompanied it.

> Maintainers made decisions to lose weight and then devised personal weight-loss plans to fit their lives. These plans usually included regular exercise or activity and a new eating style of reduced fat, reduced sugar, more fruits and vegetables, and much less food than previously eaten. Maintainers reported being patient, setting small goals that they could meet, and sticking to their personally devised weight-loss plans. Some used ideas from earlier weight-loss experiences, some used diets from books, but all persisted until new eating patterns were established.... However, they did not completely restrict favorite foods and made efforts to avoid feelings of deprivation while changing food patterns.
>
> In contrast, few relapsers (36 percent) had exercised to help lose weight. They had lost weight by taking appetite suppressants, fasting, or going on restrictive diets that they could not sustain. They took diet formulas and went to weight-control groups and programs many times. While dieting they did not permit themselves any of the special foods they enjoyed....[77]

Most maintainers (90 percent) reported exercising at least three times a week for thirty minutes or more while relapsers who exercised at all did so less often than maintainers and less vigorously, according to the study, which appeared in the *American Journal of Clinical Nutrition.* And while women in both groups reported snacking almost every day, relapsers ate considerably more snacks a day. Relapsers were also more likely to skip breakfast.[78] This is bad news for the country as a whole, since the percentage of Americans eating breakfast has dropped from 86 percent in 1965 to 75 percent in recent years.[79]

COMPARISON OF WEIGHT-LOSS METHODS USED BY RELAPSERS AND MAINTAINERS OF REDUCED WEIGHT

Weight-Loss Method	Relapsers (percent)	Maintainers (percent)
Devised personal eating plan	39	73
Exercised	36	76
Attended Weight Watchers	43	10
Attended other programs or groups	29	10
Followed doctor's orders	34	20
Took pills, shots	47	3
Fasted	11	3
Underwent hypnosis	9	—
Followed book, magazine diet	25	10
Total methods used	121	28

Source: *American Journal of Clinical Nutrition.*[80]

These are your blueprints. If you want to succeed, try to imitate the maintainers' lifestyles as closely as possible. If you wish to fail and refatten, just follow the pattern of the relapsers—which is to say the pattern of the great majority of people who lose weight.

If you do change your lifestyle, you may well find that the rewards are a lot greater than simply losing weight and regaining your health. As one of Fletcher's "masters," who kept off sixty-two pounds, put it: "The how-to's of maintaining my weight spilled over into other aspects of my life. I've become a more assertive person and am willing to take risks now—be it speaking up for myself or trying things I would never try before. Losing weight has not only rid me of my fat shell, but it also stripped me of some of my inhibitions and fears. I can handle almost anything now because of all the things I've learned."[81]

Carol A. Johnson has written a fat acceptance book called *Self-Esteem Comes in All Sizes.*[82] As you would guess, her size is XX-Large. But no, real self-esteem doesn't come from acceptance but from accomplishment. For my part, I won't say that I don't sometimes envy people who have always been thin even though they've always eaten all they want of whatever they want. But the way I see it, my achievement in losing my extra pounds and keeping them off gives me a sense of accomplishment and pride that I treasure.

Don't think that losing weight is the impossible dream that some would have you think it is. Like anything worthwhile, it takes effort. But for some of us, the successful effort is one of the most important things we will ever accomplish in our lives.

8

The Fiber Factor

It has been called the "Cinderella of nutrients,"[1] though in a sense it's not a nutrient at all. Until fairly recently it was practically ignored by the medical community. Serious proponents of its benefits were often dismissed as cranks, though one author made a best-seller out of it, giving it a mysterious-sounding name: the "F-Factor."[2] But there's nothing dirty about this F-word at all, and it may be a key in preventing a tremendous range of diseases, including obesity.

Only in the late 1960s did fiber begin to gain respectability, though by 1987 the healthful effects were obvious enough that the American Dietetic Association declared "that the public be encouraged to increase consumption of dietary fiber from a variety of foods."[3] The catalyst was the work of three scientists who noted that while Africans as a whole tended to be (and alas continue to tend to be) a highly diseased lot in terms of infections, when it came to degenerative diseases, they were in many respects far healthier than Europeans and Americans.[4] On the other hand, in urban centers of Africa where lifestyle and diets were more Westernized, the incidence of these diseases was much higher. Evidence increasingly pointed to their high-fiber diets.[5]

Fiber is only found in food from plants. It's the portion of plant cells not digested by humans. Fiber is classified broadly on the basis of its solubility in water. If it forms a gel-like substance it's called soluble; if not it's called nonsoluble. Most fruits, vegetables, and grains have a combination of these two types, though some plant products contain a greater amount of one or the other. Wheat bran is the foodstuff with the highest percentage of fiber, about 40 to 50 percent.

Related to fiber, at least for our purposes, is something called "resistant starch." Not the stuff that builds up on your clothes iron and is hell to remove; rather, it's created when grains, such as rice, and legumes, such as peas and beans, are cooked. It's called this because it resists enzymes that normally digest starches in the gastrointestinal tract and is excreted intact. Some scientists regard it as a form of dietary fiber and perhaps even superior in the benefits it confers.[6] Old nutrition tables ignored resistant starch but newer ones, such as appear in this chapter, include it.

What helped bring fiber out of the medical world closet was the broadening realization that it makes an excellent laxative in high amounts, albeit generally not the kind that makes you knock over your loved ones en route to the bathroom. To this day, no doubt the vast majority of fiber supplements are sold for this very reason. The way fiber eases constipation is by bulking up the stool and speeding it through the colon.[7]

But constipation prevention aside, fiber in recent decades has proved to be one of the greatest unsung heroes in health maintenance. Little wonder that whoever came up with the expression "an apple a day keeps the doctor away" seized on a fruit with a high level of fiber. Fiber won't watch the kids while you're at the theater and it won't shovel the snow from your driveway. But practically nothing you put down your throat—or don't put down there—will have more impact on your health. Among the diseases now widely associated with a lack of dietary fiber are diverticulosis, colon cancer, diabetes, heart disease caused by high cholesterol, and finally obesity.

The following chart looks at disease levels among South African blacks who continue to live in rural areas and have an extremely high-fiber diet; blacks who have moved to the cities and eat considerably less fiber; and whites in South Africa who eat the least fiber. The disease differences are stark. Below is a chart rating them in terms of level of seriousness.

DISEASE COMPARISON BETWEEN
SOUTH AFRICAN BLACKS AND WHITES

SERIOUSNESS RATED ON A LEVEL OF ONE TO FIVE

	Rural Blacks	Urban Blacks	Whites
Obesity	1	3	5
Hemorrhoids	—	2	3
Appendicitis	1	2	5
Ulcerative Colitis	—	1	5
Irritable Bowel Syndrome	—	2	4
Diverticular Disease	—	2	5
Colon Cancer	—	1	5
Diabetes	1	3	3
Hypertension	1	4	3
Stroke	1	2	2
Coronary Heart Disease	—	2	5

Note: A (—) indicates that occurrence is rare.

Source: *CRC Handbook of Dietary Fiber in Human Nutrition.*[8]

Fiber is by no means the only difference between the diets of rural South African blacks, their urban cousins, and white South Africans. Rural South Africans also have more carbohydrates and less fat in their diet, and presumably fewer calories overall.[9] In any event, a salesman would starve to death trying to sell Ex-Lax or Preparation H to rural South African blacks. Once these same blacks start adopting urban eating patterns, though, they start to become susceptible to the same diseases that plague white South Africans who are on a full Western diet.

Let's take various diseases one at a time and see how fiber helps.

Most Americans by the time they reach sixty have developed diverticular disease, although most don't have symptoms.[10] The illness occurs when feces push against the wall of the large intestine, causing the formation of pockets or pouches. Once formed they apparently never go away. That's unfortunate, because these are pockets you don't want to carry anything in. Once you have this condition, you have diverticulosis. When the colon becomes infected, it's called diverticulitis. This happens when the stool or something in it pushes through the weakened little pockets. Now you have all that bacteria from your feces pouring into your own body, poisoning you just as if you had eaten contaminated food. The result is a flu-like illness that, unless treated with antibiotics, can lead to death.

It appears that a high-fiber diet can prevent these pouches from forming in the first place because it prevents the formation of small, hard stools that push out the pouches. But even if it's too late and you already have the pouches, a high-fiber diet can keep them intact. This is again because fiber keeps the stool big and soft. It just keeps working its way down the intestine rather than sitting there and then deciding to force its way out the side.[11]

Numerous other illnesses are more common in persons with diverticular disease including hiatal (esophageal) hernias, abdominal hernias, hemorrhoids, and varicose veins in the legs.[12] The link is probably fiber. Lack of fiber often allows the stool to pass only with great straining, popping veins and creating hernias.

Colon cancer is the second-leading cause of cancer death in the United States. While it is by no means entirely diet-related, diet is clearly an important factor. Numerous studies have found an association between high fiber intake and a lower level of colon cancer. While the reason for this involves some speculation, one suggestion is that by speeding the feces through the intestines, carcinogens in the stool have less time in which to do their dirty work against the colon wall. A low-roughage carcinogen-producing American diet allows the fecal mass and its chemical contents to wash over the colon for three days or even longer. In one British study, stool was found to stay in patients for as long as two weeks.[13]

Another possibility is that simply by adding benign bulk, fiber reduces the level of carcinogens in the stool. A third theory suggests that the fiber is fermented by intestinal microbes and that fermentation products influence epithelial cells in the colon to reduce tumor development.[14]

While some of the research surrounding the benefits of fiber is still speculative, its ability to help sufferers of Type II diabetes has been thoroughly documented. One way fiber benefits these persons is through its ability to aid in weight loss. But it also acts directly to slow the release of sugar into the bloodstream. The best fiber for this is water soluble.[15] Since complex carbohydrates also regulate insulin flow, and fiber usually accompanies such carbohydrates, together they can have a strong impact in the regulation of insulin and in improving the health of Type II diabetics while reducing their need for medication.[16]

Heart disease is the number one killer of Americans. A recent study showed that among middle-aged to elderly men, adding ten grams of fiber to the diet resulted in a 20 percent decrease in heart attacks.[17] High cholesterol levels are often implicated as a strong factor in causing heart disease. Studies have repeatedly shown that soluble fiber can significantly lower cholesterol amounts, at least when consumed in large quantities. As Judith Marlett, a University of Wisconsin researcher, puts it: "soluble fiber . . . drains cholesterol out of the blood."[18] The fibers from fresh fruits, vegetables, legumes, oat bran, and barley appear to have the most potential. Insoluble fibers such as wheat bran appear to have no effect at lowering cholesterol levels.[19]

One medical journal review compared the American Heart Association's recommended low-fat, low-cholesterol diet with various other diets high in fiber. While the Heart Association's diet lowered blood cholesterol levels only 3 percent, guar fiber supplements lowered cholesterol about 8 percent, pectin fiber supplements lowered it 15 percent, and psyllium (pronounced "silly-um") fiber supplements decreased it 16 percent over a short-term period. Incorporating oat bran or beans into the diet lowered cholesterol 19 percent over the short term. Over the long term the results look even better, with studies showing a 25 percent reduction in the bad kind of cholesterol—low-density lipoprotein—among men who previously had high levels. At the same time, fiber increases the good kind of cholesterol—called high-density lipoprotein—by 10 percent.[20]

Unfortunately, the current obsession with removing fat has greatly obscured the benefits of adding fiber. A 1995 study by the Center for Media and Public Affairs in Washington, D.C., found that while the media cited dietary fat as a cancer risk factor forty-seven times in a three-month period, it mentioned the cancer risk associated with a low-fiber diet not once.[21]

SURE, BUT CAN IT HELP CONTROL MY WEIGHT?

As long as a millennium ago, Arab physicians—then the world's leaders in medicine—saw the value of fiber in weight control. One of the leading Arab physicians and authors was Avicenna, who wrote in his *Canon of Medicine* that to reduce obesity one should "procure a rapid descent of the food from the stomach and intestines, in order to prevent absorption," and take food "which is bulky but feebly nutritious."[22]

Remember that soluble fiber is the type that forms a gel in liquid. This makes it expand greatly in the stomach, helping to give you a feeling of fullness. Numerous studies have shown that supplementing a diet with fiber reduces feelings of hunger.[23] Hunger is an extremely complicated thing, and involves a lot more than whether or not there's something in your stomach. But it certainly appears that having something in there can reduce hunger pangs. Further, this gooey mass slows down the emptying of food from the stomach, adding to the feeling of fullness. Oat products and oat bran, dry beans, peas, lentils, and barley are rich sources of soluble fiber. Fruits usually contain similar amounts of both soluble and insoluble fiber. Psyllium, the primary ingredient in Metamucil, Perdiem, and other popular fiber supplements, is a soluble fiber.[24] Try putting just a teaspoon of Metamucil in half a glass of water and soon you'll have a glass of gel. You can see how this would help fill your belly.

Insoluble fiber, that which doesn't dissolve in water, is also often referred to as "roughage." Such fiber comes from the outer hard shell of grains, and some is also found in most fruits and vegetables. Foods such as bran muffins and raisin bran cereal are excellent sources, as are celery, corn bran, green beans, green leafy vegetables, potato skins, and whole grains.[25]

Together, soluble and insoluble fiber are a great team, slowing the exit of food from the stomach when you want it slow, and speeding it up in the intestines and bowels when you want it to go fast.

But fiber is effective in weight control for other reasons, as well. Fiber slows down eating and adds to satisfaction. Food cannot be swallowed comfortably unless it is soft and moist. Until it is so, we usually chew it. Chewing slows down intake because it adds effort to eating. It also stimulates the secretion of saliva and prolongs secretion in the stomach. These secretions temporarily expand the stomach, and distension of the belly induces satiety.[26]

That fiber slows down the intake of starch has been established experimentally. Six people were asked to eat a 300-gram meal of whole wheat bread and on a separate occasion an equivalent meal of white bread. All subjects took far longer to eat the whole wheat bread.[27]

Also, by its very presence, fiber reduces the caloric value of food. If you eat five ounces of food and an ounce of that is fiber, then you've only eaten four ounces of calories.

Yet another way that fiber apparently aids weight loss or prevents weight gain is on the other end of the consumption process. Fiber wraps up food and prevents its contact with the calorie-absorbing mechanisms. It also speeds the nutrients through the body. Through both effects, food consumed with fiber is less likely to provide energy than food without. One study of ten young women gave them first a high-fiber diet, then a lower-fiber one, then one that was lower still in fiber. With the lowest amount of fiber, 97 percent of their food was absorbed. With the highest amount, it was only 92.5 percent.[28] Earlier studies with men as subjects[29] and with rats[30] showed similar results.

You've probably heard about the report showing that adding bread to a diet led to significant weight loss and may have wondered if it weren't a rumor started by the Wonder Bread company. In fact, there was such a study published back in 1979. It comprised sixteen overweight college-age men, each of whom had to eat twelve slices of bread a day. Half the men ate standard enriched white bread while the other half ate whole wheat bread with twenty times the fiber content. That's a lot of bread but in the name of science they ate away and all found they could no longer eat nearly as many calories as they were accustomed to consuming. On average, the men eating the high-fiber bread ate 159 fewer calories *aside from* the fewer calories in their bread. At the end of the two-month experiment period, all the men had lost substantial weight. But the men eating the high-fiber bread lost the most. While the white bread men dropped on average fourteen pounds, the other men lost on average over nineteen pounds. The men eating the whole wheat bread who had high cholesterol levels also experienced a major drop in those levels.[31]

In a separate study, twelve men were asked to eat either whole wheat or white bread to a point of comfortable fullness. Ten of the twelve ended up eating less whole wheat than white bread. And again, since the whole wheat bread contained fewer calories they got a double benefit.[32]

Beyond simply what we know about the effects of fiber there is direct evidence linking obesity and lack of fiber. For example, a 1994 study comparing the self-reported diets of lean and obese men and women found that the lean men's reported diet contained 29 percent more fiber than their obese counterparts', while the lean women's diet contained 45 percent more fiber than the obese women's diets.[33]

So if a lack of fiber is linked to obesity, can adding fiber help prevent it? That very much appears to be the case. A typical study of the effect of fiber showed Swedish and Danish women on a low-calorie diet for three months given a small citrus and grain fiber supplement losing about four and a half pounds more weight than the control group of women. Additionally, the women with the fiber supplement reported fewer problems with bowel movements and claimed to be less hungry on their diets. They also saw a significant reduction in blood pressure.[34]

Another study looked at the effect of cereals with different fiber contents to see if they would influence how much the subjects ate later at lunch. Subjects were given five different cereals, each with different fiber contents. Three and a half hours later they were given lunch with a broad variety of food and told to eat as much as they desired. The researchers found a direct correlation between how much fiber the subjects consumed at breakfast and how much they ate at lunch: the more fiber for breakfast, the less food for lunch. What made this all the more remarkable was that the higher fiber cereals also contained fewer calories. So eating the lower calorie cereal at breakfast resulted in fewer calories at lunch, as well.[35]

In case you're wondering if fiber supplements containing psyllium such as Metamucil can reduce appetite and lead to weight loss, the answer appears to be yes. For example, one study found that subjects ingesting the psyllium from crackers ate on average about 150 calories fewer a day than the control subjects who ate crackers without fiber. This translated into about a pound of weight lost after two weeks.[36] Psyllium is also an oddity, the University of Toronto's David Jenkins points out, in that "It's all soluble fiber, but bacteria in the gut don't break it down as rapidly as they do other soluble fibers." The result is that it lowers cholesterol like a soluble fiber and increases stool bulk like an insoluble one.[37] This study and others convinced me to start using a fiber supplement even though I was already loading my diet with high-fiber foods.

There's little in the way of studies on childhood obesity and fiber but there's no reason to think that children will be different from adults. One study did find that children who skipped breakfast or ate noncereal breakfast foods had significantly higher cholesterol levels than children who ate breakfast, especially ready-to-eat cereals.[38]

FIBER CONTENTS OF VARIOUS FOODS
(EXPRESSED PER HUNDRED GRAMS OF DRY WEIGHT)

CEREALS

Kellogg's All-Bran	31.6
Corn bran	85.19
Oat bran	15.72
White bread	3.22
Whole wheat bread	9.26
Kellogg's Corn Flakes	1.65
Graham crackers	2.47
Saltine crackers	3.08
General Mills' Fiber 1	44.02
White flour	3.96
Whole wheat flour	12.39
General Foods' 40% Bran Flakes	15.88
Rolled oats	10.51
Kellogg's Product 19	4.47
Puffed rice	1.4
Puffed wheat	7.2
Kellogg's Rice Krispies	1.21
Kellogg's Special K	3.24
General Mills' Wheaties	8.29

VEGETABLES

Asparagus, canned	32.23
Beets, canned	24.27
Broccoli, frozen	30.4

Brussels sprouts, frozen	26.94
Cabbage, raw	23.24
Carrots, raw	23.76
Cauliflower, frozen	26.7
Corn, canned, whole kernel	9.43
Kale, frozen	33.48
Lettuce, raw	21.02
Potato, white, raw	9.48
Spinach, frozen	19.79
Sweet potato, canned	7.08
Tomato, raw	13.3

LEGUMES

Garbanzo beans, canned	10.21
Green beans, canned	33.97
Kidney beans, canned	20.9
Lima beans, canned	14.4
Navy beans, dried, cooked	23.02
Pinto beans, canned	19.11
Pinto beans, dried, cooked	24.1
Pork and beans, canned	15.67
White beans, canned	20.97
White beans, dried, cooked	18.16
Lentils, dried, cooked	15.73
Black-eyed peas, canned	11.06
Green peas, canned	21.3

FRUITS

Apple, raw	12.73
Applesauce, canned	13.29
Banana, raw	7.35
Grapefruit, raw, Florida yellow	11.9
Orange, raw, seedless, Calif. navel	11.45
Peach, canned	18.8
Pear, canned	32.18
Pineapple, canned	9.54
Purple plum, canned	22.81

Source: *American Journal of Clinical Nutrition.*[39]

Sadly, fiber has steadily been squeezed out of our diets. A national survey in the early 1990s found that most people who ate any whole-grain food at all ate it less than once a day. A fifth of the persons surveyed consumed absolutely no whole-grain products in an entire two-week period, while more than half the persons consumed no whole-grain cereals during that period.[40] A 1996 survey of shoppers found that for 80 percent, the first item they looked for on a label was fat content; only 3 percent said fiber.[41]

WHERE HAS ALL THE FIBER GONE?

Ironically, there is a parallel between the history of fiberless bread and the history of obesity in that at one time both were status symbols. Most bread at one time by necessity contained coarsely milled flour. This is because mills used stone grinding wheels with rough surfaces that couldn't completely smash the wheat berries. The rich, on the other hand, could pay to have their flour whitened by sifting it through cloth. Buying white bread then was like buying a $5,000 Rolex watch is now. Rolex watches aren't necessarily more efficient at telling time than a $40 watch; you're mostly paying for the status. But in the 1880s the steel rolling mill was introduced.

Now the grains of wheat could be smashed finely and millers could easily extract most of the fiber, producing the prestigious "pure" flour at prices anyone could pay.[42] It was as if everybody could suddenly afford a Rolex and, of course, that's just what people wanted.

The white flour had an additional advantage, however. One big problem in the flour trade was the large losses of stored flour to insects. The highly refined flour had so many of the nutrients removed that it was barely able to keep bugs alive, thereby greatly reducing insect infestation.[43] Of course, those nutrients were no longer there for humans, either. So eventually bakeries began introducing vitamins into bread to replace those milled out. This is why white bread is usually referred to as "enriched." But while the vitamins are put back, the fiber continues to be left out.

The ultimate irony of all this, of course, is that bread made from high-fiber grains is today more associated with wealth. This is because such bread is made in smaller batches, hence pushing up the price and reducing its availability. Whole wheat bread has enjoyed a resurgence in grocery stores in recent years, but bread made of other whole grains continues to be a specialty item available in most cities only in health food stores and specialty bakeries, places where costs are higher and wealthier people tend to shop.

It isn't just bread that has gone this route. Numerous other foods such as potatoes have also had the white insides associated with wealth and exclusivity, even though most of the fiber, nutrients, and indeed taste is in the skin. But something had to differentiate the potatoes consumed by the Irish landlord and those eaten by his tenants. That something was the skin. The landlord could feel superior because he could afford to throw away the skins. Then even poor people could afford to toss the skins, so they did so in imitation of the rich. And yet again, we continue to toss the skins just because that's the way it's been done for so long. The rich, of course, are now no longer able to differentiate themselves by virtue of their ability to toss away the skins. So what do they do? Yes, that's right—they buy Rolexes.

Although the process of removing the fiber from our foods began over a century ago, we keep finding new ways to reduce the little bit left. A study comparing children's fiber intake from 1977–78 to 1987–88 found a significant decrease. Fiber intake of preschool children dropped from 8.9 to 8.2 grams a day, that of six-to-eleven-year-olds declined from 12.1 to 11.5 grams a day, while that of adolescent boys fell from 15 to 14 grams a day. Only that of adolescent girls remained the same, at about 11 grams daily. The primary sources of fiber shifted away from fruits and vegetables to bread, cereal, and combination foods.[44]

Part of the problem is that manufacturers fool people into believing they're getting fiber when they're not. There has been a trend in recent years, for example, to label plain old white bread as "wheat bread," add a little caramel coloring to make it brown, and let consumers think they're buying *whole* wheat bread. Similarly, other types of breads labeled with the names of coarser grains also turn out to have nothing other than defibered wheat flour as their main ingredient. Of three muffins that I recently picked off a grocery store shelf, one labeled "corn," one "bran," and one "oat," all three actually had as their prime ingredient plain old white flour. The second ingredient was sugar and the grain that provided the muffin's name—the corn, bran, or oats—were somewhere way down the list. They could more accurately have been labeled "baking soda" or "sugar" muffins. Likewise, the pumpernickel, rye, and all other types of bread I looked at had as their first ingredient not pumpernickel or rye but, again, plain old white flour. It reminds me of how Dr. Seuss's mean old Grinch "created" a reindeer: He tied a horn that looked like antlers to the head of his poor little dog, Max.[45] Likewise, add a dash of rye to a loaf of wheat bread and now you have a loaf of rye bread. Right? No, no more than a dog with a horn tied to his head is a reindeer.

But why do manufacturers engage in such deceptions? To a great extent, it's just giving people what they want. Americans feel virtuous about buying whole-grain products but are accustomed to the taste of white flour. So the baking companies deliver up to them white flour products with whole-grain names. It's up to you to look carefully at the labels and find the baked goods that truly are whole grain. My guess is that when you locate and start eating them, you will soon learn to prefer the whole-grain product.

No Such Thing as Too Much

The National Cancer Institute recommends that Americans eat twenty to thirty-five grams per day of fiber, which is approximately twice what Americans eat per day. The American Academy of Pediatrics Committee on Nutrition has recommended a dietary fiber intake of half a gram per kilogram (2.2 pounds) of body weight.[46] That translates into a range of 6.8 to 34.5 grams a day for three-to-nineteen-year-old boys of average weight and 6 to 28.5 grams a day for three-to-nineteen-year-old girls of average weight.[47] A newer recommendation from the American Health Foundation proposed that a reasonable goal for fiber intake during childhood and adolescence may be approximately equivalent to the child's age plus 5 grams a day. This would mean a range from 8 grams a day at age three to 25 grams a day by age twenty. Based on current levels of fiber intake, 55 percent to 89 percent of two-to-eighteen-year-old American children consume less than this goal.[48]

For most children, fiber goals will be met if the daily diet contains two vegetables and three fruits, a sandwich made with two slices of whole wheat bread, a serving of breakfast cereal containing at least three grams of fiber, and one or two other foods containing fiber such as a baked potato, popcorn, beans, peanuts, or whole wheat crackers.[49]

In general, converting the average American diet to a high-fiber one would mean:

1. switching to whole-grain products such as whole wheat, rolled oats, and brown rice;
2. consuming fresh or barely cooked fruits and vegetables with as much of the skins and strings attached as possible;
3. reducing the consumption of meat and refined sugar.

By switching from the cereal I had been eating to a high-fiber one (Shredded Wheat'N Bran), I started getting eight grams of fiber where before I was getting practically none. Thus, before I even begin my workday I've eaten considerably more fiber than the average American does all day long. A mere third of a cup of cooked beans can provide half of the government's daily twenty-five-gram recommendation and three times the fiber of the average American's diet. Pay attention to food labels and you should find you can get fifty grams or more of fiber into your daily diet without any difficulty.

In addition to the kind of supplements you take directly, you can add fiber to your diet by adding oat bran. Since it has little flavor of its own and dissolves in liquids, it can be readily added to a variety of foods such as spaghetti sauce and stews as a thickener, in hamburger as a binder, in chili and sloppy joes, and in meat loaf instead of bread crumbs. Another fiber, pectin, can be purchased in powdered or liquid form at the grocery store. It is used in the making of jams and jellies, being the stuff that makes the fruit mixture thick and spreadable. It's a soluble fiber that's naturally found in some vegetables such as sweet potatoes, beans, raw carrots, and raw onions, as well as fruits such as apples, apricots, peaches, pears, plums, grapes, raisins, and the peels of oranges, lemons, and grapefruit.

You needn't have seen the hilarious bean-eating scene in the Mel Brooks movie *Blazing Saddles*[50] to know that if you switch quickly to a high-fiber diet you may have—*ahem!*—problems. That's because the bacteria in your gut haven't had a chance to adjust to breaking down that type of food. One way to avoid much of this is to switch slowly, adding a little more fiber each day. There are also products at the drugstore that can help, such as Beano. That aside, if you do insist on switching quickly, try to stay out of crowded elevators for a while. Also, if you're really pumping up on fiber it's wise to start drinking a lot more liquids, or all that bulk may cause constipation. So long as you have enough liquids, it's practically impossible to eat too much fiber.

There's no reason anybody shouldn't be able to get enough fiber in his or her diet for most purposes without using supplements such as Metamucil and Perdiem. The American Medical Association Council on Scientific Affairs says such supplements "are not generally recommended."[51] Nonetheless, it says for those who won't increase their fiber content through their foods, there's nothing wrong with supplements. I would further encourage such supplements for persons who need to lose weight. Based not only on the aforementioned studies but on my own personal experience, I think they can be a real help.

The American experience with fiber is to some extent a microcosm of all that's wrong with our feeble efforts to combat obesity. Steps that would be so easy to take are simply ignored. Habits so deadly yet so readily broken remain intact. Two of the easiest things people can do to lose weight are to eat more fiber and to consume less sugar, yet fiber is systematically stripped from our food and sugar is systematically added. In bread, the food that is called "the staff of life," both are done.

YOUR MOTHER WAS RIGHT, EAT YOUR VEGGIES (AND FRUITS)

This is as good a time as any to emphasize a point that, at some level, you must already know: fruits and vegetables are a terribly important part of the diet, even aside from the benefits of the fiber they contain. Most of the vitamins and many of the minerals we need are found in these plants. Further, in recent years an impressive body of evidence has been amassed indicating that large amounts of some of these vitamins and minerals, called antioxidants, appear to have powerful anticancer properties.[52] Unfortunately, some people think they can get everything that fruits and vegetables provide by taking vitamin pills. Wrong. I take some antioxidant supplements myself, because there's some evidence that amounts of these antioxidants much greater than you can get from eating may be helpful. But not only do pills provide no fiber, they also don't provide myriad other chemicals (called phytochemicals) in foods that may also have benefits in protecting against cancer and other disease.

"That's why you need the food itself," says American Council on Science and Health Director of Nutrition Ruth Kava. "Trying to pack the benefits into a pill just isn't enough."[53] New York nutritionist Josephine Connolly-Schoonen agrees: "We're just starting to understand the nutrients in food—how much we need and how they interact. The research isn't anywhere near the point where we can safely rely on [vitamin and mineral] pills."[54]

It is a sad sign of the times that when medical researchers started to get through to the public that vitamin supplements weren't enough, pill companies started to actually grind up vegetables and pack them into capsules. So now, if you want the benefits of broccoli but feel toward it as former President George Bush does, you can just pop capsules. Lots of capsules and at a wicked cost. According to Kava, to get the equivalent amount of a half cup of chopped frozen broccoli, you'd have to take seventeen pills.

That would be $2.04 in pills, while for the frozen vegetable it would be 32 cents. For spinach, it will cost you $2.28 to get a half cup's worth from nineteen pills.[55] I'm sure even President Bush would agree these capsules are silly. In any case, if you want the benefits of vegetables and fruits, you have to eat vegetables and fruits.

Sadly, this prescription is not being followed, especially among children. A 1996 National Cancer Institute survey of food records from children between the ages of two and eighteen found:

- Only one in five children eats five or more servings of fruits and vegetables a day, the dietary recommendation;
- One of the most common ways of getting a "serving" of fruit is actually drinking a glass of high-sugar, low-fiber fruit juice;
- Of the few vegetables children do eat, a fourth of these are French fries.[56] Let's hope another fourth of the "vegetables" wasn't ketchup.

The Department of Agriculture's Food Guide Pyramid (located a few miles down the road from its Food Guide Sphinx) recommends three to five servings of vegetables and two to four servings of fruit a day. For vegetables, a serving size is one-half cup cooked or raw vegetables, one cup leafy vegetables, or three-fourths cup vegetable juice. In other words, yes, you could have had a V-8, but remember that while vegetable juices will give you vitamins and phytochemicals, they will have little fiber in them. For fruits, a serving size is one banana or orange or apple or other thing of that size, half a grapefruit, half a cup of melon, half a cup of strawberries, and so on. (Having half a grapefruit smashed into your face like James Cagney did to Mae Clarke in *Public Enemy* counts as a half a serving, but only if you swallow.[57])

Oh, I know that vegetables have gotten a bad rap in this country. Part of that is because we have this strange aspect of our culture that says we have to make fun of things we know are good for us. Part of it is because so many of us can't remember the last time we got within spitting distance of a cabbage or a celery stalk. Part of it is because television and billboard advertising is awash with commercials designed by people on Madison Avenue paid gazillions of bucks to make you crave burgers and chicken nuggets, not peas and carrots. But trust me on this, when you start giving your body good food and exercising it, your body will start dictating to you that it wants stuff that's good for it. And nothing's better for it than fruits and vegetables.

9

Exercise: Move It and Lose It

> Better to hunt in fields, for health unbought,
> Than fee the doctor for a nauseous draught.
> The wise, for cure, on exercise depend;
> God never made his work for man to mend.[1]

No, that's not a quote from Richard Simmons. Rather, it's from author-poet John Dryden, born 300 years before the first *Sweating to the Oldies* videocassette was taped or the first NordicTrack machine sold.

Nobody bad-mouths exercise in print, though it is something in which most of us rarely engage. Even the fat acceptance people say exercise is good, though they insist it won't help you lose weight because, after all, nothing can. But in any case, the more research done on exercise, the more good stuff we learn it can do. A 1992 national fitness survey for England concluded, "The high prevalence of physical inactivity suggests that it may be even more important for public health than attention to cholesterol, arterial blood pressure, or smoking."[2]

Exercise, especially that which gets the heart really going, has been directly related to improving your chance of living long enough to play with your grandkids,[3] not to mention having the strength and energy to do so. Recent research also indicates that aerobic exercise can shape up the brain, raising IQ levels in younger people and slowing the aging of the brain and sharpening mental function in older people.[4]

But are the fat activists right that exercise is not effective for weight loss? They are not alone in this belief.[5] And in all fairness, the case for exercise for weight control has become established only in more recent years. But what has been found is surprising. Not only is exercise one way to this desired end but, for many people, it may well be the best way.

How often have you heard that the best exercise for losing weight is to lift both hands up to shoulder level and push against the supper table, thereby shoving what's left on your plate out of reach? There's clearly wisdom in those words. No matter how much exercise we get, it's always possible to make up the calorie deficit at the table. But if reasonable moderation is employed at the table, exercise can be the difference in effective weight loss.

Consider the study of Grant Gwinup, M.D., at the Irvine Medical Center in Southern California. He took "minimally to moderately obese" women and separated them into three categories: stationary cyclists, walkers, and swimmers. The women were given no advice or admonishments on food intake, so it was assumed they continued to eat the way they always had. The women gradually worked up from as little as five minutes a day of exercise to a full hour a day over a period of six months. The swimmers for some reason lost no weight and apparently no fat. But the walkers lost fully 10 percent of their initial weight (averaging seventeen pounds total weight loss), while the women who cycled lost 12 percent of their initial weight (averaging nineteen pounds total weight loss).[6] This is just the sort of slow and steady weight loss that doctors and nutritionists recommend. Further, all these women were chosen because they had failed at dieting.

If you're using swimming to lose weight, I wouldn't get all panicky over this single study. It is generally agreed that swimming is a fine way of burning calories and of exercising the heart. "Swimmers lose weight just as well as anyone," says Lewis G. Maharam, M.D., who practices sports medicine in New York City. "You *can* swim yourself thin," he maintains.[7] Indeed, I have known friends who have lost weight and attributed it to adding swimming to their exercise regimen. Doing a fast crawl stroke burns about eleven calories per minute, compared with thirteen calories for running at a moderate nine-minute pace.[8] (Don't forget to subtract a few more calories for the effort of blow-drying your hair afterward.)

In any event, some studies are even more encouraging than this one. One such study at Laval University in Quebec had five slightly overweight but otherwise healthy young males exercise on stationary bicycles twice a day at 53 minutes (nice round number) for six days a week. After 100 days the men lost an average of 17.6 pounds, with more than 80 percent of the loss from fat.[9] In a sense this is almost a best-case scenario. Few of us have 106 minutes a day, six days a week, to work out. On the other hand, the men only exercised at 55 percent of capacity, whereas one can work at up to 80 percent of capacity and still be exercising aerobically. But the point is that these men were able to lose 1.2 pounds a week through nothing but exercise. Further, these men being only slightly overweight had very little fat to get rid of. Obese persons certainly would have lost at a much greater rate. Which brings up one more point. Considering that these men were only slightly overweight, this means that in that 100-day period they lost everything they had to lose. Clearly exercise is a valuable means to lose weight.[10]

Despite such encouraging studies as these, other studies have shown no weight loss associated with exercise. How can that be? We'll look at factors that can contribute to this phenomenon later. For now, we have seen that regular, vigorous exercise can cause steady weight loss, albeit more slowly than dieting. What if we combine the two?

"While exercise alone does not appear to be as potent an initial weight-loss strategy as caloric restriction alone," state Stanford University researchers Abby King and Diane Tribble in a 1991 medical journal review article, "when exercise is added to a weight-loss program involving caloric restriction initial weight loss is often much greater than with diet alone."[11] One study cited found that those who combined diet and exercise lost fourteen pounds more over a twenty-five-week period than those just dieting. Another showed those combining the two lost about twice as much as those just dieting.[12] Yet a third showed dieting exercisers to have lost more than twice the body fat of dieters alone in a twelve-week period.[13]

One reason losing weight through exercise is better than through calorie restriction is because weight lost through diet inevitably leads to loss of muscle as well. The reduction of muscle during dieting has ranged from as little as 15 percent of overall weight lost for mild caloric restriction to as a much as 50 to 70 percent of overall weight lost during semistarvation.[14] The more muscle you have, the faster your metabolism and the more calories you burn, therefore, during any weight-loss regimen, you want to keep muscle loss to the lowest possible level.

Exercise not only leads to less muscle loss as fat comes off; it often leads to no muscle loss or even muscle gain. One review surveyed fifty-five medical reports of weight loss with exercise and found that in fifty of them there was less loss of muscle than there would have been through dieting.[15]

Yet if it's true that exercise can be helpful in promoting weight loss, it appears that where it's really essential is in maintaining that loss. Exercise is one of the few factors correlated with long-term maintenance. For example, vigorous exercise was one of the principal strategies for weight maintenance reported by a group of men and women who had lost at least 20 percent of their body fat and maintained that loss for two years. Especially interesting was that while most of the men had also used exercise to lose the weight initially, the overwhelming majority of women lost weight by diet alone and only later increased their exercise to maintain the loss.[16]

These studies looked back at what successful maintainers had done. Other studies have looked ahead to see what they *would* do. In one, during the initial eight-week segment all subjects attended weekly exercise sessions that included instruction in behavior modification, diet, general nutrition, and exercise. In addition, half of the participants were required to attend a supervised exercise program consisting of aerobic activity, calisthenics, and relaxation. Although the initial weight loss was similar in exercise and non-exercise groups, upon follow-up there was a striking difference between the groups. The average weight of the non-exercise group went right back to where it had been before dieting. But exercisers maintained their losses indefinitely, or at least to the last follow-up check at thirty-six months. These exercisers worked out at least three times per week with an average per-week expenditure of approximately 1,500 calories, meaning their workouts were about an hour long.[17]

Numerous other studies have shown similar findings, note King and Tribble, "indicating that a change in lifestyle including an increase in exercise will likely provide the most successful long-term weight-loss outcome."[18]

The most recent study as of this writing appeared in the *Journal of the American Dietetic Association* in 1996. It looked at three groups, one of whom sought to lose weight through diet only, one through diet and exercise, and one through exercise only. After one year, the diet-only group had lost fifteen pounds; the exercise-only group, a little over six pounds; the combination group, almost twenty pounds. During the second year the diet-only group regained a pound more than it had lost, the combination group regained most of what it had lost, but the exercise-only group regained less than half a pound.[19]

"We were shocked," said Baylor College's John Foreyt, who worked on the study. "We'd put our money on the diet-plus-exercise group, but apparently the negative effects of restrictive dieting—feelings of hunger and deprivation—eventually lead to overeating."[20]

Why did the exercise-only group keep the weight off when the others couldn't? Was it the exercise itself, or to some extent could the willingness to keep exercising indicate the type of person who's going to continue to make an effort to keep weight off? "That's the unanswerable question," Foreyt told me. "What are the characteristics of people who exercise? It may be a marker for highly motivated, driven, tenacious people. Whatever that drive is we may just be measuring that through exercise."[21]

So why didn't the diet-plus-exercise group maintain their loss? "When they gave up dieting they also quit exercising," says Foreyt. "Presumably they got depressed over the weight they regained." With the exercise-only group, though, there was virtually no regain at all, hence no motivation to give up.

According to Yale obesity expert Kelly Brownell, M.D.: "The key is that when people exercise, no matter how much of it they do, they feel better about themselves. It raises their self-confidence. They feel virtuous. I think when people exercise, the psychological benefits are triggered and that helps them stick to their diet better."[22] Peggy Keating of Duke University's Diet and Fitness Center in Durham, North Carolina, appears to agree. "Exercisers have higher levels of self-esteem and therefore may make better lifestyle choices," says the exercise physiologist. "If you go for a run in the morning, then you're offered a doughnut later in the day, you're more likely to think, 'I've already busted my butt. Why blow it?' "[23]

DOES EXERCISE INCREASE EATING?

One concern you may have with exercising is whether it will make you eat more. A lot of people will use this as an excuse for couch-potatoism, saying the exercise will just make them so hungry that they'll eat that much more and cancel out the effect. "Gosh, if I work out for half an hour I'll burn off 250 calories, and then, wolf down a 450-calorie slice of pie. For my health's sake I better stay on this couch and watch *Gilligan's Island* reruns!" But the studies are extremely consistent on this point: Exercise does not increase appetite and food consumption for obese persons.[24]

How can it be that burning off more calories doesn't result in eating more? This sounds counterintuitive. Certainly, in a more primitive society in which eating is closely related to hunger, more exertion would lead to more eating. But in a society like ours in which the connection between eating and hunger is very tenuous, it's not so. Let's say you eat three times a day out of genuine hunger. Then you eat two more times a day because you're bored or because Dave Thomas appears on the boob tube and tells you all about his new giant Wendy's sandwich consisting of two cows, a pound of bacon, three slices of pasteurized processed cheese food product, and that wonderful "secret sauce" that's always just salad dressing. You're already taking in calories you don't need. Those will do quite nicely for the amount of extra calories you'll need to sustain that exercise. The only people this doesn't apply to are those who eat only when truly hungry and are already lean. They do, in fact, eat more when they exercise.[25] Otherwise, the body goes to its fat reserves before urging you to load up on new calories.

This is not to be confused with the person who goes to the gym and works out for five or ten minutes then rewards herself with an ice cream sundae. The studies I've cited looked at people who engaged regularly in serious amounts of exercise, not people who figure that pedaling their bicycles five minutes to McDonald's gives them license to eat a Big Mac and a giant cup of milkless milk shake. As overweight comedienne Beth Donahue puts it, "The only good thing about going to the gym, or partaking in any other form of exercise, is that you feel good afterward . . . sort of. You've given yourself such a good workout and burnt off all those calories—at least three or four—that you feel like you deserve some sort of reward."[26] Actually, Donahue makes it clear she's just kidding that this is the "only good thing" about exercising, noting that persistent, regular exercise is the only thing that's helped her lose weight.

COVERT BAILEY AND HIS "MAGIC PILL"

Every aspect of weight loss and weight control has its assortment of hucksters taking an idea that's basically good and twisting it completely out of shape. They thereby sell you a magic formula that says you can practically suck up food like a vacuum cleaner so long as you take their nostrum. Exercise is no exception. And here the huckster shamelessly even hawks his magic as just that.

His name is Covert Bailey and he's a slick pitchman whose face graces a variety of infomercials. He is the author of numerous bestsellers, with the one that started it all called *Fit or Fat?*,[27] later revised to *The New Fit or Fat*. Like other weight-loss gurus, Bailey attempts to convince his readers that fat people eat no more than thin ones. Indeed, both books have chapters titled "Fat People Eat Less than Skinny People."[28]

By completely de-emphasizing the intake side of obesity, he convinces the reader that the only hope for weight reduction is on the output side. But that's the good news, says Bailey. His solution is practically as easy as taking a drug. "If I were offering a pill to decrease the tendency of the body to make fat, fat people would be lining up to buy it," he writes. "I AM OFFERING SUCH A PILL; IT TAKES JUST TWELVE MINUTES A DAY TO SWALLOW IT [emphasis original]."[29] Indeed, the original *Fit or Fat?* even has a graphic on the cover representing twelve minutes of exercise.[30]

Bailey's "pill" utilizes what he calls "fat-burning enzymes." "Why do I emphasize a minimum time of twelve minutes?" he writes.

"The answer is that you are trying to produce *growth* of fat-burning enzymes, and a minimum of 12 minutes of continual, gentle activity seems to be the time trigger necessary to stimulate the difference between actual fat burning and growth of fat-burning enzymes."[31] He goes on about these miraculous "enzymes," saying, "While you DO burn fat during aerobic activity, the growth of fat-burning enzymes is the real purpose for exercising. You want more and more 'butter-burning' enzymes so that a year from now a greater proportion of the calories you use up during exercise are fat calories instead of sugar (glucose) calories."[32]

Bailey then goes on to reinforce this notion, saying, "There seems to be something magical about doing 12 minutes of an aerobic exercise. . . ."[33] Using the pitchman's obnoxious practice of referring to himself in the plural to give himself more authority, Bailey adds, "For this reason we urge beginners to do 12 minutes of exercise six days a week rather than a 30-minute exercise three days a week."[34]

Well, hell's bells, jest sign me right up! Jest twelve minutes a day and I'm burnin' the fat off my rump faster than a possum bein' chased by a pack of starvin' Dobermans!

Actually, I did "sign up" in that I bought Bailey's book many years ago and followed the regimen. I lost no weight and now I know why. Bailey's promises are scientifically bankrupt. There's nothing in the medical literature to support him. There's nothing magical at all about twelve minutes of exercise. Twenty-four minutes of vigorous exercise is twice as effective in burning calories as twelve; thirty-six minutes three times as effective, and so on. In any event, twelve minutes is at least eight minutes shy of the twenty minutes of vigorous exercise that many experts say is necessary for cardiovascular conditioning.*

Having made his name with his "magic" twelve minutes, Bailey now hawks a $499 piece of equipment called the "HealthRider." It's obviously magic, too, because—still invoking the "fat-burning enzymes"—he says that with his overpriced device (you can buy an

---

*If cardiovascular aerobic fitness is your goal, you should work out for at least 20 minutes a day, four times a week, at a level of intensity high enough to raise your heart rate to 50 to 70 percent of its maximum. To determine the maximum, subtract your age from 220. Thus if you are 30 years old, your maximum is 190, and you should exercise in the range of 95 to 133 beats per minute.

identical unit for less than half the cost) twenty minutes three times a week is all you need. Alas, like his advice, apparently his equipment is useless. In its evaluation of the HealthRider, *Consumer Reports* noted that the unit was the most expensive version of that particular type of equipment and went on to say that none of their staffers were "able to get even a moderately challenging aerobic workout" with the machine.[35] Still, I understand they're great for throwing your clothes onto at the end of a long day.

How Much and How Often?

Thus we see yet again that there is no magic in weight loss and maintenance. But that doesn't tell us how often and how long we should exercise. NordicTrack, originally a maker of just a single type of machine imitating cross-country skiing but now a manufacturer of a huge line of products, entices purchasers with a promise of losing their guts with just twenty minutes of exercise three times a week. Yet the people in their ads always look like they're having so much fun you'd think their spouses have to rip them off the devices to get them to go to bed at night. Nonetheless, even the National Exercise for Life Institute says that "aerobic exercise should be performed three to five days a week for twenty to sixty continuous minutes per session."[36] What is the National Exercise for Life Institute? Apparently it's a front group for the Nordic-Track company; their literature subtly pushes indoor cross-country skiing and is distributed where NordicTrack devices are sold. NordicTrack's marketers just decided to go with the bottom of the range for both duration and frequency.

Competitors, including Bailey's HealthRider, have been forced to match the claim. After all, who wants to spend twenty-five minutes exercising when there's a piece of equipment that will do it for you in twenty? For some people, namely those who are just a couple of pounds overweight, twenty minutes three or four times a week may be enough. But most of us are a lot more than a couple of pounds overweight and, for us, sixty minutes of exercise a week is better than nothing but not nearly good enough.

Ultimately, it's up to each of us. Weight reduction and maintenance is a matter of balancing energy intake with output. For some rare people—Anne Fletcher's 15 percent—no increase in output is necessary. Conversely, some people will choose to lose weight and maintain that reduction entirely through exercise. For most people, there will be some sort of medium. I lost weight and have kept it off with four hours of aerobic exercise a week.

One delusion under which I long labored—because I didn't bother to think it through—concerned the length of exercise sessions. It suggests you won't "burn fat" unless you exercise for long periods of time, anywhere from twelve to forty minutes depending on whose advice you're taking. "Exercise," says Debra Waterhouse in her best-selling *Outsmarting the Female Fat Cell*, "is not cumulative. The thirty minutes must be done all at once. Exercising in the morning for fifteen minutes and in the evening for fifteen minutes adds up to thirty minutes—but you won't be using fat energy."[37] This just isn't true. Daniel Kirschenbaum in his excellent book, *Weight Loss Through Persistence*, explains:

> When you begin exercising, you begin using calories immediately. The energy consumed by your body initially comes from glucose stored in the muscles. As you exercise for longer periods of time, your body begins dipping into its energy reserves (fat). However, your body must replenish the energy supply it uses. This means that when you consume energy in the form of stored glucose from the muscles, your body will use its stored energy supply to replenish the glucose taken from the muscles. It makes no difference whether you exercise for short bursts of 10 or 15 minutes or for longer periods of 30 to 60 minutes per session. You burn fat both ways.[38]

Thus, if it's better for your schedule to have two 15-minute sessions a day than one for 30, go for it. You won't be handicapped in calorie burning and you may find it more palatable psychologically. A 1995 study put this to the test, telling one group of women to get their exercise in ten-minute bouts and another to take all their exercise at once. Each group was to work out five times a week. It found that the women prescribed short bouts of exercise were far more likely to keep it up. It also found that their cardiovascular improvement was just as good as the improvement of the women doing longer bouts of exercise.[39]

Interestingly, a five-day-a-week schedule might actually be easier to maintain than something less frequent. "If you ask people to exercise five or six days a week, you get better adherence over the long term than if you have them do three or four days," says Rod Dishman, a professor in the department of exercise science at the University of Georgia. "A possible explanation is that an every-other-day program isn't constant enough to become a habit but five or six days is."[40]

The time of day may be important as well. "Statistically speaking, we find that people who work out in the morning are more likely to have better long-term adherence than those who wait until evening," says Tedd Mitchell, M.D., medical director of the Cooper Wellness Program at the Cooper Aerobics Center in Dallas, Texas. "Primarily, it may be because morning schedules are a little easier to control than evening ones, where a late meeting at work, an unexpected trip with your child to the doctor, or any number of other unforeseen problems can put [exercise] on the back burner."[41]

It's important to resist the impulse to go whole hog into an exercise routine for two reasons. First, it can be harmful or even fatal. When I worked at the U.S. Commission on Civil Rights I lost a boss and friend when he suddenly embarked on a rigorous exercise program and dropped dead on a health club exercise bicycle. The poor man was extremely overweight and probably hadn't consulted with a doctor, a prerequisite to any vigorous exercise program for older or seriously overweight people. The second reason is the potential for burnout. Many people make the mistake of exercising too intensely for their current fitness levels. In their efforts to burn more calories they just burn out and end up back on the couch, tortilla chips in one hand and remote control in the other. Placing consistency above all else will yield the best results.

"It's been found that people who start out exercising moderately are twice as likely still to be exercising at the end of a year as people who start out at high intensity," according to William McCarthy, M.D., director of science at the Pritikin Longevity Center in Santa Monica, California. "And we only suggest starting out at even a moderate level if it feels comfortable. The best way to make the best beginning is a step approach. Do what feels good and build from there. That way you won't scare yourself off the program."[42]

Spousal or other outside support may also be helpful. Indiana University psychologist John Raglin presented a study to the Society of Behavioral Medicine of sixty-five adults divided into two groups. In one group were married people who exercised alone; half of them quit the program within a year. In the second group were married people who exercised together. Of these, 92 percent stayed with it. "Social support is very important," Raglin says. "And we've found that exercising with your spouse is one of the most effective ways to maintain a regimen."[43] I called my friend Diane Medved, author of *The Case Against Divorce*, to see if she knew about this. "Oh, yes," she said. "It's just one more reason to keep the knot tied."[44]

But how about people who have simply no time for exercise? Often that's just an excuse for laziness, bringing to mind the comment of the university president who said that whenever he got the desire to exercise he would lie down until it went away. Cute. Real cute. But many of us feel we really are too harried to set aside time for a workout. To them I commend the observation of John Foreyt and his colleague G. Ken Goodrick: "Regular exercise requires only about five percent of your waking hours [and] if you can't fit that into your schedule, your life is probably very stressful and you really need exercise badly to help you unwind."[45]

If you make time, you'll have time. My guess is that 90 percent of my readers who say they have no time fall into the category of those described by Geoffrey Godbey, a leisure-time expert at Pennsylvania State University, as "people [who] say they have no time and then watch three to four hours of TV a day."[46] That's no excuse. Set up an exercise bike or rower or ski machine in front of the tube. If you use it just every time you watch *Roseanne* you won't end up looking like her. And if you use it just every time you watch *Home Improvement* you'll be amazed at the improvement you're making in your health and looks. As I have discussed previously in this book, TV is the enemy of weight control. Putting a piece of exercise equipment in front of it is the way to convert the enemy into an ally.

WHICH MACHINES ARE BEST?

Ah, there's nothing like going for a bike ride or a run in the great outdoors! On the other hand, there's nothing like being warm (or cool) and dry in the great indoors. More and more Americans have turned to various machines to help keep them in shape. If you're wondering whether some machines burn more calories in a given time period than others, the answer is yes. According to a 1996 *Journal of the American Medical Association* study, the king of stationary exercisers is not the ski machine, as so many of us were led to believe, but the lowly treadmill. Here are calories burned per hour for the various machines tested:

Treadmill: 700

Stair Machine: 627

Rower: 606

Cross-Country Ski Machine: 595

Stationary Bicycle with Arm Rower: 509

Stationary Bicycle without Arm Rower: 498

Source: "Energy Expenditure with Indoor Exercise Machines," *Journal of the American Medical Association.*[47]

Still, the best machine for you is the one you like the best and therefore are most likely to use. The difference in calories burned between one type of machine and another is irrelevant if you don't exercise at all.

HOW VIGOROUS SHOULD AEROBIC EXERCISE BE?

Since most of the diet industry is built around telling us what we want to hear, as opposed to what is true, it's not surprising that we are bombarded with messages that easy exercise is as good, if not far better, for you than vigorous exercise. Many women's magazines have been sold on the basis of a cover story saying that less-intense exercise (say, walking rather than running) is better at burning off fat calories. The best-selling *You Count, Calories Don't* proclaims it a "myth" that "exercising vigorously burns more fat."[48] And if I see one more article on how many calories you can burn off while having sex, I'm going to take a vow of celibacy.

There are two essential facts here. First, the vast majority of the calories we burn daily will not be in exercise sessions because we burn calories all day long and the most dedicated of us exercise for only a few hours a day. It is important to try to maximize calorie burning while not exercising, say, by walking more, eschewing labor-saving devices, and so on. But when it does come to exercise for exercise's sake, there's no substition for vigor. It certainly may be good advice to tell beginning exercisers to start out by walking and then work their way up. It's also true that walking can in some cases provide enough exercise for weight control. But jogging burns more calories than walking, and running fast burns more than jogging.

Additionally, it appears that intense exercise may result in more body fat lost than less intense exercise that burns the same number of calories. That was the conclusion of researchers at Laval University in Quebec. They put two sets of volunteers on different exercise patterns on indoor bicycles. The first set engaged in steady exercise at an aerobic pace, while the second set interrupted their pace with occasional bursts of high-intensity exercise. At the end of the study it was found that even though the steady exercisers had burned twice as many calories as the high-intensity ones, the high-intensity ones had lost more fat. Indeed, calorie for calorie the high-intensity exercisers lost an amazing nine times the amount of fat as the steady exercisers.[49] If other studies bear this out, the message to exercisers will be clear. While any exercise is better than none, the more intense the better. Instead of just a steady jog, try tossing in a few sprints. Instead of a steady pace on the bicycle or ski machine, work in the occasional burst of speed. This is something I've always done just to help avoid boredom.

Again if you can't do high-intensity exercise because of health conditions, then don't worry about this. Or maybe you can't because you're just too heavy right now. In that case, do the low-intensity until such a time as you're in shape enough to begin high-intensity bursts.

GETTING OFF OUR DUFFS

As I've noted, most of our calorie burning will necessarily take place during those hours we aren't exercising. Thus, those who need to keep their weight down need to think creatively about how to burn as much energy as possible during the course of the day. We also need to think about what can be done as a society. One tool is urban planning. There is a relatively new school of thinking, called the "new urbanism," that seeks to reverse the trend toward wide-open spaces that only cars can traverse. It seeks to get suburbanites to accept smaller lawns, narrower streets, more through streets, and fewer cul-de-sacs. Much of this will promote bicycling and walking. Developers and zoners can help bring back the corner store so that people can once again walk to the store for the proverbial loaf of bread, rather than piling into the minivan for a trek to the closest superstore.[50] Author James Howard Kunstler has recently argued that city zoning laws established since World War II have had much to do with suburban spread and that repealing these laws can help bring back tighter but more comfortable living.[51]

One example is the Walt Disney Company's new planned community outside Orlando, Florida. Called Celebration, it uses new urbanism planning, with homes of many styles clustered around a central business district that is within walking distance.[52] A loaf of bread, a quart of milk, and a set of Mickey Mouse ears will never be more than a short stroll away.

Already-established suburban communities can make improvements in this direction, as well. One Chicago suburb, the name of which has come to be synonymous with the kind of place you can only get around by car, is now trying to remedy that. Schaumburg, Illinois, is actually building a ready-made downtown, complete with shops, restaurants, a library, ponds, parks, and waterfalls.[53] Exercise aside, I know that when I go to Europe one of the things I enjoy most is how every city and town has such areas. People sit at outdoor cafés with their chairs pointed out so they can watch other people stroll by. True, there's an ambience generated by sitting in the shadows of buildings hundreds of years old that Schaumburg will never be able to duplicate in its "Olde Schaumburg" downtown. But a little imagination can work wonders.

Public information campaigns can also encourage Americans to get out of their cars whenever possible and use human power instead. Likewise for using stairs instead of elevators. In one experiment, signs saying "Stay Healthy, Save Time, Use the Stairs" were placed in a Glasgow, Scotland, tube (subway) station next to a stairway consisting of two flights of fifteen steps. Before the signs went up, only 8 percent of subway passengers used the stairs. After the signs were posted, this doubled to about 16 percent. Not a fantastic increase, by any means, but definitely worth something.[54] On the down side, it is rather pathetic that given the option of saving time and improving their health, 84 percent of those given a choice chose the lazy route. (Handicapped persons were excluded from the data, by the way.)

But most of all, Americans are going to have to start thinking in terms of getting every little bit of exercise they can. As *New York Times* health reporter Jane Brody encouraged her readers:

> Chop food and mix dough by hand instead of throwing everything into a food processor. Push a power mower instead of using a rider mower. Carry your clubs around the golf course. Use a hand saw to cut up wood for the fireplace. Shovel snow and rake leaves instead of blowing them off the walk with a machine. Do some or all of your own gardening and yard work. Play ball with the children. And walk: up stairs, to stores, to work, to social engagements, wherever and whenever it is possible and safe to walk.[55]

Other ideas include using fewer telephones in the house, standing instead of sitting, parking your car on the far side of lots (and definitely not in other people's handicapped spaces), and perhaps the most important exercise of all—pushing the "off" button on the television set. I'm told that having children—and thus later chasing after them—is also an effective means of getting in extra daily exercise. You could also try getting a dog that insists on being walked three times a day, else he soils your carpet.

Nonetheless, for many of us even this won't be enough. Energy-saving devices are just too efficient and prevalent. A generation ago, the only "automatically" sliding doors where those on the original *Star Trek* series—in which a man behind the set manually pulled them open and closed. Today, it's darned hard to find a grocery store door that doesn't open automatically. For many of us, nothing short of planned exercise sessions will work to control our weight problem. And the first part of that session requires placing your hands on both sides of your hips and pushing downward—thrusting yourself up from the couch.

THE "AB" FAD

As I write this, the current fitness fad concerns abdomen exercisers. At any given time I can flip through the range of channels on my TV and see two or three different infomercials for them. "Turn on your television," writes humor columnist Dave Barry, "and you will see the Abdominals People. I do not wish to generalize here, but these people display the intelligence of sherbet—selling abdominal devices, demonstrating abdominal devices, and of course proudly showing off their abdominal muscles, which bulge and writhe beneath a thin, sweaty layer of skin, so that the people look as though they're smuggling pythons down there."[56]

Ponytailed fitness guru Tony Little tells you in one infomercial, "If you don't have an Ab Isolator, you're like, *weird*."[57] But if you don't mind being, like, *weird*, you can also buy an Abflex, Abs of Steel Abdomen Machine, Pro-Form Ab Resister, Abworks, AbCoach, AB Blaster, Abs by HealthRider, Weider Ab Shaper, Power-Tek Abdomen System, Ab Roller Plus, FlexaBall, Trim Roll, Trim Roller, EZ Crunch, Weslo Crunch Force, Ab Trainer, Body by Jake Ab and Back Plus, ABSculptor, ABToner, ABRock'it Plus, Perfect Abs, and for you saggy-bellied patriots, the AbFlex U.S.A. Even my grocery store has gotten in on the act. Now when you buy a pint of Ben and Jerry's Chubby Hubby ice cream to devour all by yourself, you can restore your virtue by picking up a Max Ab for $39.95 on your way out. And I'm ABsolutely sure I've missed more than a few, so consider this an ABridged list—and excuse my ABominable puns. In any case, I think that if Bob Dole had thought to promise voters an abdomen machine for every pot(belly), the 1996 election might have had a far different outcome.

I don't blame people for liking the so-called washboard look. While I harbor no doubts about my heterosexuality, I must say that when I'm at the beach I find myself admiring both good-looking women and hard male stomachs. (The women I admire head to toe.) If you look at ancient Greek art (all or virtually all done by males), you'll note the same sort of admiration. But the abdominal exerciser thing is just a mania. In 1995, makers of an estimated 2.75 million ab thingamajigs racked up about $145 million in sales. And 1996 shaped up to be an even bigger year. In the last week of May of that year, four of the top ten infomercials pitched ab machines. QVC, the home-shopping channel, reported that in one remarkable fifteen-hour sales period, its viewers ordered 41,000 Weider Ab Shapers, for about $40 apiece.[58]

Some of these devices are better than others. Indeed practically all are better than the AbFlex, which resembles nothing so much as a model Stealth bomber. You hold it by handles on either "wing" and it just presses against the stomach. This is something you can do with your own hands or get your dog to do to you if you lie on your back with a pork chop sticking out of your mouth. Anyway, there's little value in pressing on your belly. The best machines are those that allow you to do some form of sit-up or crunch while relieving the strain on the neck and back that these exercises normally entail.

Some of these pieces of equipment, like that NordicTrack's Abworks, are honestly advertised as just being able to firm up and accentuate abdominal muscles. Others, however, make such false claims as Ab Roller Plus's "Get a Flat, Sexy Stomach in Five Minutes Flat." Ab Sculptor's infomercials guarantee that with their $80 device you'll lose ten pounds and four inches off your waist in thirty days. AbRock'it Plus's full-page ads in *USA Today* claim: "You'll be surprised at how soon you'll lose inches at your waist in just minutes a day."[59]

Yes, be surprised. Be very surprised. I guarantee you'll lose no pounds and no inches in thirty days simply using the Ab Sculptor or any of its competitors. Building the body's muscles in general can lead to weight loss, but just toughening up the belly won't. Further, there's no such thing as spot reduction. When you lose fat, it comes off the last place your body put it on, wherever you happen to be focusing your exercise. If you want your ab muscles to appear, you need to lose total body fat through diet and exercising the whole body.

A healthy man who is already in shape has about 12 percent to

15 percent body fat; a woman, 15 percent to 18 percent. But James Rippe, M.D., author of *Fit Over Forty*,[60] estimates that the models used in most of the advertising for abdominal machines have less than 10 percent. "To look like some of them, you would have to be around 6 percent or 7 percent," he says.[61]

As for me, you'll never see my stomach on the cover of a muscle magazine but I have something of a washboard and I do all of about ten minutes of stomach exercises a week. And I don't do it on any device promoted on TV. Unfortunately, the ab machine obsession is just another bad sign of the times. The same Americans who buy books with titles like *The Five-Day Miracle Diet*; *Eat More, Weigh Less*; and *Why Women Need Chocolate* desperately want to believe that some $40 device used for five minutes a day will completely make up for twenty-three hours and fifty-five minutes of bad eating habits and couch-potatoism. It's hardly coincidental that so many of these devices are sold via television. But pudgy people who think they're going to get stomach muscles resembling Ruffles potato chips from any kind of sit-up or other abdominal device are just engaging in the same mass self-deception that keeps fueled the weight-loss industry.

THE "HOOVER OPTION"

If you're not going to get washboard abs simply from using some device with the letters "ab" in it, how about with another device, the kind that's long and hollow and sharp at the end? Liposuction has now become one of America's most popular forms of plastic surgery. In 1995 alone, 51,000 procedures were performed just by board-certified plastic surgeons alone, not to mention those done by dermatologists and other doctors. Liposuction techniques continue to improve and it's easy to find a doctor who will tell you just what you want to hear about it. Glowing testimonials are easy to come by, such as that of a woman who used it to combat her "middle-age spread" and concluded an article on the subject declaring, "While liposuction was no day at the beach, I sure look better at the beach."[62] The problem with all these testimonials is that they are made fairly soon after surgery. What about a few years later? Ah, and there's the rub. Many in the media will tell you, as

Maclean's told its readers in 1996, "One appeal of liposuction is that it not only eliminates fat—it appears to keep it off."[63] But this just isn't true. It *can't* be true.

Consider: When you eat more calories than you need for energy, cell repair, and so on, a bit of the excess burns off and the rest goes to fat somewhere on your body. If it didn't return to wherever you had it sucked out, it would have to go somewhere else. In my case, my excess fat tended to go first to my belly and then to my face. If it were permanently removed from my belly, yet I kept eating excess calories (which is what put the fat there in the first place), then it would just go to my face. I would have "love handles" hanging off my cheeks.

In one extreme case, a terribly obese woman went on a diet and lost more than 150 pounds. She then demanded that the doctors do something about the huge apron of deflated flesh that now sagged from her midsection. Surgeons performed a lipectomy, which involved using a scalpel to cut away the "apron," then drawing the woman's stretched skin tight at the waistline. But the woman could not maintain her new weight, and when she ballooned out again the fat went to her remaining adipose cells, in her thighs and upper arms. Once fat but proportionately so, she was now both fat and a freak.[64]

With liposuction it's not at all clear that the fat doesn't just go right back whence it came. The liposuction experts whom I consulted say it does. "We suck the fat out of the fat cells, but the fat cells remain and if one eats at the preoperative pace, they'll just fill the fat cells back up," said Paul Gardner, M.D., of the Plastic Surgery Division at the University of Alabama at Birmingham.[65] If you eat at your old level, Charles Billington, M.D., from the University of Minnesota's Obesity center agreed, "Inevitably the weight will come back." He told me, "I think evidence shows it will come back in roughly the same place."[66]

Thus we see that liposuction, far from being a permanent fix like a nose or breast job, is really rather more like changing your oil. Unless you change your eating and/or exercise habits, it's just a temporary fix. And if you do change your eating and/or exercise habits, you will probably find you have no need or desire for liposuction. Yet again we see that when it comes to weight loss, magic is very much in short supply.

RESISTANCE TRAINING

Until now, this chapter has concentrated entirely on aerobic exercise. As the chapter winds down, it's time to pull out a surprise. One of the most important types of exercise for losing weight and maintaining the loss involves vigor, to be sure, but no huffing and puffing and disturbing your makeup and neatly coiffed hair and all that. It is resistance exercise.

It is commonly understood that metabolism slows as we age and that this is one reason people tend to get fatter as they enter their third decade and continue to grow fatter thereafter. But what's less understood is that the metabolism isn't slowing of its own accord, but rather because the body is losing muscle.[67] "We know that resting metabolic rate goes down 3 percent per decade, and the limited research we have suggests that's mostly due to the loss of muscle mass," says Jack Wilmore, an exercise physiologist at the University of Texas, Austin. "That's why we hear so much more emphasis on resistance training. The resistance training helps to regain some of that lost muscle mass."[68]

Resistance training means using weights or something else that pushes against you as you push it. Resistance training itself doesn't use that many calories. One study found only 139 calories burned during a forty-two-minute workout.[69] The way it works is through building up the size and weight of the muscle, which burns calories day-round and, yes, "even while you're sleeping" as the ads for weight-loss potions like to put it.

In one study, Wayne Westcott, M.D., strength-training consultant for the national YMCA, found those who performed fifteen minutes of strength training and fifteen minutes of aerobics three times a week for two months lost more than twice as much fat as those who did just half an hour of aerobic exercise during the same period.[70] In another study, researchers took eight men and four women, ranging from ages fifty-six to eighty, and put them to work with what is popularly known as a Universal machine that uses a system of steel plates. The people lifted three times a week for twelve weeks. At the end of this time their metabolic rates were measured and it was found that on average they had a 15 percent increase. Years of muscle shrinkage were erased in just twelve weeks.[71] If these people consumed on average 2,000 calories a day before they began the study and if their resting metabolic rate accounted for about 70 percent of this, then they could eat an additional 210 calories each day without gaining weight. Conversely, if they didn't eat an additional 210 calories a day, they would lose weight.

Another study of strength training in older men (average age sixty) found that after sixteen weeks of such exercise they had gained 4.4 pounds of muscle and lost 4.4 pounds of fat.[72]

If you're not as old as these people were you may not get the same results from resistance exercise as they did since they had probably lost more muscle than you have. On the other hand, their study ended at twelve weeks. It's possible that they could have continued to gain muscle for some time more. So a metabolic boost of 15 percent may not be unreasonable even for younger people who begin resistance exercise.

As far as how much resistance training you should do, eight to twelve repetitions is considered ideal. If you can pump the weights easily this number of times, add more weight. Twelve should be doable but never easy. It is commonly believed that three or even more sets of repetitions (known in macho terminology as "reps") are optimal. For professional power lifters or bodybuilders, that's no doubt true. But a major study at the University of Florida Center for Exercise Science in Gainesville followed fifty people over a fourteen-week training period and found that measurements of muscle strength and thickness revealed little difference between those who did one set and those who did three.[73] "Studies on bench presses show that you may not find two sets better than one, and three are a little more effective," says Michael Pollock, Ph.D., at the University of Florida. "But the extra is something like a 27 percent increase in strength, compared to 23 percent."[74] This is significant because one set is not only easier but that much quicker than three sets, meaning more people can stick to a program.

As far as how many times one should work out per week, never more than three (or every other day), because muscles need a day off to recover and grow, but as often as every other day. Nevertheless, apparently you can get about 75 percent of the benefit from working out just twice a week.[75]

As any patent official will tell you, there's no such thing as a perpetual motion machine. But habits come close. And they don't call habits "habits" for nothing. Once started, they can be very hard to break. So it is with exercise. Get used to the rush, get used to the added strength, get used to the all-around good feeling, and you may never want to go back. You've got nothing to lose but perhaps some fat.

10   **Pill Talk**

It is the obese person's lament everywhere: "If only they could invent a pill!" Well, they have. Lots of them. Many Americans don't know about them, but for some they may offer real hope.

Let me state from the outset what I don't like about weight-loss drugs:

1. I don't believe anybody "needs" drugs to lose weight in any physiological sense. Americans didn't need drugs thirty years ago to be thin. The Dutch don't need them now. Drugs are only for people who have convinced themselves that exercise and a proper diet will not work for them, as indeed I was convinced before I did the research for this book.

2. No weight-loss drug currently in use, nor probably any in experimental stages, enables you to bring your weight down as low as proper nutrition and exercise can. Without using drugs, I lost about 20 percent of my weight. Very few persons using drugs have had that kind of success. A drug can keep you from looking like Roseanne or Eddie Murphy's 400-pound character in *The Nutty Professor*; it will not give you the waistline of David Hasselhoff or Pamela Anderson Lee.(Incidentally, neither diet nor exercise nor a drug will give the bust of Pamela; only a qualified surgeon can.)

3. No prescription weight-loss drug currently available is labeled by the FDA for non-obese persons. This means that if you are just five or ten or even fifteen pounds heavier than you want to be, you may have difficulty getting a doctor to prescribe a drug for you. And no, I don't advise that you gain ten pounds to become officially obese just so you can get on an anti-obesity drug.

4. All weight-loss drugs in use or in experimental stages will probably have to be taken for life. Over time, even the cheapest drug may add up to a considerable expense. More importantly, over time and spread over a large enough population, even the safest drug will prompt some dangerous side effects in some people. For example, the quintessential "safe" drug, aspirin, is thought to cause about 1,000 deaths per year and causes many more cases of painful stomach ulcers.

5. No weight-loss drug in use or in experimentation will provide the health benefits of exercise such as strengthening the heart, lungs, and limbs. "Unless the (weight-loss) pill exercises the heart muscle, I'm not really interested," says G. Ken Goodrick, of Baylor College in Houston, co-author of *Living Without Dieting*.[1]

6. No weight-loss drug in use or in experimentation will provide the benefits of vitamins and minerals in preventing chronic illness, heart disease, and cancer.

7. Even what is generally considered the "perfect" or "ultimate" weight-loss drug, one that allows the consumption of absolutely everything while allowing people to be perfectly thin, is hardly perfect in that it prevents the psychological advantages and attainment of self-esteem through accomplishment.

8. Drugs are not going to solve the national obesity problem. You can't lace the country's drinking water supply with fenfluramine like we do with fluoride.

All that said, some of my readers will have convinced themselves that they cannot accomplish weight loss through proper nutrition and exercise and even those who don't fall into this category are probably going to be very curious about what the world of pharmaceuticals has to offer. Indeed, by 1996 about 4.4 million Americans were already using prescription diet medications[2] and nobody knows how many were using nonprescription ones. To these people, I have an obligation to explain what these drugs are, how they work, and how effective they are. I also have an obligation to tell you that I am not your doctor. Each drug interacts at least slightly differently with each taker. If you want to go down to Mexico and buy these things over the counter for less than you'd pay for a prescription, that's fine, but you should still consult a doctor. The more overweight you are now, the poorer your health, the more important that advice is for you.

While Americans clamor for weight-loss drugs, in the medical community, pharmaceuticals have a real PR problem. There are a couple of reasons for this. First is the bad track record of the original weight-loss pills, amphetamines. Available since the 1930s, amphetamines *do* work. The people who used them did lose weight. Unfortunately, the drug often also made them frantic, and many users became addicted to them.[3] Today these drugs are listed as controlled substances and no doctor who isn't a blockhead would prescribe them for weight loss.

The other reason for the prejudice against weight-loss drugs is that while they may offer a fairly quick fix, in that the pounds usually come off rapidly, they do not offer a permanent fix. Assuming you have success with them, you'll probably need to take them for life. Of course, that's also true of many other drugs. For most obese people, overweight is a chronic problem, like high blood pressure or diabetes, and unlike tuberculosis or a yeast infection. With an infection, a series of drugs taken anywhere from a few days to a few months can often promote a complete cure. But a chronic disease is lifelong and requires lifelong treatment.[4]

Herewith a rundown of the latest science has to offer.

CIGARETTES

What? Cigarettes? This guy is recommending smoking, the leading cause of preventable death in this country, as a way to help reduce the second-leading cause of death, obesity? No. Cool your jets. Smoking causes lung and various other types of cancer, emphysema, heart disease, yellow teeth, and, worst of all, whenever anybody smokes anywhere near me it always goes right in my face. I'm merely pointing out that cigarettes are the most common drug used in America today to control weight.

Everybody believes that cigarette smoking can keep weight in check, and especially that quitting smoking often leads to weight gain. What everyone believes is occasionally true, and the medical literature indicates this is one such case. Quitting the habit causes weight gain in perhaps 80 percent of ex-smokers. Body weight increases on average from five to ten pounds, with females slightly more likely to gain more weight than males.[5]

Sadly, it appears a lot of people use cigarettes expressly as a form of weight control. A survey of female college students found almost 40 percent of them listed weight control as a reason for smoking.[6] Once the habit is acquired, a fear of weight gain discourages many smokers from trying to quit.[7]

As to why smoking causes weight loss, here is where the popular beliefs are wrong. Most studies indicate that smokers don't eat less food.[8] In fact, it appears smokers' consumption may be somewhat higher. As one would guess, there is also no evidence that smokers have a higher level of physical activity.[9] Instead, the medical literature indicates that smoking appears to raise people's metabolism, specifically their resting energy expenditure.[10] One study found that smoking twenty-four cigarettes a day raised resting energy expenditure by about 10 percent.[11] This explains why you never see Joe Camel with a potbelly.

The reason for this increased metabolism, if you haven't already guessed it, is the most controversial ingredient of cigarettes: nicotine. Administration of a fairly small amount of nicotine with a nasal spray was found to raise the resting energy expenditure of test subjects by 6 percent, while another study found the level doubled to 12 percent in persons engaged in light physical activity.[12]

Obviously this points to one possible way of counteracting the weight gain that often accompanies quitting cigarettes: using a nicotine replacement in either gum or transdermal patch form. Indeed, one yearlong study of nicotine gum users found that they gained 4.4 pounds less than former smokers who weren't long-term gum users—this though the gum users had tended to be the heaviest smokers and therefore could have been expected to gain the most.[13] Thus, nicotine supplements not only make it easier to quit smoking; they also make weight gain less likely.

Drugs other than nicotine have proven effective in countering the weight gain associated with smoking. Phenylpropanolamine, thankfully abbreviated to PPA, which sells over the counter under such names as Dexatrim and Acutrim, may be useful in preventing the weight gain that often accompanies quitting smoking. One study found that among persons who had just quit smoking, those who took nothing gained about two pounds in two weeks, while those on a placebo chewing gum gained about a pound and a half, and those who chewed gum containing twenty-five milligrams of PPA divided into three pieces per day had a gain that was barely even measurable.[14]

One trial of quitting smokers who took the drug dexfen-fluramine found that in addition to preventing an expected increase in anxiety and irritability in the weeks following cessation, the drug users went on to lose almost two pounds in the next four weeks. In contrast, those on placebos gained three and a half pounds in the four-week postquitting period.[15]

HELP IN YOUR MEDICINE CABINET?

Another drug available over the counter that causes weight loss and doesn't have the nasty effects of cigarette smoking is ephe-drine. Most of today's weight-loss drugs fall into the anorexiant category; meaning, they chiefly reduce your appetite so you *take in* fewer calories. Some are "thermogenic agonists"; meaning, they rev up your metabolism so you *burn* more of the calories you do take in. (Thermogenic *agnostics* are people with high metabolisms who question the existence of God.) Ephedrine appears to be both an anorexiant and a thermogenic agonist. In various forms, such as the Chinese herb Ma Huang, it has been used for centuries as a stimulant and more recently has been used widely for asthma, bronchitis, and nasal congestion.

Though stories about sham diet pills often question ephe-drine's effectiveness and some books such as Laura Fraser's 1997 *Losing It* have gone so far as to say it's worthless,[16] study after study has found quite the opposite.[17] For example, a 1993 study in the *International Journal of Obesity* looked at four groups of individuals. One group was given 20 milligrams of ephedrine three times a day. Another was given 200 milligrams caffeine (the equivalent of about two cups of coffee) three times a day. A third group was given both drugs together, while a fourth group was given a placebo. All groups were on a low-calorie diet. At the end of a twenty-four-week period, the researchers found that the placebo group had lost twenty-nine pounds; the ephedrine-only group, a little over thirty-one pounds; the caffeine-only group, twenty-five pounds, but the ephedrine-plus-caffeine group lost more than thirty-six pounds. Thus the ephedrine-plus-caffeine group lost about a third of a pound per week more than the placebo group. The study was carried out for a full fifty weeks but was marred by a large number of people dropping out because they reached their goals. Nonetheless, the weight loss in the ephedrine-plus-caffeine group was maintained.[18] Curiously, the FDA claims there is no evidence that caffeine aids weight loss and has therefore banned its being advertised or packaged for such purposes.

That caffeine would add to the effect of ephedrine is hardly surprising. Caffeine has been found to be a tremendous energy booster, because it blocks natural tranquilizers the brain emits. In one treadmill test, for example, runners had a 30 percent improvement in performance. Runners who normally tired at forty to sixty minutes could go sixty to eighty minutes.[19] There is also evidence that in high enough doses caffeine can significantly speed up metabolism and burn off calories. One study administered 100 milligrams (about the equivalent of a cup of coffee) to volunteers six times a day. It found a daily increase in energy expenditure of 150 calories, which translates into a bit less than a pound lost every three weeks.[20]

While coffee and caffeine have repeatedly prompted various reports of adverse health indications, time and again these have proven either completely false or greatly overstated. To quote the title of a lengthy article on the subject by Jane Brody in *The New York Times*, "The Latest on Coffee? Don't Worry. Drink Up."[21] Caffeine is also thought to act as a brain booster, which is one reason I use it a lot. (I figure I can use all the brain-boosting I can get.) "The clearest effect of caffeine on cognition is its ability to enhance vigilance," says U.S. Army psychologist Harris Lieberman. It helps sustain attention during performance of various deep-thinking tasks for long periods of time.[22] On the other hand, it's also a diuretic, meaning it draws the water out of your cells and makes you have to urinate more often. (When I took my Law School Admission Test I thought I was going to be really sly and take caffeine to pump up my cranial capacity. Unfortunately, I had neglected my bladder capacity, and probably actually lowered my score as a result of several trips to the bathroom.)

It turns out that when aspirin is added to the ephedrine-caffeine cocktail, the results get better yet. At the beginning of a companion study to the one discussed above, one set of subjects ingested the equivalent of a standard aspirin per day (330 milligrams), plus 150 milligrams of caffeine, plus 75 milligrams of ephedrine. The ephedrine was later bumped up to 150 milligrams. After eight weeks the placebo group had lost a mere pound and a half, while those using the real cocktail lost almost five pounds.[23]

Obviously results will vary from person to person and study to study. But to use one of the better case scenarios, one 1994 study even found that after fifteen weeks persons using an ephedrine-caffeine combination lost more than eighteen pounds compared with fifteen pounds for the subjects taking prescription dexfenfluramine.[24]

While there's no doubt that both ephedrine and caffeine boost the metabolism, there's some evidence that in combination they also reduce the appetite.[25] How long the effects of these drugs last isn't known, since none of the studies went on for more than fifty weeks. Stimulants in general tend to be less effective the more you use them. This effect is called tachyphylaxis, and it means that your body responds to a foreign substance by reacting against it. Repeated exposure blunts the reaction mechanism, and you become more tolerant of the substance. That may be the case here.

Also, just because it's available without a prescription doesn't mean that ephedrine doesn't have potential side effects if too much is taken. These tend to be similar to those of too much caffeine. Thus, subjects given 150 milligrams of ephedrine a day complained of such symptoms as agitation, insomnia, headache, weakness, palpitation, giddiness, tremor, and constipation.[26]

Obviously, at doses higher than this you're asking for trouble. There have been deaths of people taking massive doses of ephedrine, resulting in some states and counties limiting the availability of the drug.[27] One short item in the *Dallas Morning News* actually told readers that ephedrine "when combined with caffeine ... delivers a dangerous one-two punch."[28] But it offered no evidence to back this up, and indeed there doesn't appear to be any. It's important to know that these overdoses aren't caused by people using low levels of the drug for either weight loss or breathing problems. Rather, the overdose is caused by people trying to get a "high" from massive amounts of the drug, amounts that are expressly packaged, advertised, and sold by companies as mind-altering. As I write this, the FDA is discussing outlawing such practices. But it's like the difference between smelling glue while building a model airplane and intentionally sniffing it until it scrambles your brain. Too much of any drug will hurt you or even kill you. (Each year, overdoses of aspirin and aspirin substitutes send about 25,000 teenagers alone to hospital emergency rooms.[29])

But taken in doses of 25 milligrams ephedrine thrice daily and 200 milligrams caffeine thrice daily, you should suffer at worst the symptoms I just listed.[30] Try to get the ephedrine from medicine in a drugstore rather than from Ma Huang, in that the amount of ephedra in Ma Huang may vary from product to product and even from package to package. If this level makes you nervous or agitated, start out lower and work up to it, but never go over that dose. Even though ephedrine has been used by tens of millions of people for decades, if you plan to start using it regularly you may wish to check with your doctor. This is especially the case if you are taking a prescription drug regularly. The material included with ephedrine pills will list some of those that may cause unwanted interactions.

I have tried the caffeine-ephedrine-aspirin combination myself. Whether it helped control my weight I can't say for sure. I trust the studies that say it does. As to its side effects, for the first few days I was a bit excitable, but after that there was little noticeable difference. The main problem I had is that if I took the drugs anywhere near bedtime, even within four hours, I had insomnia.

Why haven't you heard about this caffeine-ephedrine-aspirin combination if it seems so successful? Probably for the same reason I hadn't until I began researching this book. There's just no money in it. All three ingredients involve drugs that in their basic form are unpatentable, hence advertising their effectiveness just isn't worth it for any company.

FOR MEN ONLY

One treatment for obesity that someday may be routinely offered to middle-aged and older men is the hormone testosterone, available through either injection or a patch. As men age, their testosterone levels decline, and some scientists believe that beefing up levels of the hormone is a way of restoring some youthful properties, including a slimmer waist. A study of eleven men averaging forty-three years of age found that after six weeks of testosterone injections, nine of them had lost significant fat off their bellies. The study found no negative side effects, but testosterone supplementation is still quite experimental[31] and in any case probably won't help men who haven't reached middle age yet.

BLOCKERS

Yet another class of weight-loss drugs is called "blockers." They are so called because they block the absorption of either fats or carbohydrates. One of these currently in testing is tetrahydrolipstatin, with the trade names of Xenical and Orlistat. They block intestinal absorption of about a third of fat consumed, according to one of the researchers who has tested it, John Foreyt.[32] This inherently produces one side effect in that stools are greasy and noxious-smelling. (Please don't forget to flush the toilet if you're using this.) It can also cause diarrhea and increased flatulence. As you would guess, this is a slow method of losing weight, since fat makes up only about a third of our caloric intake, and therefore, what's being blocked is about a third of a third, or one ninth of total calories.

One carbohydrate blocker is acarbose, which under the name Glucobay is being considered by the FDA for treatment of diabetes. It's already marketed for this use in Europe and Japan. Like other blockers, it can cause gas, bloating, and diarrhea, though generally this disappears after six months. On the other hand, with symptoms such as these, it can be a long six months.

A problem with any kind of blocker, though, is that they may encourage people to eat even more than they otherwise would. If you know that a third of your fat is sliding out of you untouched by the digestive system, you may increase your fat intake by another third or even more. This leads us to one of the major problems with what has been touted by some as a miracle food, Procter & Gamble's (P&G's) olestra.

OLESTRA: NEITHER SATAN NOR (SIGH) SAVIOR

One way of decreasing calorie intake is to use artificial fat that the body doesn't recognize and hence doesn't digest. Although there are many forms of fat substitutes on the market, they tend to have little impact on obesity because they're only available in peripheral products, things you shouldn't be eating too much of anyway, like ice cream. Chief among these is Simplesse, which, because it breaks down when exposed to heat, is only available in frozen desserts. As such it isn't going to help fat people too much because these desserts tend to remain high in calories despite the addition of Simplesse.

But what if there were a fat substitute that could be baked into food or used for frying? That's what olestra is. Olestra is P&G's brand name for sucrose polyester, though it tastes nothing like sugar and also has nothing in common with those embarrassing clothes we wore in the seventies. According to most taste testers, foods made with olestra taste identical to those made with real fat. But to the body, olestra may as well be Teflon, since it literally slides trough the intestines without stopping off to visit arteries, hips, or waistlines. P&G petitioned the FDA to approve olestra only for salty snacks such as potato chips, nacho chips, and crackers, but it can also be baked into cookies and cakes. As such, it has potential to break through the "peripheral food" barrier.

Early in 1996 the FDA approved olestra over the objections of some scientists and consumer advocates, who warned that it has unusual risks.[33] Some studies have shown that as little as two ounces of olestra chips can act as a laxative. It can also cause other gastrointestinal difficulties including a condition called—*ahem!*— "anal leakage." But as such it will hardly be alone among favorite foods. If you eat more than a few prunes or other dried fruits at one sitting you may well find yourself doing several more sittings somewhere else.

In any event, the FDA approval requires labeling the product to this effect. My guess, though, is that the label will often be ignored by overzealous consumers—though probably ignored only once.

More alarming, perhaps, is olestra's ability to wash out of the body certain nutrients believed important for preventing disease. While P&G will fortify olestra with vitamins A, D, E, and K, it will not add back a controversial class of nutrients known as carotenoids, which many believe protect against cancer. P&G says evidence for that is lacking.

This nutrient depletion "could potentially produce a large number of deaths annually and major morbidity in the U.S. population," wrote Meir Stampfer, M.D., of Harvard University to the FDA.[34] But numerous recent studies have shown that the most popular carotenoid, beta carotene, appears to have no cancer-fighting effects.[35] Certainly one factor that boosts P&G's position is that for the most part, olestra can only wash out whatever went in with it. Eat spinach and Pringle's potato chips with olestra and you're going to lose the benefit of the spinach. Alas, people are a lot more likely to combine the potato chips with dip and a beer or soda pop than with nutritious vegetables.

But if olestra isn't the anti-Christ, it may not prove much of a savior, either. "By replacing the fat in snacks, Olean [the name under which P&G will license olestra] can help millions of Americans cut excess fat and move closer to achieving an important dietary health goal," said John Pepper, chairman of P&G.[36] I'd say more like thousands of Americans, and here's why. True, if you ate two ounces of potato chips cooked in olestra rather than fat, you'd have just 120 calories instead of 300. But if Americans ate that amount of chips, they wouldn't need fat substitutes in the first place and we wouldn't be the fattest industrial nation on the earth. Overeating is our problem, and olestra, far from curing it, will only encourage it among many people.

Consider the experience with artificial sweeteners such as saccharin and aspartame (NutraSweet), which provide virtually no calories. Their use tripled in the 1980s and should have caused sugar consumption to decline and caloric intake to decline. Instead, even as artificial sweetener consumption has increased, so has sugar intake, caloric intake, and Americans' waistlines.

Then there's the even newer fat substitute Z-Trim, developed by a very clever government scientist in Peoria, Illinois. All signs are that the food will not only "play in Peoria," but elsewhere in the United States as well. It's made by grinding "agricultural byproducts," which unlike dog food doesn't mean horse and pieces of cows nobody will eat, but rather oat and corn hulls. In other words, it's made of fiber. That makes Z-Trim not only not bad for you, but good for you. There's no indication that it has the gastrointestinal side effects of olestra, either. On other the hand, it can't be used for frying but supposedly works very well for baking. It can cut the calories of a brownie or cookie by half.[37] But again, many—and perhaps most—users will respond by eating at least twice as much.

That said, if you have the discipline to simply swap equal amounts of olestra- or Z-trim-containing foods for their fatty counterparts, you come out ahead of the game. It's a matter of free will and having the strength to exercise it.

BELAY THAT BINGE!

Binge eating is the consumption of a huge number of calories at one sitting. As discussed in chapter seven, it appears to be a major cause of diet failure and obesity in general. DuPont's antagonist drug naltrexone, an opium derivative, has promise in controlling binge eating. The drug is currently used in treating alcoholism, and Wayne State University pharmacologist Mary Ann Marrazzi reported in a 1995 issue of the *International Journal of Obesity* that it seems to interrupt bingers' cravings just as it does those of alcoholics.[38]

A cousin of naltrexone is naloxone, which is used in reducing the terrible side effects of heroin withdrawal. It made the newspapers in 1995 when University of Michigan nutritionist Adam Drewnowski and his colleagues gave the drug to binge eaters and found it made them eat an average of 160 fewer calories per meal.[39] But what really caught the media's attention was that the drug appeared to selectively block the craving for chocolate and other sweets in bingers, though not in normal eaters. At last, a cure for chocolate addiction! There's only one problem, though, and it's a big one. Currently naloxone can only be taken by injection. Only the most dedicated dieter is going to opt for a self-administered shot the next time a chocolate craving hits. Drewnowski says he's hoping that an ingestible form will eventually be made available. That is, unless the Nestlé, Cadbury, and Hershey companies buy the patent and kill the drug. (Yes, I'm just kidding. I think.)

THE CHROMIUM CAPER

In 1989, Minnesota researcher Gary Evans gave chromium supplements to football players and weight lifters and discovered absolutely phenomenal results, with both groups gaining vast amounts of muscle and losing gobs of fat. Thus began the chromium fad. The supplement is now hyped mercilessly by health food stores, "alternative" magazines, and original Brady Bunch mom Florence Henderson. You could call it a Very Brady Supplement. There's even a drink called "Fat Burner" that justifies its name on containing a bit of chromium. The metal also has its own book, Jeffrey Fischer's *The Chromium Program.*[40] It's another one of those diet books that could be summed up in a single sentence: Make sure you get enough chromium in your diet. That a lot of people shelled out $19.95 for the hardback shows that we truly are a wealthy nation.

The problem with the chromium hype is that repeated studies have failed to verify Evans's work. Notwithstanding this, he refuses to give in. This could be a result of his having been retained as a consultant by the chromium supplement industry, but far be it from me to suggest there may be a connection.

One problem with Evan's studies (he did two others) is that he used hand-held calipers to measure the students' fat, an inexact method. More importantly, his results were just *too* phenomenal. After just six weeks, those who took the chromium in Evans's main study had seemingly added six pounds of muscle and lost seven of fat. "Changes like that in such a short period of time are preposterous, as anyone familiar with training effects knows," says Robert Lefavi, who studies the mineral requirements of athletes at Armstrong State College in Savannah, Georgia. "You can't even get results like that using anabolic steroids."[41]

At least five studies have found no impact from chromium

supplements on fat loss or muscle gain.[42] And the studies continue to come in. The most recent such to appear in the journals as of this writing was in 1996 in *Medicine and Science in Sport and Exercise.* It put sixteen sedentary men, whose average age was twenty-three, through a twelve-week strength training program. Half received the standard recommended chromium supplement of 200 micrograms, while the others got a placebo. The result: No difference in strength, muscle tissue, or body fat. The only difference was that the men getting the supplement had high levels of the mineral in their urine, indicating they were just urinating away the excess.[43] Research on chromium for problems other than obesity (especially diabetes) have shown some promise. But if you think it's going to make you lose weight, you're just tinkling away your money.

Another widely sold diet supplement is something called hydroxycitrate, or hydroxycitric acid, or HCA for short. Since it's got such a long, scientific-sounding name and it comes all the way from India, naturally you figure it has to be effective. There is a bit of evidence that it may help rats slim up. That's a blessing if you know the heartbreak of having an overweight pet rat. But there appears to be nothing in the medical literature to indicate HCA causes human weight loss.[44] Apparently it's sort of like a dieter's urban legend. People think it works because it's sold; it's sold because people think it works.

ANOREXIANTS

Recall that anorexiants are drugs that reduce appetite. The word is obviously entymologically related to "anorexia" and "anorexic," but anorexiants do not cause anorexia. The most widely sold of these—indeed, the only one sold over the counter in the United States—is PPA. An amphetamine derivative, the anorectic effect of PPA was first described in 1939,[45] though it wasn't marketed widely until 1972 when it became available without a prescription. Numerous clinical trials have demonstrated it can help, at least a little. One recently showed patients on seventy-five milligrams of PPA a day losing over five and a half pounds over the study period versus less than two and a half pounds for those on a placebo.[46] A

1992 combination study of seven individual PPA studies found that PPA caused a weight loss of half a pound a week more than did placebos up to the fourth week. For the entire length of the studies the weight loss was slightly less than a third of a pound per week.[47]

The other over-the-counter drug sold in the United States for the express purpose of weight loss is benzocaine, which is thought to act by numbing taste, smell, and perhaps the sensations from the stomach that signal hunger. But the medical literature indicates it's nearly or completely worthless.[48] And at least one study comparing benzocaine to PPA found that the benzocaine users lost no weight. That same study also looked at a combination of PPA and benzocaine and found that the combination users lost no more than the placebo users.[49] So benzocaine can't be recommended.

Many anorexiants are what's known as serotonin reuptake inhibitors. Serotonin is a brain chemical that appears to govern a number of physical and emotional responses, especially the craving for carbohydrates. By inhibiting its reuptake (absorption and disposal by your system), it's possible to keep serotonin levels high and cravings low. The best known of all the drugs in this class is fluoxetine, commonly known as Prozac, the extremely popular antidepressant. Prozac itself has been tested for weight-loss purposes, but didn't work out.[50] On the other hand, older antidepressants such as Lithium can cause major weight gain, whereas Prozac does not.

Yet another anorexiant is mazindol, sold under the names Mazanor and Sanorex. I actually tried this drug and found it very effective—while it lasted. The first day I took it I simply forgot to eat. I lost weight rapidly. But after about three weeks the effect just quit and the pounds went right back on. Apparently the drug quickly induced tolerance; that is, my body started to counteract its effects. Nonetheless, it's apparent from clinical studies that some patients have had good effects for fifteen months or longer.[51]

REDUX RIDICULOUSNESS

The anti-obesity drug that everyone's talking about as I write this is dexfenfluramine, sold in the United States under the brand name

Redux. The reason for all the fuss is that it's the most recent weight-loss pharmaceutical to be approved by the FDA. Just as Steven Lamm and Gerald Couzens built a whole book around the weight-loss drug combination of phentermine and fenfluramine (phen/fen) in 1995,[52] in 1996 Sheldon Levine managed to produce a whole book about dexfenfluramine, called the *Redux Revolution: Everything You Need to Know About the Most Important Weight-Loss Discovery of the Century*.[53] He even refers to the drug as a "magic pill."[54] But let's get a couple of things straight right away.

First, the most important weight-loss discovery of the century is the one you make yourself when you discover there is no magic out there—no magic foods, no magic exercise devices, and no magic pills.

Second, to talk about Redux as revolutionary is sheer nonsense. It is a close chemical relative of fenfluramine, which has already been available in the United States for decades. It is believed to cause fewer side effects than fenfluramine, but already fenfluramine is a relatively benign drug, so there's only so much room for improvement. There is, so far as I know, no published evidence that it is more effective than the phen/fen combination that was widely prescribed in the United States for years. Levine doesn't tell you any of that. Nor does he tell you about the study I previously mentioned showing that a combination of ephedrine and caffeine may be more effective than dexfenfluramine. To the contrary, in a question-answer section of the book he responds to the question: "Does ephedrine cause weigh loss?" by citing a single 1985 *International Journal of Obesity* study that concluded in a trial that it didn't.[55] Note, he doesn't say outright that it's ineffective. He simply goes back eleven years to find one study that supports his position and ignores the myriad ones since then, even in the same journal. Why? Because it's darned hard to sell something as "revolutionary" when it may be inferior to drugs that have long been available and are far cheaper.

Levine's book is also reprehensible in that he appears to blame all obesity on "the obesity gene" (apparently ignorant that there are several known obesity genes), saying in the first few pages that its discovery means that saying " 'eat less and exercise more' is no longer a viable treatment for overweight people."[56] Taking in fewer calories and burning off more is in fact the *only* way to compensate for any genetic predisposition a person may have toward excess weight. I have written elsewhere in this book that people pushing exercise will often downplay the nutrition side of obesity while people pushing nutrition will often downplay the exercise side. Here we see someone pushing pharmaceuticals downplay both. In fact, Levine flat out tells you that "there is ample evidence that exercise does not cause weight loss."[57] This is not to say that Levine is trying to sell Redux the drug, merely his book about Redux.

Everybody's trying to sell you something, aren't they? Later on in his book, by the way, long after saying that eating less and exercising more doesn't work for fat people, Levine tells you that the way to lose weight is by eating less and exercising more—so long as you do it while taking Redux.[58]

So what is the truth about this drug? A review of dexfenfluramine studies has found that overall it appears to reduce daily energy intake by about 10 to 15 percent in most patients and alters the size of meals and the pattern of meal taking and snacking.[59] There is evidence that it reduces the consumption of fat and carbohydrate particularly in snacks, and that it may especially inhibit the eating of fatty foods. It doesn't make your body do anything special with the food you eat; it just makes you eat less. In obese patients it appears to continue to reduce body weight even after significant weight reduction has already taken place on a low-calorie diet.[60]

In a one-year clinical trial carried out in sixteen clinics across Europe, dexfenfluramine gradually reduced body weight over six months and maintained the weight loss for a further half year. When the drug was withdrawn, patients' weight began to climb, indicating that the drug had still been working after twelve months of continuous use.[61]

During the FDA hearings, dexfenfluramine came under fire from people who feared it may prove harmful. In 1994, George Ricaurte, M.D., and his associates at Johns Hopkins University in Baltimore published a study indicating that doses of dexfenfluramine twenty times higher than what humans use produced brain damage in squirrel monkeys after use had stopped.[62] A short while later, though, a second study—conducted on mice by the Environmental Protection Agency—refuted the Johns Hopkins results.

"We noted no neurotoxic effect," said James O'Callahan, M.D., who performed the research.[63]

Another doctor who has expressed concern about dexfenfluramine is Lewis Seiden, a pharmacologist at the University of Chicago. He was one of several critics who testified against approval of the drug before the FDA advisory panel. He said his studies have shown that lab animals had depleted levels of serotonin for months after they had stopped taking the drug. In humans, that could be expected to produce a sudden severe depression or bursts of impulsive behavior, he said. In rats, he said, the levels of serotonin "stay down weeks and months after we stopped giving the drug."[64] Still, the FDA is an extremely conservative organization. If it considered all the evidence and approved dexfenfluramine, that carries a lot of weight.

After the FDA approval, further evidence came out that Redux when used for three months or longer may greatly increase the risk of developing something called primary pulmonary hypertension, a sort of high blood pressure in the lungs that can cause heart attacks. An August 1996 study in which most of the persons looked at had used dexfenfluramine (though some had used fenfluramine and some had used other weight-loss drugs) found they had twenty-three times the chance of developing the disease as those not on the drugs.[65] The good news is that the condition is extremely rare, and multiplying a rare condition even by such a high number still gives you something that doesn't happen too often. Using the study's numbers, I calculated that risk of contracting the illness from weight-loss drugs as being around 1 in 17,000. By comparison, your lifetime risk as an American of *dying* in a car crash is about 1 in 70. An accompanying editorial by Harvard's JoAnn Manson, M.D., the chief researcher of the Nurses' Health Study, and by Gerald A. Faich of the University of Pennsylvania took issue with some of the study's methodology but, more important, calculated that for every life lost because of using the drug, probably twenty would be saved.[66] What I would really warn you about isn't so much the health risks of Redux but the hype risks.

Baylor's G. Ken Goodrick told me: "I'm not recommending [Redux] to any of my patients until research shows that it's better than phen/fen." I agree. Phen/fen is far cheaper, has been tested far longer in this country for safety, and may be as effective or more so than Redux. Even Sheldon Levine deep enough into his book admits, "It is still premature to assume that Redux should be used on a daily basis for more than a few months at a time."[67] Now he tells us! I don't think there's any cause for going on Redux unless you've tried phen/fen and have had no success.

THE PHEN/FEN PHENOMENON

So let's talk more about this phen/fen stuff. This combination of drugs also has its own book, *Thinner at Last*, authored by the afore-mentioned Lamm and Couzens. This one at least is honest, but it's just a little science with a whole lot of silly padding.[68] Save yourself $23 and just read what I have to say about it.

Fenfluramine, sold under the brand name of Pondimin, appears to partially inhibit the reuptake of serotonin and to release serotonin from nerve endings.[69] Approved by the FDA in 1972, the drug makes users feel less hungry before eating and feel full after eating less food. Its major side effect appears to be causing a chronic dryness of the mouth. Less often, patients report diarrhea, short-term memory loss, sleepiness, and lethargy. If the drug is withdrawn suddenly it may also prompt depression.[70]

Phentermine, sold under the brand names of Fastin and Ion-amin, was also approved by the FDA in 1972. It is a mild stimulant that boosts a different brain chemical called norepinephrine. Apparently this action causes users to eat less. Phentermine has been reported to cause anxiety, sleeplessness, heart palpitations, tremors, and irritability in some users.[71] It may also raise blood pressure. It is not recommended for patients with glaucoma, high blood pressure, or cardiovascular problems.

Both drugs may be effective separately but appear to be far more effective in combination. Not only do their weight-control characteristics seem to enhance each other but their side effects to an extent are balanced. That is, the slight stimulation that phen-termine gives makes up for the slight depressive effect of fenfluramine.

Way back when the FDA approved these drugs, it did so only for three months of continuous use. Since then it has become apparent that if the drug is stopped after three months or any other period, the weight lost will probably come right back. As a result, doctors commonly prescribe it for longer periods or even indefinitely. This is legal and probably because it's already so common the FDA hasn't bothered to go back and review whether it should drop the three-month limit.

The person most widely associated with advocating phen/fen is Michael Weintraub, formerly with the University of Rochester and now with the FDA. In a landmark 1984 study in which he put obese patients on a combination of a half dose of each drug, he found they met with more success than previous groups had when using full doses of either drug. The subjects, who ranged from 130 to 180 percent ideal body weight, lost twice as much of that excess weight during a twenty-four-week test period as similar patients on a placebo.[72]

Other studies have continued to show the promise of the drug combination. In a 1992 study, which Weintraub also headed, obese patients receiving the combination lost during a period of thirty-four weeks almost 16 percent of their body weight, averaging thirty-one pounds lost. This compared to those on the placebo who lost just 5 percent of their body weight, averaging ten pounds lost.[73]

Many persons absolutely swear by the drug combination. "I used to go crazy for certain foods. I'd want ice cream or Mexican food. And I'd want it immediately," one woman told a reporter. "Now I've completely lost the urge to eat between meals." According to the woman, she'd lost forty-six pounds in the year and a half she'd been on the drugs.[74] Such anecdotes have limited reliability—unless, of course, they're your own. And I have my own because I tried this drug combination. It really did work. By the second day my appetite was noticeably curbed and within a week it was clear I was losing weight. I can't say that there were specific foods I was craving less, just that I seemed to eat less frequently and in smaller portions. I only noticed two side effects. One was dry mouth—*very* dry mouth. It was irritating at first, but gradually subsided. The other was that for the first week I was definitely euphoric. In fact, I almost got in trouble at a fair because somebody mistook my giddiness for being drunk. But that subsided. Too bad.

Then I went off the drug and watched with horror as my weight went back up just as quickly as it had gone down, if not more so. I was eating everything I could lay my hands on. So why did I quit? First, because I didn't want to spend the rest of my life on a drug unless it was absolutely necessary. Second, I had just begun researching this book and was coming to believe that even in this day and age, an overweight American could bring himself or herself down to the proper weight and maintain it and do it without drugs. I would be a guinea pig. And as I've noted previously, my belief was right. The more I learned, the more weight I lost. Not so quickly as with the drugs, but eventually I got considerably lower than I had with the drugs.

It does appear there's a limit to how much weight you can lose with these pharmaceuticals. A 1994 medical journal review of phentermine, fenfluramine, and dexfenfluramine found that all these drugs were effective in bringing about more weight loss than placebos and more weight loss than dieting alone, but it also found that weight loss didn't continue past the six-month mark. This isn't the same as developing tolerance to the drugs, since true tolerance means the drug doesn't work anymore and the weight would be regained. Such was my experience with mazindol. In most of the studies reviewed, with most of the patients the weight loss just stopped at some point and the drug simply helped people maintain that new level.[75]

In any case, I know phen/fen works. So why aren't more people using it, especially now that it's been getting tremendous publicity? And why are some people who have been using it successfully quitting? Said Baylor's John Foreyt of his phen/fen study that began with 1,200 people: "We're finding enormous numbers of people dropping out and we don't know why." He says it may be the cost, but as far as drugs go, phen/fen isn't really that expensive and you could easily save more money from reduced grocery and restaurant bills than you spend on the pills. In any case, "If it's working you'd think people would pay the money," Foreyt told me, adding, "They [the drugs] clearly do work, there's no question."[76]

I think the answer to this puzzle is a sad one. My guess is that Americans by and large don't want a drug that makes them eat less. They want a drug that allows them to eat *more*, but not gain weight. In one case I tried hard to make an obese friend in his fifties (meaning heart attack range) try phen/fen, to no avail. I gave him articles filled with glowing testimonials about the drugs. I told him it worked for me and he saw for himself the evidence on my own body. But nothing doing. He's a gourmet; food is an integral part of his life and he wasn't going to give up any part of it. With drugs such as phen/fen, the pharmaceutical industry has brought the horse to water, but it can't make him drink. Americans continue to hold out for a drug that allows them to eat like pigs and look like storks. They're not going to get it any time soon, but that doesn't stop them from dreaming. Then came leptin.

LUCKY LEPTIN?

"Researchers have discovered what they hope will be a magic bullet for obesity, or at least the forerunner of major new therapies. . . ." So began a front-page *New York Times* piece on the "miracle" hormone leptin.[77] The article discussed a study that appeared in *Science* magazine in July 1995. High doses of the synthesized hormone caused mice to go from Jackie Gleason to Art Carney in a matter of weeks.[78] This sparked a celebration throughout the media. "Just think: You could gorge yourself on ice cream, potato chips, tacos," gushed a *St. Petersburg* (Florida) *Times* editorial. "Then just pop a miracle pill, and your worries are over. . . . The world would be couch-potato heaven."[79]

Ah . . . Eat, drink, and be merry, for tomorrow there's a drug, right? Reality check.

The first little problem with leptin is that the "pill" is actually injections, possibly daily, for life. No big deal? Ask any insulin-dependent diabetic. Diabetics die every day or lose limbs because they didn't take their shots as often as they should, or not at all. Shots hurt and you never get to a point where they don't. The difference between leanness and simple obesity is about the equivalent of a McDonald's Big Mac. Probably few of us would cherish trading sandwiches for shots.

Then there's the efficacy issue. Leptin works wonders on rotund rodents and perhaps Mickey will soon have heard the last of Minnie's teasing about his "beer cheese belly." But mice are not small men. Medical literature is replete with instances of drugs that cured or killed rodents yet had no effect on humans.

Recent research by José Caro, M.D., and his colleagues at Thomas Jefferson Medical Center in Philadelphia has found that obese people actually already have far higher levels of leptin than do lean ones.[80] This could mean that leptin is useless as a weight regulator in humans. Or, as Caro told me, the situation could be like Type I diabetes, in which sufferers have high levels of insulin but are resistant to its effects and therefore must be given much more insulin. Maybe a massive dose of leptin would work on obese humans, says Caro. "But that is an optimistic view. It may also not work."[81]

Indeed, a month after the leptin headlines, *The New York Times* carried an article beginning, "A natural substance that made headlines last month for slimming down overweight mice may not do the same for highly obese people, new research suggests."[82] The article cited two studies in the September 1995 issue of *Nature Medicine*.[83] In them, it was estimated that fat people might have twenty to thirty times the amount of leptin that lean people do. Researcher Bradford Hamilton, a Ph.D. candidate at the Sunny-brook Health Science Center in North York, Ontario, suggested it was possible that the receptors in very fat people are so defective they cannot respond to leptin. If so, injecting them with even more would be futile. "If the receptor is expecting Chinese, it doesn't matter how much you scream at it in English, it's still not going to understand the message," he put it colorfully.[84] At this writing, two studies have looked at this problem, one seeming to find such a defective receptor and one not.[85]

So "couch-potato heaven" is a long way off, at the very least. But then, the couch just isn't heaven. The human body was meant to be exercised. It's not meant to become a trash receptacle for any amount of any gunk that any food manufacturer can come up with. Big waists and fat thighs aren't just a problem in and of themselves; they are also a marker for other problems—those not necessarily caused by obesity but accompanying them. As Yale researcher Kelly Brownell commented upon hearing of leptin's possible efficacy, "Even if a person could eat all the bad food he wants and be thin, what about diet's contribution to heart disease and cancer?"[86]

In the meantime, for those of us who need help right now in controlling our appetites, the help is there with the drugs and drug combinations I've discussed. But it has yet to make any impact on the national obesity problem and quite possibly never will. The use of pharmaceuticals to control weight will probably parallel the use of birth control pills. Although the Pill is remarkably effective, out-of-wedlock pregnancies have nonetheless skyrocketed since its introduction. Why? Because the culture that discouraged such pregnancies broke down. Likewise, so long as we live in a culture that encourages overconsumption and under-exertion, Americans will become fatter regardless of what the drug companies produce.

11

Defatting the

Land

Not long ago I was standing outside my podiatrist's office wearing a postsurgical wooden shoe. The doctor was late and soon another patient showed up, a woman about five and a half feet tall weighing about 300 pounds. She asked me about my foot. "They had to remove a piece of nerve," I said. "It's actually the third time. The first two times it regenerated. Yes, I know nerves aren't supposed to regenerate; just call me a freak of nature." I then asked, "Why are *you* here?" She answered that she had a mysterious pain on her right foot. "Lady," I said. "Your feet appear to be about two-thirds the size of mine and yet you weigh probably more than twice as much as I do. With all that pressure you're putting on your feet, maybe you should be thinking the real mystery is why your left foot doesn't hurt."

No, I didn't actually say that part. That was up to her doctor to point out, and I hope he did.[1] For he may be able to help her somewhat with the foot problem, but in a few years it's probably going to be knee problems. Then maybe diabetes. Then heart disease. Then maybe cancer. Medical science can only do so much to protect us from ourselves, as smokers find out when the doctor tells them they have lung cancer and their odds of surviving it are slim. Even though I proclaim this book to be the first trade (popular press) book dealing with obesity as a *national problem,* I don't think that I am being inconsistent in saying that the most important factor in solving this national problem is the action of individuals. Yes, we live in a society that's a conveyor belt to obesity. But some of us have gotten off, and all of us have an obligation to try.

Remember that obesity is a socially contagious disease. If you improve your eating and exercise habits, there's an excellent chance other members of your family will, too. Other people will see you and if they are fat they will no longer be able to take comfort in thinking, "Oh well, there goes another person who's as fat as I am." You will serve as proof that, even in the America of the late 1990s, it is possible to be in good shape.

We have to realize also that there will be no quick fixes, that our personal weight problems and the obesity epidemic can't be stopped with a five-day miracle diet or working out three minutes a day with an "ab" device or just "eating, breathing, and moving" or by simply adjusting the amount of fat, protein, and carbohydrates in diets. And we need to spread the word. If you have a friend who's in the process of buying into the latest fad, you have a responsibility to set him or her straight, not just roll your eyes toward the ceiling.

RECOGNIZING THE PROBLEM

If the first step is looking after ourselves, the next is recognizing how great a national problem obesity is and that it's not going away on its own. Unfortunately, we are only now getting to that point. A huge number of us are still in denial about the health risks of obesity. As I write this, three new denial books have appeared recently.[2] Others acknowledge obesity as a personal health problem but deny its importance nationally, thereby relegating it to a simple matter of choice and assumption of the risk.

Australia's Dale Atrens, in his 1988 book *Don't Diet*, insists those who warn of the growing national and international obesity problem are part of the "fascist, orthodox medical establishment" you see.[3] "Instead of fatness being a new epidemic," he writes, "we are probably merely witnessing a gradual shift to a new body-composition profile for most of our species."[4] Those who object to this change he accuses of imitating Adolf Hitler's attempts to create an *Übermensch,* a master race.

But the analogy doesn't work. Those of us who decry industrial societies getting fatter by the year aren't trying to create a trend; we're trying to *stop* one. Far from trying to build an *Übermensch,* we're just combating those who, like Atrens, celebrate the coming of an *Untermensch (über* means "above"; *unter* means "below"): a species that requires ever greater volumes of medicine to survive, that can't walk more than a hundred feet without huffing and puffing, that gets worn out after just a few minutes of playing with the children, that suffers from poor hygiene from places on the body that can't be seen or reached. Already there are people who ride in electric wheelchairs and motorized scooters for no other reason than with their great bulk they find it easier to do so. As the population fattens, more and more of us will find we can do nothing without the aid of mechanics. As the population fattens, we will hear more and more stories about thousand-pound men being cut out of their homes and taken to the hospital. And then we'll stop hearing about it because it will become too common-place to make the news. What Atrens also doesn't acknowledge is that this new *Untermensch* isn't just settling in at twenty or thirty pounds overweight. It appears that half a ton may indeed be the upper limit for human obesity and every year more of us move ever closer to that limit.

The Institute of Medicine (IOM), an arm of the National Academy of Sciences, in its 1995 book *Weighing the Options,* says its "first policy recommendation is that there be a change in thinking in this country by the public and health-care providers alike to treat obesity as an important chronic, degenerative disease that debilitates individuals and kills prematurely."[5]

STOP PLAYING GAMES WITH PEOPLE'S FEARS

Obesity continues to get short shrift as a problem, in great part because so many other things get disproportionately "long shrift"— an expression I probably just invented.[6] There were two major themes running through both of my previous books, one on AIDS and one on environmental scares.[7] First, if you overemphasize smaller risks, you underemphasize larger risks; you then end up losing more lives from the risk you underplayed than you saved from the risk you overplayed. Second, if you lie to people by exaggerating lesser risks, they're not going to believe you when you jump up and down and turn red in the face and swear that *this time* you're telling the truth. It is with no sense of self-satisfaction to see that with the obesity epidemic, the chickens are coming home to roost on both counts.

Thus, in my environmental book I talked about how expenditures on tiny or even non-existent risks denied funds for much higher but non-environmental risks. I provided the story of how I and my girlfriend were driving in a car that went off a cliff on California's Pacific Coast Highway. She suffered massive head injuries and a broken neck, and came within a hair's width of death, retardation, and paralysis. All this because a state that spends more per capita on environmental regulations than any other state in the nation didn't have $1,000 for a 100-foot stretch of guard rail where, I later learned, there had been previous fatal accidents.[8]

As to the issue of lying, many critics of my AIDS book said it was perfectly OK to lie so long as it fulfilled whatever particular end they desired, whether increasing research funds for the disease, making heterosexuals more sensitive to the plight of homosexuals and drug users, or getting heterosexuals to postpone sex until marriage. I replied that in addition to lying being simply wrong, if you lie about this major health problem, people aren't going to believe you in the future when you try to tell them about a health risk that has a very real chance of killing them.

But scares of the week continue to fly at us unabated, with virtually nobody bothering to engage in any risk analysis and with lots of special interest groups and reporters justifying wild exaggerations on the basis that a little white lie here and there will accomplish good ends. Yet all of these sap the nation's funds, harm the credibility of scientists and science in general, and destroy the ability of people to make intelligent risk-avoiding decisions.

The IOM cites a classic example. In 1989, the government issued its Diet and Health report recommending more consumption of fruits and vegetables. At that time, however, the Natural Resources Defense Council (NRDC) launched an all-out campaign to convince the public that children were being excessively exposed to chemicals on fruits and vegetables, especially Alar on apples.[9] The NRDC had the full support of the media, especially CBS's *60 Minutes*, which first aired the allegations.[10] The panic was so great that parents flooded their family physicians with calls.[11] Two weeks later the shipment of all fruit from Chile was halted when two Chilean grapes were found to have been injected with cyanide. Grapes followed apples into the trash. Thus, by not giving their children fruit, parents ended up raising the risk of their children getting cancer and other illnesses in an effort to lower it.[12]

In 1995, the Gallup organization found that more than half of women surveyed named cancer as their greatest health threat. Yet heart disease kills almost twice as many women as cancer. Women "fear breast cancer more. They worry more about getting AIDS. They hear more about domestic violence," said Debra Judelson, a spokeswoman for the American Medical Women's Association, commenting on the poll.[13] There are no heart disease activist groups. But there is an AIDS activist group on every corner and a breast cancer activist group on every other block. Environmental groups are always trying to tie this or that manmade chemical to cancer. But heart disease and obesity, because they are so universal, don't have activist groups.

And the media can always be counted on to take its cues from the activists. So it was that on a September 1996 *ABC Nightly News* broadcast, in a segment focusing on a women's health, this same 1995 Gallup poll was discussed. Yet even though the segment began with a camera shot of five or six extremely obese female survivors of heart attacks, nowhere in the entire segment was obesity mentioned as a risk factor.[14]

Meanwhile the nation's largest consumer group, Consumers Union (publisher of *Consumer Reports*), has done little to combat obesity. What they have done is to scare the hell out of people over much lesser or non-existent risks such as Alar, passive smoking, and household radon. *Consumer Reports* repeatedly warned readers of the threat of Alar, saying it could result in one child in 20,000 contracting cancer.[15] This, while scientists were insisting that Alar posed no threat whatsoever.[16] But don't look for the magazine to warn its readers about the dangers of obesity any time soon: Its editorial director is Joel Gurin, co-author of the highly influential 1982 fat acceptance book *The Dieter's Dilemma*.[17]

When it comes to what health problems they should be worried about, people—and especially parents—are simply overwhelmed. They know that some of these scares are real and others false, but have little ability to tell one from the other. Too often they simply end up ignoring them all.

Efforts to mobilize the population against obesity are even crippled by campaigns against what are clearly serious, population-wide problems. For example, smoking is the main cause of self-inflicted disease in this country and as such deserves constant attention. On the other hand, in 1996 the Alexandria, Virginia-based Media Research Center counted every evening news story during the first six months of the year that had to do with tobacco or with obesity and dietary fat. Given that tobacco prematurely kills 400,000 Americans and obesity 300,000, the center opined, "It's reasonable to assume that there are three news stories about [dietary fat and obesity] for every four news stories about tobacco and the tobacco industry, right?" Wrong. Instead, they counted 138 stories about tobacco and the tobacco industry, "all of which portrayed tobacco as a risk product. There were only 38 stories about dietary fat and obesity" that discussed the risk to consumers.[18]

In an August 1996 edition of the Sunday newspaper supplement *USA Weekend*, an interview with David Kessler, then the FDA administrator, showed a photo of him at a 1995 press conference with HHS Secretary Donna Shalala. Next to where they're standing is a large bar graph labeled, "Annual Deaths from Smoking and Other Preventable Causes." There's a huge bar for smoking and tiny bars for the other seven causes listed. Where's the bar for obesity? It's not there.[19] An obesity bar on the graph would destroy the nice imagery of one huge, preventable cause of death against seven tiny ones. In other words, it might prove a distraction from Kessler's war on tobacco. Indeed, in the public policy sphere Kessler has done practically nothing about obesity, even though on a personal basis he took it seriously enough to lose fifty-five pounds. It doesn't help when the head of the FDA and the nation's top health official ignore obesity because it isn't convenient to the crusade at hand.

OBESITY AS A REFLECTION
OF SOCIETAL PROBLEMS

The next step is acknowledging that long before our waistlines began to balloon we were building a society that promotes values that themselves promote obesity. "This population-wide problem [of obesity]," editorialized Northwestern University epidemiologist Jeremiah Stamler, M.D. in the *Archives of Internal Medicine*, "like others of its kind, is best comprehended as a *societal* problem, rooted in what was referred to earlier as '. . . disturbances in human culture.' "[20] Likewise, stated the IOM's *Weighing the Options*, "The root of the problem . . . must lie in the powerful social and cultural forces that promote an energy-rich diet and a sedentary lifestyle. But if social and cultural forces can promote obesity, these same forces should be able to control it. Therein lies the still unrealized potential for preventing obesity."[21]

The obesity epidemic isn't just an isolated problem in America; it's also the symptom of various problems, of various trends that continue to gain steam. One is the cult of victimization, in which everything not right in our lives is somebody or something else's fault. The British magazine *The Economist* observed with bemusement that in the United States, "If you lose your job you can sue for the mental distress of being fired. If your bank goes broke, the government has insured your deposits," even if you didn't pay for that insurance, as was the case with the S&L bailout. "If you drive drunk and crash, you can sue somebody for failing to warn you to stop drinking. There is always somebody else to blame."[22] But you can't sue your ancestors, so you just curse them for giving you a "fat gene" that you've never been tested for but you "just know" you must have it. It's not your fault that there's three hours of TV programming every night that you simply *must* watch. It's not your fault that the restaurant serves portions big enough for a Boy Scout troop and since it's there you *have to* eat it all. It's not your fault that you're fat; that's just the way it is.

Another trend is the self-esteem movement, in which we are told that we must not do anything to make anyone have anything less than a glowing opinion of himself or herself. This cult has made its greatest inroads in education. Some schools now have as many as twenty-six valedictorians.[23] Twenty-eight percent of college-bound seniors in 1972 reported having an A or B high school average, while by 1993 it was 83 percent—even as the average SAT score fell by 35 percent during the same period.[24] "Feeling good is an inalienable right," Steven Muller, former president of Johns Hopkins University, said sardonically. "Negative characterizations such as stupid, lazy, or dumb are offensive violations of the newly defined American right to individual self-esteem."[25] The result is such anomalies as American students who rank last in international comparisons of math abilities yet rank first when asked how they feel about their math abilities.[26] But the cult is moving into the obesity world, too, with books like *Self-Esteem Comes in All Sizes*,[27] and fat activist groups calling themselves "The Network for Self-Esteem."

The underpinning of the cult is that there's clearly a connection between high self-esteem and accomplishment, but the cultists have the causality switched around. High self-esteem no more leads to accomplishment than opening an umbrella makes it rain.[28] The basis for all self-improvement and advancement is a perceived *need* to improve or advance. Telling people that, whatever their current condition, all they need do is feel good about it locks them firmly into place. False self-esteem for schoolkids leads to dumbness and dead-end jobs; false self-esteem for the obese simply leads to death.

The whole notion of self-esteem being all or nothing is also foolish. A normal, healthy-minded human being has certain things about which he is proud and others which he wishes to change. Myself, I have a lot to be proud of. I've become a success in a very tough field, I'm really a nice guy once you get to know me, and I've got a Claudia Schiffer calendar that she personally signed for me. On the other hand, for the longest time I was disgusted with my inability to get my weight down to a healthy level. But for that disgust, I wouldn't have lost the weight and you wouldn't be reading this book. Not long ago I had a terrible yelling problem, the brunt of which was borne by my girlfriend. Oh sure, I could have blamed my upbringing; after all, in my parents' house yelling was the main form of communication. I could have blamed my genes; they're finding a gene for everything else these days, why not one for yelling? I could have blamed my Italian-American heritage. (I'll probably get a nasty letter from Mario Cuomo or some anti-defamation league for saying this, but it does seem like a lot of us shout and lose our tempers.) Or I could have smiled sweetly and said, "That's just the way I am, and if you say anything negative about it you'll harm my self-esteem."

What's wrong is that none of these reasons solved the underlying problem of my girlfriend being yelled at. Instead I took full responsibility for my own actions, I got therapy, and today I only yell when my computer crashes—for which no apology is requested or offered. Yes, perfection is an impossible and foolish goal, but a goal that says "Tomorrow I want to be a better person than I am today" is both obtainable and worthwhile. The touchy-feely self-esteem cult does for personal progress what emphysema does for deep breathing.

Yet another harmful trend is the overveneration of personal autonomy. America has always placed great value on individuality and personal freedom of choice. It's no coincidence that we lead the world in entrepreneurialism. On the other hand, we're also at the top when it comes to all sorts of nasty things like killing each other. What we have increasingly forgotten in recent decades is that because we are allowed to do something, it doesn't necessarily make it right. Because there is no school dress code forbidding you to wear pants ten sizes too big and expose your boxer shorts to the world doesn't make it OK to do so. It's great that we don't live in a country where the government can punish you for looking or acting like an idiot; but that doesn't mean you should go ahead and look or act like an idiot.

Nobody's arguing that it should be illegal to be such a glutton and such a sloth that you can't get around without an electric scooter. But neither should we pretend that it's a choice on a par with picking a red car over a blue one. Actions that we all agree should be perfectly legal and tolerated nevertheless can be wrong.

The absurdity of these trends is most apparent when we apply them to our own children. Families were never meant to be democracies. It is the duty of parents to continually exert pressure to bring up their children to be intelligent, well behaved, responsible, thrifty, and compassionate. And, yes, healthy. Rosemary Green, author of *Diary of a Fat Housewife*, told me that parents are always saying to her that their children won't eat healthy food. Her reply? "I advise them to hold out a hand to their child and say, 'Put your hand next to mine. Now, whose is bigger? Mommy is going to tell you what you can eat because Mommy is bigger.' "[29]

It would be one thing for me to just sigh when I see my super-sized neighbor lying next to the pool with a super-sized bag of potato chips next to him and a super-sized soda balanced on his belly. It would be quite another to do the same with my son or daughter. We are sacrificing our children in the names of such fads as self-esteem and overveneration of personal freedom. A 1996 poll showed that a teenager's likelihood of using drugs was directly related to how resigned the parent was that the child was going to go ahead and use them, no matter what.[30] "What is infuriating," said Joseph Califano, director of the National Center on Addiction and Substance Abuse, which group commissioned the poll, "is the resignation of so many parents to the present mess."[31] I hear you, guy. And it's the same with obesity.

How ludicrous it is that the director of nutrition for a school district in southern California says one of her "biggest" problems is that high school kids want their French fries fried, when baked ones are so much healthier.[32] Lady, you tell them that baked fries are all that's on the menu. Problem solved. Now the schools can concentrate on the "little" problems, like violence and teenage pregnancies.

Somewhere along the way, Western societies, especially America, have forgotten that there is a value in both moderation and setting limits. "Controlling of appetites is a fundamental role of religion because without that no civilization can flourish," a rabbi friend told me. "The mugger, robber, murderer, and rapist are all in the grip of their appetites. Hence, God's very first commandment was a dietary law—not to eat the fruit of the special tree. Which tree? Who cares? Just so you can start learning limits."[33]

One needn't be Jewish or Christian or religious at all to see the value in setting certain limits, or to see that setting limits can, in fact, be liberating. But we as individuals often falter, which is why society has traditionally played a role. "Communities of all sorts and sizes make and keep their members moral by harnessing their fear of rejection or disapproval by other members of the group," wrote contemporary British philosopher Linda Woodhead.[34] Unfortunately, society continues to move steadily away from its traditional role.

At some point, society is going to have to step in and say enough of this nonsense. "Society cannot exist," said eighteenth-century British statesman Edmund Burke, "unless a controlling power upon will and appetite be placed somewhere, and the less of it there is within, the more there must be without."[35] It's ironic for our purposes that he chose the word "appetite." Baylor's G. Ken Goodrick, who treats obese patients, has come up with a related observation. Obesity is "a sociocultural condition," he says. "We need to change society. I see obesity as a subset of the problem that a democratic free society can't exist unless people in it believe in self-respect and certain moral principles. If we move away from self-respect toward self-pity, we're going to end up as fat slaves of thin hordes from the east."[36]

But I think the tide is beginning to turn against rampant self-indulgence and the various cults of victimization, self-esteem, and false tolerance. It wasn't all that long ago that it was fashionable to reject out of hand any attempt to speak in terms of right and wrong. "Isn't that a value judgment?" people would sneer at you. But by the mid-1990s it was rapidly becoming more accepted that "value judgments" have value.

Let me emphasize that this doesn't mean oppressing fat people. During World War I, the British government had pretty young women hand white feathers to men on the street who weren't in uniform. In Britain, the white feather is a sign of cowardice. Surely many a young man ended up in the trenches out of shame over being handed one of these. I'm not saying we should now employ pretty young women and handsome young men to hand obese people of the opposite sex little plastic pig figurines. (I even turned down a bribe from the ACME Little Plastic Pig Figurine Company, Inc., for not making this recommendation.)

On the other hand, as I've already noted, society has built-in biologically based prejudices against obesity, especially extreme obesity. We should not use our laws or the media to try to break those down. Articles in *GQ* magazine that try to make employers look oppressive when they ask 600-pound men not to sit on their sofa do not help. Laws that would force the military to accept women who weigh twice what they should do not help. Hollywood producers who glorify obesity and treat it as just another handicap, like a leg that was blown off in Vietnam, do not help. Morning news shows that put fat acceptance people on opposite obesity scientists to discuss medical aspects of obesity do not help. Television ads urging owners of overweight dogs to put them on special diets, which nonetheless show the owner as being obese, do not help. Huge HMOs like Kaiser-Permanente allowing fat acceptance people to indoctrinate their doctors do not help. *Newsweek* magazine cover stories that get their information from fat acceptance advocates and urge, "Don't Worry. Be Fat and Happy!" do not help.[37]

THE ANTI-TOBACCO PARADIGM

I think perhaps the best model for a societal campaign against obesity should resemble that of the anti-smoking campaign prior to late 1993. At that point I think the anti-tobacco campaign got out of hand, with sweeping—almost vicious—legislation across the country designed to put smokers on a level just above child molesters and force them to sneak cigarettes like schoolchildren. But well before these draconian measures, in the course of a couple of decades, we cut the number of smokers in half. We did it with barrages of warnings, we did it by limiting tobacco advertising, but mostly we did it by making smoking gauche, uncouth, nasty. We didn't take away the right to smoke; we took away the right to not be embarrassed about smoking.

We need to make overeating gauche. We need to learn to sneer at twenty-four-ounce steaks, sixty-four-ounce sodas, monster muffins, and chocolate bars that pretend to be health foods because they have 30 percent less fat than the average amount found in the ten leading brands.

We need to make TV addiction gauche. The standard response to somebody who can outline the plots of the last ten episodes of *Friends* and *Melrose Place* should be "Get a life." Or to put it more politely, perhaps, to ask with a concerned tone of voice if that's really setting a good example for the kids. In short, gluttony and sloth ought once more to become things of which people are made to feel ashamed.

We also need more nutrition activist groups. For practically any cause you can name, there are numerous such groups: animal rights, human rights, homeless rights, abortion rights, anti-abortion, gay rights, antigay rights, free speech rights, spotted owl rights, kangaroo rat rights, ad infinitum. There are so many anti-tobacco groups it's utterly impossible to list them. But the number of anti-obesity activist groups? All of two of them: the Center for Science in the Public Interest (CSPI), and the more recently formed C. Everett Koop's Shape Up America, which so far hasn't been very active. Unfortunately, in the last couple of years I believe CSPI has steadily progressed in the direction of irresponsible grandstanding and has moved away from its original intent of protecting consumers. Its campaign against the fat substitute olestra had nothing to do with science and nothing to do with public interest.[38] They need to get back to the basics. At this time I would like to see two consumer groups for whom I have done work, Consumer Alert and the American Council on Science and Health—both of whom have been severe critics of CSPI—commit major resources to the fight against obesity. If they don't like CSPI's tactics, what better way to undercut them than by approaching the same issue from a different angle?

We need people who will instigate letter-writing campaigns against fast-food restaurants that keep coming up with devilishly larger sandwiches. Arby's needs to be told that its new Giant Beef 'n' Cheddar sandwich *isn't* better, just bigger. McDonald's stores need to be put on notice that when they double the number of quarter-pound hamburger patties on a bun, they're hurting people—or rather helping people hurt themselves. Likewise, 7-Eleven should be shamed into abandoning sixty-four-ounce Super Big Gulps and instead offering thirty-two-ounce drinks at half the price. Wendy's needs to be told that packing commercials with obese people—while perhaps more honest than indicating that people who eat 1,000-calorie sandwiches regularly are always svelte—is still sending the wrong message. Activist groups need to enlist the food makers in the campaign against overeating, just as they have managed to enlist beer companies and tobacco companies in campaigns against underage drinking and smoking.

We can also learn a lesson from the way teenage smoking rates vary by race. Since 1976, there has been a slight drop in white teenage smoking, from 29 percent to 25 percent. Yet in that same time, black teenage smoking has fallen from 27 percent all the way to 7 percent.[39] Why? "Religion, lack of resources, and strong peer pressure not to smoke seem to be factors," says John Wallace of the School of Social Work at the University of Michigan. "What it all points to is this: For many of them, it is just not accepted."[40] In other words, the attitude of young blacks toward cigarettes is rather opposite their attitude toward obesity. Cigarette smoking in young black society is far more deeply frowned upon than in young white society, hence young blacks do it far less. Overeating and being a couch potato is far more accepted in black society, hence they do it far more.

Yet the difference between obesity in whites and blacks is just a matter of degree. Among both, as well as among Hispanics, overeating and underexerting is considered not only respectable but sometimes downright entertaining. Think about it: *couch potato, lounge lizard, pigging out, scarfing down*—these are all humorous terms. That needs to change. Gluttony and sloth need to be demonized to the extent that cigarettes have been.

You've Got to Accentuate the Positive

The tobacco paradigm emphasizes a negative approach. But that's not to say we can't throw in many positive aspects in the battle against obesity. Hollywood should be pressured to depict eating less, snacking much less, and to show people eating healthier foods. Suggests the IOM, "Bill Cosby, for example, idly munching a stalk of raw broccoli as he talks to one of his kids (or nuzzles his wife who is chewing an apple) would convey a much more powerful message than would any amount of explicit dietary advice."[41]

I have now seen two movies in which women wore T-shirts with "Support Abortion Rights" in huge letters. It had nothing to do with the plots; the producers were trying to send a message. Well, let them send messages about healthful eating. Further, obesity should be worked into plot themes. For example, one of TV's top-rated (and smartest) shows, *NYPD Blue*, had two separate plotlines going over several episodes concerning characters suffering from alcoholism. Both plotlines showed unequivocally that alcoholism is a bad thing and is treatable. Ironically, one of the recovering alcoholics, Detective Sipowicz, is quite obese. In the first draft of this chapter, I suggested that the show could work the hazards of such obesity into its plot. Imagine my delight when I saw that prior to my completing the final draft, it had done just that.

The help of the Ad Council is needed. Says the IOM: "The goal should be to increase consumer awareness of the health benefits of fruits and vegetables; to motivate people to eat more of them while emphasizing their convenience, taste, great variety, and relatively low costs; and to provide tips on how to incorporate at least five servings of these foods into the diet each day."

We should also encourage more workplace fitness programs and centers. The proportion of workplaces offering physical activity and fitness programs has grown in recent years, from 22 percent in 1985 to 42 percent in 1992. Not surprisingly, the rates are highest at the biggest companies, which can best afford the facilities. Of the largest companies, more than 80 percent claimed to offer such programs, while at ones with between 50 to 100 employees it was only a third.[42] There is some evidence that such workplace programs have been effective in achieving at least short-term improvements, especially among high-risk individuals.[43]

Education campaigns should encourage adults to not question children who leave food on their plates. Restaurants should worry less about adding "healthy" meals to their menus that often are as fatty and caloric as the other meals, and instead offer smaller portions as alternatives. Food companies should follow the lead of Entenmann's and others in offering individual-size packages so that a person who just wants a couple of cookies doesn't end up buying three dozen and eating all of them over guilt at wasting food.

Society needs to change its attitude that wasting food is a sin (formed at a time when food was extremely expensive and often hard to come by) and dump the "waste not, want not" in favor of one that says, "better to waste it than have it go to the waist." Restaurant patrons need to be able to feel comfortable telling fellow patrons or their waiter that, no, they aren't going to eat everything on their plate and, no, they're not going to take the leftovers home. People need to feel it's OK to buy a big piece of cake and simply eat a little. When it comes to food, our society is one of plenty and becoming ever more plentiful. If food wastage did go up substantially, farmers could produce enough to cover it without blinking an eyelash. Far better for half a plate of fettuccine Alfredo to end up in the garbage disposal than wrapped around the internal organs of someone who didn't really want the second half anyway.

WHAT ROLE SHOULD THE GOVERNMENT PLAY?

I think we have long since passed a point where anybody thinks the government can do anything particularly well. Show me somebody who thinks that the Post Office does as good a job delivering packages or overnight letters as any of its competitors, and I'll show you somebody who wears a light-blue uniform with an eagle on the shoulder. But let's face it, the resources to which the government has access utterly dwarf anything private industry can come up with. It also makes the laws. That means power.

So what can a government like ours do to help hold back the growing tide of obesity, short of replacing the pyramid on the back of the dollar bill (the one with that weird eyeball) with the Agricultural Department's Food Guide Pyramid? Well, first it can follow the Hippocratic Oath, the part that goes, "first do no harm."

For example, government programs that dole out food—such as the school lunch programs—should discourage high calorie foods, especially those we call "junk food." If the government is going to take on the responsibility of giving away food, it has a duty to make sure it's of high nutritional value.

Far more harmful, though, has been the government's misleading campaign to get Americans to reduce fat intake to 30 percent of calories. Emphasis should be on avoiding the fats that are worst for your heart, and on reducing caloric intake. Instead of saying eat foods with less fat, government programs should be saying eat less calorically dense food, period, meaning food with high fat *or* high sugar. Britons, the only other people I know of beside Americans who have laws requiring calorie and nutrition labeling on their food packages, have a label that includes calories on a per 100-gram basis. Our labels should be similarly modified to show calories per ounce. This avoids the problem of food makers arbitrarily deciding what a portion size is. The special distinction of number of calories coming from fat should be removed from the label; it just encourages people—as indeed it is intended to do—to think there's something special about fat calories.

Another example of gross government failure is the public school systems. Just as our schools have steadily moved away from the basics in learning,[44] so have they done in health. When I was a kid in the 1960s, physical education was required and it was real. It was wind sprints, circuit training, long-distance running, push-ups, pull-ups. But more and more, physical education is becoming elective or not offered at all. By 1990, only 42 percent of high school students had physical education and by 1995 that had fallen to 25 percent. Somehow this happened despite Congress passing a resolution in 1987 urging every school to offer physical education every day to every student from kindergarten through twelfth grade.[45] That shows you the value of a congressional resolution. If the government is going to insist on taxing us to put our children in a building for seven hours a day, five days a week for the ostensible purpose of instructing them, we have a right to demand that it actually instructs them and helps keep them in shape. Because the diet culture now reaches well into elementary school, children should also be taught about weight-loss fads and why they never work. Everything in my chapter on weight-loss quacks could be conveyed to kids within the space of a single hour-long class.

Now to some ideas I *don't* like. One is to subsidize certain foods, primarily fruits and vegetables. Already with few exceptions, the fruits and vegetables we eat the most of are really quite cheap. I eat far more of these than the average American, yet the amount that I spend on them in a whole month is practically negligible. I am price sensitive to a point where I always buy the store's brand of frozen vegetables rather than one of the national brands. You save a few cents and—as Shakespeare would have put it while strolling through the Ye Not Yet Olde Supermarket—sweet corn by any other name would taste as sweet. But at my middle-class income level, stores could literally give away fruits and vegetables and I wouldn't eat a bit more than I do now. Of course, for poorer people that may not be true, but Americans as a whole spent 16 percent of their food bills on fruits and vegetables in 1993, down considerably from 21 percent in 1980. Since their overall food bills are only about 8 percent of their income, fruits and veggies just don't account for a lot.[46]

If not subsidies on the "good foods," why not taxes on the "bad" ones? Sales taxes clearly affect people's purchases, something government planners always rediscover (to their chagrin) when they raise taxes on items to increase government revenue, only to find that people buy so many fewer of those products that the government ends up with less income than before.

Yale obesity researcher Kelly Brownell offered on the Op-Ed page of *The New York Times* the idea that "Congress and state legislatures could shift the focus to the environment by taxing foods with little nutritional value. Fatty foods would be judged on their nutritive value per calorie or gram of fat. The least healthy would be given the highest tax rate."[47]

Obviously, I share Brownell's concern over obesity, but I don't agree with him here. For one, I'll be honest, I just don't like taxes. I don't like subsidies either, because one person's subsidy has to be paid for by another's taxes. Most Americans work hard for every dollar they earn and those dollars should be left alone whenever possible. The only subsidies I'll ever favor are those that clearly help us as a whole, such as children's vaccination or education. Beyond that, I think such taxes on specific types of food are politically untenable. A few years ago, California tried to impose a special tax on snack food. It was horribly unpopular and pounded into oblivion in a referendum.[48]

But even these considerations aside, the problem with singling out certain foods for taxation is that it sends the wrong message. It says that brownies are bad, soft drinks are insidious, doughnuts are diabolical, muffins are malicious, pecan pie requires penance, and—well, you get the point. Yet we had access to all these things back when we as a nation were so much thinner. The thinnest Americans have as much access to these foods as the fattest. Europeans, who on average are much thinner than Americans, have ready access to these foods. The key word in controlling caloric intake is moderation. A brownie isn't bad; a brownie the size of a brick is bad. A soft drink isn't insidious at eight or twelve ounces; at sixty-four, it's a nightmare. Americans used to value moderation; now they treat it as a joke. Both the food and the advertising industry are waging war against the idea of moderation. "Eat what you like," urges an advertisement for Healthy Choice luncheon meats. After all, it's 97 percent fat-free by weight.[49] Any successful anti-obesity campaign (or personal plan) must emphasize that you cannot eat as much as you might like of most foods, including any type of luncheon meat, while at the same time pointing out that no food need be completely forbidden. Taxing certain products will only harm that end.

WE CAN PREVAIL

Many factors of fairly recent development have led to the obesity epidemic. Food has become so cheap that not only can the poorest Americans be fat but indeed it appears the poorest Americans are the fattest.[50] Labor-saving devices continue to proliferate. Television has more variety than ever and has now been joined by web-surfing as a major sedentary activity. And with any major introduction of something that affects our culture, there is a "shakeup" period in which we learn to adjust. Consider, for example, automobiles. Even though they were much slower when they started to come into wide use about a century ago, their per capita accident and death rates were appalling by today's standards. But over time we adjusted. Traffic laws were passed, roads were improved, myriad safety devices appeared. The result is that death rates have steadily declined and continue to do so.

Another drawback with cars was the tremendous amount of air pollution they produced. By the 1960s, the situation was becoming critical. By the 1970s, however, it was improving thanks to one good law (the Clean Air Act of 1970) and many improvements in technology. Today the air over our cities is as clean as it's been since anyone began measuring.[51]

There is hope. I noted earlier the tremendous progress made against cigarette smoking. Illegal hard drug use among adults has gone down as has use of hard liquor.[52] Americans have also been persuaded to change their eating and drinking habits. There has been a 4 percent decline in cholesterol in the American diet today from 15 years ago. As one essayist put it, though, "It's one thing to switch from martinis to white wine or from saturated fat to unsaturated fat, and quite another to adopt moderation as a permanent lifestyle."[53]

Eventually, I think we can adjust to the factors that have caused the obesity epidemic. We can adjust to the modern lifestyle without becoming gluttons and sloths. After all, if we can put a man on the moon, surely we can get him through a doorway without greasing down his sides.

Notes

1. William Langley, "Size Is Everything," *Sunday Telegraph* (London), 13 November 1994, p. 1.
2. JoAnn E. Manson et al., "Body Weight and Mortality Among Women," *New England Journal of Medicine* 333 (11[11 September 1995]): 677–85.
3. Robert J. Kuczmarski et al., "Increasing Prevalence of Overweight Among U.S. Adults," *Journal of the American Medical Association* 272 (3[20 July 1994]): 205–11.
4. Centers for Disease Control and Prevention, "Prevalence of Overweight Among Adolescents—United States, 1988–91," *Morbidity and Mortality Weekly Report* 43 (44[11 November 1994]): 818–20.
5. Institute of Medicine, *Weighing the Options* (Washington, D.C.: National Academy Press, 1995), p. 51, fig. 2-6, and p. 52, fig. 2-7.
6. John Foreyt and G. Ken Goodrick, "The Ultimate Triumph of Obesity," editorial in *The Lancet* 346 (8968[15 July 1995]): 134–35.
7. Hartmann von Aue, "Poor Henry," as quoted in Emily Morison Beck, ed., John Bartlett, *Familiar Quotations* (Boston: Little, Brown and Company, 1980), p. 138.
8. See Mark S. Warnick, "The Price of a Tasty Lifestyle," *Pittsburgh Post-Gazette*, 24 July 1994, p. A1.

1. The Perils of Poundage

1. Hippocrates, *The Genuine Works of Hippocrates Translated from the Greek with a Preliminary Discourse and Annotations*, translated by Francis Adams (London: The Sydenham Society, 1849), as cited in George A. Bray, "Obesity: His-

torical Development of Scientific and Cultural Ideas," *International Journal of Obesity* 19 (11[November 1990]): 909–26.

2. Benjamin Franklin, *Poor Richard's Alamanack* (New York: Doubleday, Doran and Co., 1928), p. 6.

3. Metropolitan Life Insurance Company, "Build and Blood Pressure Study: 1959," vols. I and II (Chicago: Society of Actuaries, 1960).

4. H. McCue Jr., "The 1979 Build and Blood Pressure Study," in H. Bostrom and N. Ljungstedt, eds., *Medical Aspects of Mortality Statistics* (Stockholm: Almquist and Wiksell International, 1981), 182–98, as cited in F. Xavier Pi-Sunyer, "Health Implications of Obesity," *American Journal of Clinical Nutrition* 53 (6[June 1991]): 1595S–1603S.

5. Lawrence Garfinkel, "Overweight and Mortality," *Cancer* 58 (8[15 October 1986]): 1826–29.

6. Edward A. Lew, "Mortality and Weight: Insured Lives and the American Cancer Society Studies," *Annals of Internal Medicine* 103 (6 pt. 2[December 1985]): 1024–29.

7. M. D. A. F. Hoffmans, D. Kromhout, and C. De Lezenne Coulander, "The Impact of Body Mass Index of 78,612 Eighteen-Year-Old Dutch Men on Thirty-two-year Mortality from All Causes," *Clinical Epidemiology* 41 (8[1988]): 749–56; Lars V. Sjöström, "Mortality of Severely Obese Subjects," *American Journal of Clinical Nutrition* 53 (supp. 2[February 1992]): 516S–523S.

8. S. Sonne-Holm, Thorkild I. A. Sørensen, and U. Christensen, "Risk of Early Death in Extremely Overweight Young Men," *British Medical Journal* 287 (6395[17 September 1983]): 795–97.

9. H. T. Waaler, "Height, Weight, and Mortality: The Norwegian Experience," *Acta Medica Scandinavia* 679 (supp. [1984]): 1–56.

10. See Natalie Angier, "Researchers Link Obesity in Humans to Flaw in a Gene," *New York Times*, 1 December 1994, p. A1.

11. I-Min Lee et al., "Body Weight and Mortality," *Journal of the American Medical Association* 270 (23[15 December 1993]): 2823–28.

12. Jayne Hurley and Stephen Schmidt, "Pound Foolish?" *Nutrition Action Health Letter*, 18 (4[May 1991]): 7.

13. Personal telephone communication with JoAnn Manson, M.D., 18 September 1996.

14. JoAnn Manson et al., "Body Weight and Mortality Among Women," *New England Journal of Medicine* 333 (11[14 September 1995]): 677–85.

15. Charles Marwick, "Obesity Experts Say Less Weight Still Best," *Journal of the American Medical Association* 269 (20[26 May 1993]): 2617–18.

16. Manson et al., "Body Weight," 677–85.

17. See Nanci Hellmich, "Don't Gain Weight as You Age," *USA Today*, 3 January 1996, p. 9D.

18. Jane E. Brody, "Personal Health: A New Study on Midlife Weight Gain Raises Concerns Among Millions of American Women," *The New York Times*, 20 September 1995, p. B7; Manson et al., "Body Weight," 677–85.

19. Manson et al., "Body Weight," 677–85.

20. J. Michael McGinnis and William H. Foege, "Actual Causes of Death in the

United States," *Journal of the American Medical Association* 270 (18[10 November 1993]): 2207–12.

21. Jane E. Brody, "Moderate Weight Gain Risky for Women, a Study Warns," *New York Times*, 14 September 1995, p. B13; John Schwartz, "Thin Women Reduce Health Risk," *Washington Post*, 14 September 1995, p. A11.

22. Jane E. Brody, "Study Rebuts Acceptable Midlife Weight Gain," *New York Times*, 8 February 1995, p. B7.

23. Robert J. Garrrison and William B. Kannel, "A New Approach for Estimating Healthy Weights," *International Journal of Obesity* 17 (7[July 1993]): 417–23.

24. For more detailed descriptions, see Suzanne Schlosberg, "How Much of You Is Fat?" *Health* 10 (5[September 1996]): 36.

25. Kathleen Keough, "Rate Your Weight," *Prevention's Guide to Weight Loss* (New York: Rodale Press, 1995), p. 14.

26. "Too Fat? Too Thin? How Media Images of Celebrities Teach Kids to Hate Their Bodies," *People* 45 (22[3 June 1996]): cover.

27. Martin A. Alpert and M. Wail Hashimi, "Obesity and the Heart," *American Journal of Medical Sciences* 306 (2[August 1993]): 117–23.

28. Ibid.

29. Dale M. Atrens, *Don't Diet* (New York: William Morrow and Company, Inc., 1988), p. 93; see also *Food for Thought* newsletter, August 1994, p. 8.

30. U.S. Bureau of the Census, *Statistical Abstract of the United States: 1995*, 115th edition (Washington, D.C.: U.S. Department of Commerce, 1995), p. 86 (table 114).

31. Francisco Javier Martínez and José M. Sancho-Rof, "Epidemiology of High Blood Pressure and Obesity," *Drugs* 46 (supp. 2[February 1993]): 160–64; see also Benjamin N. Chiang, Lawrence V. Perlman, and Frederick H. Epstein, "Overweight and Hypertension: A Review," *Circulation* 39 (3[March 1969]): 403–21.

32. Theodore Van Itallie, "Health Implications of Overweight and Obesity in the United States," *Annals of Internal Medicine* 103 (6, part 2 of 2[December 1985]): 983–88.

33. Roland E. Schmieder et al., "Obese Hypertensive Patients Are Less Effectively Treated than Lean Hypertensives," *Journal of Hypertension* 11 (supp. 5[December 1993]): S348–S349.

34. Kathryn M. Rexrode et al., "A Prospective Study of Body Mass Index, Weight Change, and Risk of Stroke in Women," *Journal of the American Medical Association* 277 (19[21May 1997]): 1639–45.

35. See Jane E. Brody, "Type II Diabetes Is an Increasingly Common Killer that Many Patients Fail to Take Seriously," *New York Times*, 15 November 1995, p. B7.

36. Bernard Gutin and Gail Kessler, *The High Energy Factor*, as quoted in Diane Epstein and Kathleen Thompson, *Feeding on Dreams* (New York: Avon, 1994), pp. 98–99.

37. K. Westlund and R. Nicolaysen, "Ten-Year Mortality Related to Serum Cholesterol: A Follow-up of 3751 Men Aged 40–49," *Scandinavian Journal of Clinical and Laboratory Investigation* 30 (supp. 127[1972]): 1–24.

38. Manson et al., "Body Weight," 677–85.

39. Graham A. Colditz, "Economic Costs of Obesity," *American Journal of Clinical Nutrition* 55 (2[February 1992]): 503S–7S.
40. M. E. J. Lean et al., "Obesity, Weight Loss and Prognosis in Type II Diabetes," *Diabetic Medicine* 7 (3[March-April 1990]): 228–33.
41. Pi-Sunyer, "Health Implications," 1595S–1603S.
42. Margo A. Denke, Christopher T. Sempos, and Scott M. Grundy, "Excess Body Weight: An Underrecognized Contributor to High Blood Cholesterol Levels in White American Men," *Archives of Internal Medicine* 153 (9[10 May 1993]): 1093–1103.
43. Glenn A. Gaesser, *Big Fat Lies* (New York: Ballantine, 1996), 5, 101.
44. Lawrence Garfinkel, "Overweight and Cancer," *Annals of Internal Medicine* 103 (6 pt. 2[December 1985]): 1034–36.
45. Pi-Sunyer, "Health Implications," 1595S–1603S.
46. Linda Morris Brown et al., "Adenocarcinoma of the Esophagus: Role of Obesity and Diet," *Journal of the National Cancer Institute* 87 (2[18 January 1995]): 104–9.
47. "Weight Gain, Cancer Link Eyed," *Cancer Researcher Weekly*, 30 May 1994, p. 6. "Weight Gain by Thirty May Raise Breast Cancer Risk," *St. Petersburg Times*, 18 May 1994, p. 4A. See also Rachel Ballard-Barbash and Christine A. Swanson, "Body Weight: Estimation of Risk for Breast and Endometrial Cancers," *American Journal of Clinical Nutrition* 63 (3 supp.[March 1996]): 437S–41S.
48. "Breast Cancer (Increased Risk): Increased Risk Associated with Weight, Not Fat Intake," *Cancer Weekly Plus* [8 July 1996]: 7.
49. Mathew J. Reeves, "Body Mass and Breast Cancer—Relationship Between Method of Detection and Stage of Disease," *Cancer* 77 (2[15 January 1996]): 301–7.
50. Deborah J. Hart and Tim D. Spector, "The Relationship of Obesity, Fat Distribution, and Osteoarthritis in Women in the General Population: The Chingford Study," *The Journal of Rhematology* 20 (2[February 1993]): 331–35; see also R. E. Leach, S. Baumgard, and J. Broom, "Obesity: Its Relationships to Osteoarthritis of the Knee," *Clinical Orthopedics* 93 (June 1973): 271–73.
51. P. H. Broomfield et al., "Effects of Ursodeoxycholic Acid and Aspirin on the Formation of Lithogenic Bile and Gallstones During Loss of Weight," *New England Journal of Medicine* 319 (24[15 December 1988]): 1567–72.
52. T. M. Mabee et al., "The Mechanism of Increased Gallstone Formation in Obese Human Subjects," *Surgery* 79 (4[April 1976]): 460–68; Gary D. Friedman, William B. Kannel, and Thomas R. Dawber, "The Epidemiology of Gallbladder Disease Observations in the Framingham Study," *Journal of Chronic Disease* 19 (3[March 1966]): 273–92; George Bray, "Complications of Obesity," *Annals of Internal Medicine* 103 (6, part 2[December 1985]): 1052–62.
53. Konald A. Prem, Nicholas M. Mensheha, and John L. McKelvey, "Operative Treatment of Adenocarcinoma of the Endometrium in Obese Women," *American Journal of Obstetrics and Gynecology* 92 (1[May 1965]): 16–22.

54. Patricia Smith Choban et al., "Obesity and Increased Mortality in Blunt Trauma." *The Journal of Trauma* 31 (9[September 1991]): 1253–57.

55. A. A. Rim et al., "Relationship of Obesity and Disease in 73,532 Weight-Conscious Women," *Public Health Reports* 90 (1[January–February 1975]): 44–51.

56. Health and Welfare Canada, *Canada Health Survey* (Ottawa: Health and Welfare, Canada, 1978).

57. Robert J. Glynn et al., "Body Mass Index: An Independent Predictor of Cataract," *Archives of Ophthalmology* 113 (9[September 1995]): 1131–37.

58. Michele M. Gottschlich et al., "Significance of Obesity on Nutritional, Immunologic, Hormonal, and Clinical Outcome Parameters in Burns," *Journal of the American Dietetic Association* 3 (11[November 1993]): 1261–68.

59. Martha M. Werler et al., "Prepregnant Weight in Relation to Risk of Neural Tube Defects," *Journal of the American Medical Association* 275 (14[10 April 1996]): 1089–92; Gary M. Shaw et al., "Risk of Neural Tube Defect: Affected Pregnancy Among Obese Women," *Journal of the American Medical Association* 275 (14[10 April 1996]): 1093–96; see also Robert L. Goldenberg and Tsunenobu Tamura, "Prepregnancy Weight and Pregnancy Outcome," editorial in *Journal of the American Medical Association* 275 (14[10 April 1996]): 1127–28.

60. Colleen S. W. Rand and Alex M. C. Macgregor, "Morbidly Obese Patients' Perceptions of Social Discrimination Before and After Surgery for Obesity," *Southern Medical Journal* 83 (12[December 1990]): 1390–95; Colleen S. W. Rand, Karen Kowalski, and John M. Kuldau, "Characteristics of Marital Improvement Following Obesity Surgery," *Psychosomatics* 25 (3[March 1984]): 221–26; Jeff Sobal, "Marriage, Obesity, and Dieting," *Marriage and Family Review* 7 (1–2[spring-summer 1984]): 115–39; M. B. Harris, "Is Love Seen as Different for the Obese?" *Journal of Applied Social Psychology* 20 (15 pt. 1[September 1990]): 1209–24; David J. Kallen and Andrea Doughty, "The Relationship of Weight, the Self-Perception of Weight, and Self-Esteem with Courtship Behavior," *Marriage and Family Review* 7 (1–2 [spring–summer 1984]): 93–114; Steven L. Gortmaker et al., "Social and Economic Consequences of Overweight in Adolescence and Young Adulthood," *New England Journal of Medicine* 329 (14[1993]): 1008–12; Stanley M. Garn, Timothy V. Sullivan, and Victor M. Hawthorne, "Educational Level, Fatness, and Fatness Differences Between Husbands and Wives," *American Journal of Clinical Nutrition* 50 (4[October 1989]): 740–45.

61. Laura Flynn McCarthy, "Keeping Your Kid Off the Fat Track," *McCall's* 123 (2[November 1995]): 126.

62. Tim Friend, "Heart Disease Awaits Today's Soft-Living Kids," *USA Today*, 15 November 1994, p. 1D.

63. J. M. Court, G. H. Hill, and M. Dunlop, "Hypertension in Childhood," *Australian Journal of Pediatrics* 10 (1974): 295, as cited in Rosenbaum and Leibel, "Pathophysiology of Childhood Obesity," *Advances in Pediatrics* 35 (1988): 73–137.

64. W. R. Clare et al., "Tracking of Blood Lipids and Blood Pressure in School-Age Children: The Muscatine Study," *Circulation* 58 (4[October 1978]): 626.

65. Rosenbaum and Leibel, "Pathophysiology," 73–137.

66. F. Javier Nieto, Moyses Szklo, and George W. Comstock, "Childhood Weight and Growth Rate as Predictors of Adult Mortality," *American Journal of Epidemiology*, 136 (2[15 July 1992]): 201–13.

67. Mary K. Serdula et al., "Do Obese Children Become Obese Adults? A Review of the Literature," *Preventative Medicine* 22 (2[March 1993]): 167–77.

68. Shumei S. Guo et al., "The Predictive Value of Childhood Body Mass Index Values for Overweight at Age Thirty-five Years," *American Journal of Clinical Nutrition* 59 (4[April 1994]): 810–19.

69. E. M. E. Poskitt and T. J. Cole, "Do Fat Babies Stay Fat?" *British Medical Journal* 1 (6052[1 January 1977]): 7–9.

70. Aviva Must et al., "Long-Term Morbidity and Mortality of Overweight Adolescents," *New England Journal of Medicine* 327 (19[5 November 1992]): 1350–55.

71. Sidney Abraham, Gretchen Collins, and Marie Nordsieck, "Relationships of Childhood Weight Status to Morbidity in Adults," *Public Health Reports* 86 (3[March 1971]): 273–84; Hoffmans et al., "Impact of Body Mass Index," 749–56; Thorkild I. A. Sørenson and Stig Sonne-Holm, "Mortality in Extremely Overweight Young Men," *Journal of Chronic Diseases* 30 (1977): 359–67; and Ralph S. Paffenbarger Jr. and A. L. Wing, "Chronic Disease in Former College Students, X. The Effects of Single and Multiple Characteristics on Risk of Fatal Coronary Heart Disease," *American Journal of Epidemiology* 90 (6[December 1969]): 527–35.

72. Must et al., "Long-Term Morbidity," 1350–55; see also J. A. Grinker et al., "Overweight and Leanness in Adulthood: Prospective Study of Male Participants in the Normative Aging Study," *International Journal of Obesity* 20 (6[June 1996]): 561–69.

73. Foreyt et al., "Ultimate Triumph," 134–35.

74. Jeremiah Stamler, "Epidemic Obesity in the United States," *Archives of Internal Medicine* 153 (9[10 May 1993]): 1040–44.

75. S. A. Richardson et al., "Cultural Uniformity in Reaction to Physical Disabilities," *Sociological Review* 26 (1961): 241–47, as cited in Rosenbaum and Leibel, "Childhood Obesity," 73–137.

76. *Leeza*, 11 May 95.

77. For example, Von T. Nguyen et al., "Fat Intake and Adiposity in Children of Lean and Obese Parents," *American Journal of Clinical Nutrition* 63 (4[April 1996]): 507–13.

78. L. F. McCarthy, "Keeping Your Kid," 126.

79. C. Klesges et al., "Effects of Obesity, Social Interactions, and Physical Environment on Physical Activity in Preschool Children," *Health Psychology* 9 (4[1990]): 435–49; Sallis et al., "Family Variables and Physical Activity in Preschool Children," *Journal of Development and Behavioral Pediatrics* 9 (2[April 1988]): 57–61.

80. L. Moore et al., "Influence of Parents' Physical Activity Levels on Activity Levels of Young Children," *Journal of Pediatrics* 118 (2[February 1991]): 215–19.

81. Leonard H. Epstein, "Family-Based Behavioral Intervention for Obese Children," *International Journal of Obesity* 20 (supp. 1[February 1996]): S14–S21.

82. Alexander K. C. Leung and W. Lane M. Robson, "Childhood Obesity," *Postgraduate Medicine* 87 (4[March 1990]): 123–30.

83. Gaesser, *Big Fat Lies*, 81.

84. Ibid., 128.

85. Laura Shapiro et al., "Is Fat That Bad?" *Newsweek* 129 (16[21 April 1997]): 61.

86. T. Kue Young and Dale E. Gelskey, "Is Noncentral Obesity Metabolically Benign?" *Journal of the American Medical Association* 274 (24[27 December 1995]): 1939–41.

87. Ibid.

88. See G. Razay, K. W. Heaton, and C. H. Bolton, "Coronary Heart Disease Risk Factors in Relation to the Menopause," *Quarterly Journal of Medicine* New Series 85 (307–8[November–December 1992]): 889–96.

89. Census Bureau, *1995 Statistical Abstract* 93 (table 126).

90. See Benjamin E. Reubinoff et al., "Effects of Hormone Replacement Therapy on Weight, Body Composition, Fat Distribution, and Food Intake in Early Postmenopausal Women: A Prospective Study," *Fertility and Sterility* 64 (5[November 1995]): 963–68. The study did, however, find that estrogen supplements could reduce this upward shift, while having no effect overall on how much fat the women accumulate.

91. Personal telephone communication with JoAnn Manson, M.D., 29 August 1996.

92. Colditz, "Economic Costs," 503S–7S.

93. Ann M. Wolf and Graham A. Colditz, "The Cost of Obesity: The U.S. Perspective," *PharmoEconomics* 5 (supp.1[1994]): 34–37.

94. IOM, *Weighing the Options*, 26.

95. Charles Dickens, "A Christmas Carol," in *Charles Dickens' Christmas Ghost Stories* (New York: St. Martin's Press, 1992), p. 111.

96. Louis I. Dublin, "Relation of Obesity to Longevity," *New England Journal of Medicine* 248 (23[4 June 1953]): 971–74.

97. Gary Borkan et al., "Body Weight and Coronary Heart Disease Risk: Patterns of Risk Factor Change Associated with Long-Term Weight Change," *American Journal of Epidemiology* 124 (3[September 1986]): 410–19; Helen B. Hubert et al., "Obesity as an Independent Risk Factor for Cardiovascular Disease: A Twenty-six-Year Follow-up of Participants in the Framingham Heart Study," *Circulation* 67 (5[May 1983]): 968–77.

98. Chad I. Friedman and Moon H. Kim, "Obesity and Its Effect on Reproductive Function," *Clinical Obstetrics and Gynecology* 28 (3[September 1985]): 645–63.

99. A. S. Dixon and D. Henderson, "Prescribing for Osteoarthrosis," *Prescribers' Journal* 13 (2[April 1973]): 41–49.

100. John Garrow, "Importance of Obesity," *British Medical Journal* 303 (6804[21 September 1991]): 704–6.

101. David J. Goldstein, "Beneficial Health Effects of Modest Weight Loss," *International Journal of Obesity* 16 (6[June 1992]): 397–415; see also Rena R.

Wing and Robert W. Jeffrey, "Effect of Modest Weight Loss on Changes in Cardiovascular Risk Factors: Are There Differences Between Men and Women or Between Weight Loss and Maintenance?" *International Journal of Obesity* 19 (1[January 1995]): 67–73.

102. Personal telephone communication with Jerry Darm, M.D., 26 April 1996.

103. Karin Franson and Stephan Rössner, "Effects of Weight Reduction Programs on Close Family Members," *International Journal of Obesity* 18 (9[September 1994]): 648–49.

104. Gaesser, *Big Fat Lies*, xviii, 23.

105. Leslie I. Katzel et al., "Effects of Weight Loss vs. Aerobic Exercise Training on Risk Factors for Coronary Disease in Healthy, Obese, Middle-Aged and Older Men," *Journal of the American Medical Association* 274 (24[27 December 1995]): 1915–21.

106. Hurley and Schmidt, "Pound Foolish?" 5.

107. Glennda Chui, "U.S. Lab Rats Eating Themselves to Death," *Denver Post*, 4 November 1995, p. 16A.

108. Edwin Bayrd, *The Thin Game: Dietary Scams and Dietary Sense* (New York, Newsday Books, 1978), 132.

109. As cited in Daniel S. Kirschenbaum, *Weight Loss Through Persistence* (Oakland, California: New Harbinger Publications, 1994), 29.

2. One Nation, Overweight

1. Larry McShane, "Half-Ton Man Cut Out of Home," *Denver Post*, 18 May 1996, p. 13A; Catherine Crocker, "Half-Ton Man Lifted from Home," Associated Press, 16 August 1996.

2. Theodore B. Van Itallie, "Health Implications of Overweight and Obesity in the United States," *Annals of Internal Medicine* 103 (6 part 2 [December 1985]): 983–88.

3. Cynthia Crossen, "Fright by the Numbers: Alarming Disease Data Are Frequently Flawed," *Wall Street Journal*, 11 April 1996, p. B1.

4. Robert J. Kuczmarski et al., "Increasing Prevalence of Overweight Among U.S. Adults," *Journal of the American Medical Association* 272 (3[20 July 1994]): 205–11.

5. For example, R. J. Roberts, "Can Self-Reported Data Accurately Describe the Prevalence of Overweight?" *Public Health* 109 (4[July 1995]): 275–84.

6. Centers for Disease Control and Prevention, "Prevalence of Overweight Among Adolescents—United States, 1988–91," *Morbidity and Mortality Weekly Report* 43 (44[11 November 1994]): 818–20.

7. Kuczmarski et al., "Increasing Prevalence," 205–11.

8. Philip Shenon, "Many Troops Are Found Seriously Out of Shape," *New York Times*, 8 May 1996, p. B1.

9. Kuczmarski et al., "Increasing Prevalence," 205–11, table 3.

10. Centers for Disease Control and Prevention, "Update: Review of Overweight Among Children, Adolescents and Adults—United States, 1988–1994," *Morbidity and Mortality Weekly Report* 46 (9[7 March 1997]): 199–201.

11. Institute of Medicine, *Weighing the Options* (Washington, D.C.: National Academy Press, 1995), p. 51, figure 2-6, and p. 52, figure 2-7.

12. Humphrey Taylor, "Americans Get Fatter, and Fatter, and Fatter," The Harris Poll, 8(5 February 1996): 1.

13. Smoking among Americans had declined from 42.4 to 26.5 percent of the population from 1965 to 1992. See Census Bureau, *1995 Statistical Abstract*, 144 (table 219).

14. Katherine M. Flegal et al., "The Influence of Smoking Cessation on the Prevalence of Overweight in the United States," *New England Journal of Medicine* 333 (18[2 November 1995]): 1165–70.

15. Tara Meyer, "CDC: Adult Smoking Rises Slightly in U.S.," Associated Press, 11 July 1996.

16. Calculated from Frederick H. Epstein and Millicent Higgins, "Epidemiology of Obesity," in Per Björntorp and Bernard N. Brodoff, eds., *Obesity* (Philadelphia: J. D. Lippincott, 1992), 334 (table 27–3).

17. James Langton, "The Right Stuff," *Sunday Telegraph* (London), 28 January 1996, Review p. 1.

18. Personal telephone communication with Robert Whelan, 13 March 1996.

19. U.S. Department of Agriculture, Agricultural Research Service, *USDA Continuing Survey of Food Intake by Individuals* (Washington, D.C.: USDA, 1994).

20. Michael Gibney et al., "Consumption of Sugars," *American Journal of Clinical Nutrition* 62 (1 supp. [July 1995]): 178S–94S.

21. Personal telephone communication with Marion Nestle, 24 April 1996.

22. Karen Baar, "To Eat: Perchance to Lie," *New York Times*, 30 August 1995, p. B6.

23. "Errors in Reporting Habitual Energy Intake," *Nutrition Reviews* 49 (7[July 1991]): 215–17.

24. Walter Mertz et al., "What Are People Really Eating? The Relation Between Energy Intake Derived from Estimated Diet Records and Intake Determined to Maintain Body Weight," *American Journal of Clinical Nutrition* 54 (2[August 1991]): 291–95.

25. Personal telephone communication with Steven Heymsfield, M.D., 22 February 1996.

26. Shirley A. Gerrior and Claire Zizza, *Nutrient Content of the U.S. Food Supply 1909–1990*, U.S. Department of Agriculture, Home Economics Research Report No. 52 (1994): 52–53.

27. Personal telephone communication with Marion Nestle, 24 April 1996.

28. Nanci Hellmich, "A Plate Full of Reasons for Eating Your Pasta," *USA Today*, 8 March 1995, p. 7D.

29. National Research Council, *Diet and Health* (Washington, D.C.: National Academy Press, 1989), 60.

30. Census Bureau, *1995 Statistical Abstract*, 148, table 227.

31. Ibid.; National Research Council, *Diet and Health*, 61.

32. Marcy Magiera, "Coca-Cola Marketing Barrage," *Advertising Age*, 21 March 1994, 43, citing data from *Beverage Digest*; Census Bureau, *1995 Statistical Abstract*, 856, table 1374.

33. U.S. Bureau of the Census, *Statistical Abstract of the United States, 1996* (Washington, D.C.: 1996), p. 148, table 228.

34. Cathy Perlmutter, Michele Stanten, and Rosemary Iconis, "How in the World to Stay Slim," *Prevention* 47 (9[September 1995]): 83, 88–89.

35. Jacob C. Seidell, "Obesity in Europe: Scaling an Epidemic," *International Journal of Obesity* 19 (supp. 3 [September 1995]): S1–S4.

36. Personal telephone communication with Robert Kuczmarski, M.D., 30 July 1996.

37. Glenn A. Gaesser, *Big Fat Lies: The Truth About Your Weight and Your Health* (New York: Fawcett, 1996), p. 22.

38. Nanci Hellmich, "Trying to Copy Adults Can Lead to Eating Disorders," *USA Today*, 12 August 1996, p. D1.

39. Marcia Mogelonsky, "Americans Are Sweet on Goodies," *Denver Post*, 11 October 1995, p. G1, citing a Roger Starch Worldwide poll.

40. American Dietetic Association, *Nutrition Trends Survey* (Chicago: American Dietetic Association, September 1995), Exhibit C and A.

41. William Langley, "Size Is Everything," *Sunday Telegraph* (London), 13 November 1994, p. 1.

42. Philip Elmer-DeWitt et al., "Fat Times," *Time* 145 (2[16 January 1995]): 65.

43. Melinda Beck and Mary Hager, "An Epidemic of Obesity," *Newsweek* 124 (5[1 August 1994]): 62–63.

44. Jennifer L. Stevenson, "Life Begins Anew without Millstone," *St. Petersburg Times*, 26 March 1996, p. D1.

45. Marjorie Rosen and Lujina Fisher, "Oprah Overcomes," *People* 41 (1[10 January 1994]): 43.

46. Alisa Bland, "I Am Waif," *Glamour* 92 (11[November 1994]): 118.

47. Ibid.

48. Michael Loewy, "All in the Family," *NAAFA Newsletter* 26 (2[July–August 1996]): 6.

49. Jennifer Steinhauer, "Retailers Find That Big Is Beautiful (Profitable, Too)," *New York Times*, 20 September 1995, p. B1.

50. Ibid., B6.

51. CNN, *CNN Presents*, "Food to Die For," May 1995.

52. Steinhauer, "Retailers Find," B1.

53. Erma Bombeck, "Go Figure: We Grow in Girth, but Sizes Get Smaller," *New York Daily News*, March 21, 1995, p. 28.

54. L. Kaufman, "Prime-Time Nutrition," *Journal of Communication* 30 (1980): 37–46, as cited in William H. Dietz, "You Are What You Eat—What You Eat Is What You Are," *Journal of Adolescent Health Care* 11 (1[January 1990]): 76–81.

55. Langton, "The Right Stuff," 1.

56. Figure applies to the peach-flavored tea. The unflavored tea has 160 calories in sixteen ounces.

57. See Dottie Enrico, "Snapple Campaign Goes Down Smoothly with Viewers," *USA Today*, 16 October 1995, p. 8B.

58. As quoted in Teri Agin, "Queen-sized Women Are a Growing Market for Fashion Designers," *Wall Street Journal*, 13 May 1996, p. A1.

59. Steinhauer, "Retailers Find," B1, B6.

60. Brody, "Midlife Weight Gain," B7.

61. Florence Fabricant, "Big Portions Still Make Big People," *New York Times*, 19 October 1994, p. B1.

62. Lisa R. Young and Marion Nestle, "Portion Sizes in Dietary Assessment: Issues and Policy Implications": *Nutrition Reviews* 53 (6[June 1995]): 149–58.

63. Bruce Horovitz, "Portion Sizes and Fat Content 'Out of Control,'" *USA Today*, 20 February 1996, p. A1.

64. "Top Fifty Growth Chains," *Restaurant Business Magazine* 95 (10[1July 1996]): 51.

65. Ibid.

66. Kathleen Keough, "Rate Your Weight," *Prevention's Guide to Weight Loss* (New York: Rodale Press, 1995), p. 22.

67. Horovitz, "Portion Sizes," A4.

68. Bea Lewis, "The Secret of Weight Loss Is Eating Less. Some Secret," *Newsday*, 8 March 1995, p. B23.

69. Horovitz, "Portion Sizes," A4.

70. "Best Quick Fix for Chocoholics," *Westword* (Denver) 19 (44[27 June–3 July 1996]): 170.

71. Mark Potok: "Handicapped Parking Abuse Mushrooms," *USA Today*, 8 February 1996, p. A1.

72. Sally Squires, "Exercise: A Little Bit'll Do You," *Washington Post*, 3 August 1993, Health, p. 9.

73. Carlos J. Crespo et al., "Leisure-Time Physical Activity Among U.S. Adults," *Archives of Internal Medicine* 156 (1[8 January 1996]): 93–98.

74. U.S. Department of Health and Human Services, *Physical Activity and Health: A Report of the Surgeon General* (Atlanta: U.S. Department of Health and Human Services, 1996), 180–81 (table 5-3).

75. Joseph Carey and Ronald A. Taylor, "Battling the Bulge at an Early Age," *U.S. News & World Report* 102 (8[2 March 1987]): 67.

76. Gregory W. Heath et al., "Physical Activity Patterns in American High School Students," *Archives of Pediatric and Adolescent Medicine* 148 (11[November 1994]): 1131–36.

77. Jennifer Steinhauer, "Teenage Girls Talk Back on Exercise," *New York Times*, 4 January 1995, p. B1.

78. Peter Jaret, "The Way to Lose Weight," *Health* 9 (1[January–February 1995]): 57.

79. Cathy Perlmutter, Michele Stanten, and Rosemary Iconis, "How in the World to Stay Slim," *Prevention* 47 (9 [September 1995]): 83.

80. *Home Alone 2*, 1992, Twentieth Century Fox, Chris Columbus, director.

81. Suzanne Hamlin, "Time Flies, but Where Does It Go?" *New York Times*, 6 September 1995, p. B1.

82. John Sedgwick, "America Is Fat!" *Self* 17 (1[January 1995]): 85.

83. Larry A. Tucker, "Television, Teenagers, and Health," *Journal of Youth and Adolescence* 16 (5[October 1987]): 415–25.

84. William H. Dietz and Steven L. Gortmaker, "Do We Fatten Our Children at the Television Set? Obesity and Television Viewing in Children and Adolescents," *Pediatrics* 75 (5[May 1985]): 807–12.

85. Steven L. Gortmaker, William J. Dietz Jr., and Lilian W. Y. Cheung, "Inactivity, Diet, and the Fattening of America," *Journal of the American Dietetic*

Association 90 (9[September 1990]): 1247–55; later studies would build the case that it wasn't just fat children hunkering down in front of the set, but rather that watching TV actually contributed to obesity. Larry Tucker confirmed the obesity-TV link in a study, first, of adult males and, then, of adult females. Like Dietz and Gortmaker before them, Tucker and another researcher found a steady correlation between the amount of TV viewing and the amount of fat on the viewer's body, such that men who watched four or more hours a day were more than twice as likely to be obese as those who watched less than an hour a day and were more than three times as likely to be "super-obese, that is, among the fattest 5 percent of men." See Gortmaker et al., "Fattening of America," 1247–55. In women there was also a steady rise in obesity coincidental with increased TV viewing. On the other hand, Tucker and his fellow researcher further found that women who watched TV tended to exercise less, and pointed out that this lack of exercise could be contributing to the women's obesity. See Larry A. Tucker and Glenn M. Friedman, "Television Viewing and Obesity in Adult Males," *American Journal of Public Health* 79 (4[April 1989]): 516–18.

86. Grace A. Falciglia and Joan Dye Gussow, "Television Commercials and Eating Behavior of Obese and Normal-Weight Women," *Journal of Nutrition Education* 12 (4[October–December 1980]): 196–99.
87. "TV Characters Spend Time Drinking and Snacking," *Environmental Nutrition* 19 (1[January 1996]): 8.
88. H. L. Taras et al., "Television's Influence on Children's Diet and Physical Activity," *Journal of Developmental and Behavioral Pediatrics* 10 (4[1989]): 176–80.
89. Leslie Miller, "Most Users See Internet as Happy Medium," *USA Today*, 18 June 1996, p. 4E (graphic).

3. The Low-Fat Myth
1. Martin Katahn, *The T-Factor Diet* (New York: Bantam, 1993).
2. Jamie Pope and Martin Katahn, *The T-Factor Fat Gram Counter* (New York: W.W. Norton and Co., 1989).
3. Susan Powter, *Stop the Insanity!* (New York: Simon & Schuster, 1993).
4. Dean Ornish, *Eat More, Weigh Less* (New York: HarperCollins, 1993).
5. John McDougall, *The McDougall Plan for Super Health and Life-Long Weight Loss* (New York: New Win Publishing, 1984).
6. Annette B. Natow and Jo-Ann Heslin, *The Fat Counter* (New York: Pocket Books, 1995).
7. Elaine Moquette-Magee, *Fight Fat and Win* (Minneapolis: Chronimed/DCI: 1994).
8. Eric Witt and Carol Worth, *Bodystat* (New York: Viking, 1996).
9. Jean Antonello, *How to Become Naturally Thin by Eating More* (New York: Avon Books, 1989).
10. Bruce K. Lowell, *Dr. Bruce Lowell's Fat Percent Finder* (New York: Perigee, 1991).
11. Joseph Piscatella, *The Fat Tooth Fat-Gram Counter* (New York: Workman, 1993).
12. Joseph Piscatella, *Controlling Your Fat Tooth* (New York: Workman, 1993).

13. Jeane Rhodes, *Fat to Fit, Without Dieting* (Chicago: Contemporary Books, 1990).

14. Victoria Moran, *Get the Fat Out* (New York: Crown Publishers, 1994).

15. Dennis Remington, Garth Fisher, and Edward Parent, *How to Lower Your Fat Thermostat* (Provo, Utah: Vitality House International, Inc., 1983).

16. Covert Bailey, *The Fit or Fat Target Diet* (Boston: Houghton Mifflin, 1984), p. 3.

17. Jamie Pope, *The Last Five Pounds* (New York: Pocket Books, 1995), p. 32.

18. Ron Goor and Nancy Goor, *Choose to Lose* (Boston: Houghton Mifflin, 1995), p. 1.

19. Powter, *Stop the Insanity!*, p. 127.

20. Annette B. Natow and Jo-Ann Heslin, *The Fat Attack Plan* (New York: Pocket Books, 1990), p. 3.

21. Ibid., p. 32.

22. Debra Waterhouse, *Outsmarting the Female Fat Cell* (New York: Warner Books, 1993), p. 71.

23. Art Ulene, *Take It Off! Keep It Off!* (Berkeley, California: Ulysses Press, 1995), p. 24.

24. Ornish, *Eat More, Weigh Less*, p. 31.

25. Associated Press, "Fear Fat? Forget Many Deli Sandwiches," *St. Petersburg Times*, 22 March 1995, p. 6A.

26. Center for Media and Public Affairs, "Food for Thought," *Media Monitor* 9 (6[November–December 1995]): 2.

27. See Gina Kolata, "Report Urges Low-fat Diet for Everyone," *New York Times*, 28 February 1990, p. A1. See also U.S. Department of Health and Human Services (HHS), *Healthy People 2000* (DHHS Publication No. (PHS) 91-50213), p. 93.

28. Food Marketing Institute and *Prevention Magazine* (FMI/PM), *Shopping for Health* (Washington, D.C., and Emmaus, Pennsylvania: Food Marketing Institute and *Prevention Magazine*, 1996), 16.

29. See Marian Burros, "Eating Well," *New York Times*, 29 April 1992, p. C4.

30. Laura Shapiro, "A Food Lover's Guide to Fat," *Newsweek* 124 (23[6 June 1994]): 53.

31. E. V. McCollum, *A History of Nutrition* (Boston: Houghton-Mifflin, 1957), as cited in Jo Anne Cassell, "Social Anthropology and Nutrition: A Different Look at Obesity in America," *American Journal of Clinical Nutrition* 95 (4[April 1995]): 424–27.

32. Martin Katahn, *The Rotation Diet* (New York: Bantam Books, 1987).

33. The basic idea of the Rotation Diet is to vary caloric intake every few days. For example, women eat about 600 calories per day for three days, then 900 calories per day for four days, and then a week at 1,200 calories per day. Even the theory was cockeyed. Only about half the slowdown in metabolism that affects dieters is from reduced caloric intake. The other half is from the muscle loss that generally accompanies fat loss. With less muscle, the body burns fewer calories. Not surprisingly, Katahn never published his alleged study. But somebody else then at Vanderbilt, clinical nutritionist James Hill, conducted his own study using Katahn's parameters. Hill set up two groups of moderately obese women, one with a Rotation Diet–like regimen alternating

600-calorie days with 1,800-calorie days and the other with a simple 1,200-calorie-a-day diet. Over the course of twelve weeks, both groups consumed the same number of calories. Both groups suffered a drop in their metabolisms and both lost the same amount of weight. "A pattern of alternating-calorie intake provided neither an advantage nor a disadvantage in weight reduction in this study," concluded Hill. See James O. Hill et al., "Evaluation of an Alternating-Calorie Diet With and Without Exercise in the Treatment of Obesity," *American Journal of Clinical Nutrition* 50 (2[August 1989]): 248–54.

34. Katahn, *The T-Factor Diet,* 3.
35. Ibid., 10.
36. Ibid., 28.
37. Ibid., 89.
38. Ornish, *Eat More, Weigh Less,* 20.
39. Katahn, *The T-Factor Diet,* 269–72.
40. Personal telephone communication with Jean-Pierre Flatt, M.D., 21 December 1995.
41. For example, Valerie George et al., "Effect of Dietary Fat Content on Total and Regional Adiposity in Men and Women," *International Journal of Obesity* 14 (12[December 1990]): 1085–94; Lisa H. Nelson and Larry A. Tucker, "Diet Composition Related to Body Fat in a Multivariate Study of 203 Men," *Journal of the American Dietic Association* 96 (8[August 1996]): 771–77.
42. For example, one study compared fat loss among two sets of dieters given equal numbers of calories but with either 40 percent or 20 percent coming from fat, finding that the "low-fatters" lost 3 percent of their fat while the high-fat group lost 2.5 percent of theirs. See William V. Rumpler et al., "Energy-Intake Restriction and Diet-Composition Effects on Energy Expenditure in Men," *American Journal of Clinical Nutrition* 53 (2[February 1991]): 430–36. Another found that after a year, women on a 17 percent fat diet lost 4.7 percent of their body fat compared with 2.2 percent lost by women on a 36 percent fat diet. See Sidika E. Kasim et al., "Dietary and Anthropometric Determinants of Plasma Lipoproteins During a Long-Term Low-Fat Diet in Healthy Women," *American Journal of Clinical Nutrition* 57 (2[February 1993]): 146–53.
43. Kasim et al., "Dietary and Anthropometric Determinants," 146–53.
44. Another study that has been wrongly said to show that eating fewer calories from fat leads to body-fat loss appeared in the *American Journal of Clinical Nutrition* in 1991. It found that after a year's time, women who decreased their fat intake (from 39.2 percent to 21.6 percent of all calories) had lost almost seven pounds, while a comparison group with only slightly decreased fat from calories (from 38.9 percent to 37.3 percent) lost just one pound. See Lianne Sheppard, Alan R. Kristal, and Lawrence H. Kushi, "Weight Loss in Women Participating in a Randomized Trial of Low-Fat Diets," *American Journal of Clinical Nutrition* 54 (5[November 1991]): 821–28. But as one of the co-authors, Lawrence H. Kushi from the University of Minnesota School of Public Health, pointed out in a later article, there was no reduction in either body fat or abdominal circumference in these women. The low-fat eaters didn't lose fat at all; they lost muscle and water. See Lawrence H.

Kushi, Elizabeth B. Lenart, and Walter C. Willett, "Health Implications of Mediterranean Diets in Light of Contemporary Knowledge," *American Journal of Clinical Nutrition* 61 (6[(supp)(June 1995)]): 1416S–27S. That may also have been true in two other studies. See Norman F. Boyd et al., "Quantitative Changes in Dietary Fat Intake and Serum Cholesterol in Women: Results from a Randomized, Controlled Trial," *American Journal of Clinical Nutrition* 52 (3[September 1992]): 470–76; and G. D. Brown et al., "Effects of Two 'Lipid-Lowering' Diets on Plasma Lipid Levels of Patients with Peripheral Vascular Disease," *Journal of the American Dietetic Association* 84 (5[May 1984]): 546–50. In both cases the low-fatters lost significantly more pounds but, unfortunately, there was no measurement of fat loss.

45. For example, James O. Hill et al., "Development of Dietary Obesity in Rats: Influence of Amount and Composition of Dietary Fat," *International Journal of Obesity* 16 (5[May 1992]): 321–33; D. M. W. Salmon and J. P. Flatt, "Effect of Dietary Fat Content on the Incidence of Obesity Among *Ad Libitum* Mice, *International Journal of Obesity* 9 (6[1985]): 443–49. These show that fewer fat calories make for leaner test animals. But other animal studies don't show this. For example, K. Steinbeck et al., "The Effect of Diet Composition on Weight Gain and Pyruvate Dehydrogenase Activity in Heart Muscle in the Gold Thioglucose Obese Mouse," *International Journal of Obesity* 11 (5[October 1987]): 507–18.

46. Alain Golay et al., "Similar Weight Loss with Low- or High-Carbohydrate Diets," *American Journal of Clinical Nutrition* 63 (2[February 1996]): 174–78.

47. Lori R. Roust, Kriss D. Hammel, and Michael D. Jensen, "Effects of Isoenergetic, Low-Fat Diets on Energy Metabolism and Obese Women," *American Journal of Clinical Nutrition* 60 (4[October 1994]): 470–75.

48. Rudolph L. Leibel et al., "Energy Intake Required to Maintain Body Weight Is Not Affected by Wide Variation in Diet Composition," *American Journal of Clinical Nutrition* 53 (2[February 1992]): 350–55.

49. Molly O'Neill, "So It May Be True After All: Eating Pasta Makes You Fat," *New York Times*, 8 February 1995, p. C6.

50. Betty B. Alford, Ann C. Blankenship, and R. Donald Hagen, "The Effects of Variations in Carbohydrate, Protein, and Fat Content of the Diet Upon Weight Loss, Blood Values, and Nutrient Intake of Adult Obese Women," *Journal of the American Dietetic Association* 90 (4[April 1990]): 534–40). The other study, from the University of Chicago, compared obese women who were assigned diets comprising 50 percent fat and 25 percent carbohydrate or diets comprising 15 percent fat and 60 percent carbohydrate. After the twelve-week program ended, it turned out the women on the high-fat diet had lost on average five and a half pounds more than those on the low-fat diet. The only guess the researchers could make at "this unexpected finding" was that perhaps the women on the diet with so little fat couldn't stick with the diet and essentially cheated. Susan B. Racette et al., "Effects of Aerobic Exercise and Dietary Carbohydrate on Energy Expenditure and Body Composition During Weight Reduction in Obese Women," *American Journal of Clinical Nutrition* 61 (3[March 1995]): 486–94.

51. David G. Schlundt et al., "Randomized Evaluation of a Low-Fat Ad Libitum

Carbohydrate Diet for Weight Reduction," *International Journal of Obesity* 17 (11[November 1993]): 623–29.

52. Kushi et al., "Health Implications," 1416S–27S.

53. Personal telephone communication with Walter Willett, M.D., 25 April 1996.

54. Survey data as collected between 1975 and 1988 as presented in Satoshi Sasaki and Hugo Kesteloot, "Value of Food and Agricultural Organization Data on Food-Balance Sheets as a Data Source for Dietary Fat Intake in Epidemiological Studies," *American Journal of Clinical Nutrition* 56 (4[October 1992]): 716–23.

55. Adam Drewnowski et al., "Diet Quality and Dietary Diversity in France: Implications for the French Paradox," *Journal of the American Dietetic Association* 96 (7[July 1996]): 663–69.

56. Natow and Heslin, *The Fat Attack Plan*, 2.

57. U.S. Department of Agriculture, *What We Eat in America: 1994–96*, February 1996, p.1.

58. Alison M. Stephen and Nicholas J. Wald, "Trends in the Individual Consumption of Dietary Fat in the United States, 1920–1984," *American Journal of Clinical Nutrition* 52 (3[September 1990]): 457–69.

59. Jacob C. Seidell, "Obesity in Europe: Scaling an Epidemic," *International Journal of Obesity* 19 (Supp. 3[September 1995]): S1–S4.

60. Gina Kolata, "Benefit of Standard Low-Fat Diet Is Doubted," *New York Times*, 25 April 1995, p. B7.

61. Ibid.

62. Although the research in this area is in great flux, with some scientists like Willett fingering trans-fatty acids as being highly dangerous and others saying otherwise, and some saying palm oils are terrible for your heart and others saying that's not the case, there seem to be a few things on which everybody agrees. First, fat from animal flesh is not good (especially if you're the animal being eaten). Animal fat is strongly implicated in both heart disease and cancer. There has been found a strong correlation between animal fat and red meat and incidence of cancers of the colon— Edward Giovannucci et al, "Intake of Fat, Meat, and Fiber in Relation to Risk of Colon Cancer in Men," *Cancer Research* 54 (9[1 May 1994]): 2390–97; R. Alexandra Goldbohm et al, "A Prospective Cohort Study on the Relation of Meat Consumption to Colon Cancer," *Cancer Research* 54 (3[1 February 1994]): 718–23—and prostate—(Edward Giovannucci et al., "A Prospective Study of Dietary Fat and Risk of Prostate Cancer," *Journal of the National Cancer Institute* 85 (19[6 October 1993]): 1571–79; Loic Le Marchand et al., "Animal Fat Consumption and Prostate Cancer: A Prospective Study in Hawaii," *Epidemiology* 5 (3[May 1994]): 276–82. Breast cancer is considered less and less likely to have a fat connection; see David J. Hunter et al., "Cohort Studies of Fat Intake and the Risk of Breast Cancer, a Pooled Analysis," *New England Journal of Medicine* 334 (6[8 February 1996]): 356–61.

All animal fat is saturated, including that from milk products, and saturated fat has long been suspected of being a particular villain in heart disease. The Department of Agriculture thus recommends that we get no more than 10 percent of our calories from saturated fats. See Gerry Oster and David Thompson, "Estimated Effects of Reducing Dietary Saturated Fat Intake on the Incidence and Costs of Coronary Heart Disease in the United States," *Journal of the American Dietetic Association* 96 (2[February 1996]): 127–31. But there are those who dissent from this view. See Sally Fallon, Pat Connolly, and Mary G. Enig, "Why Butter Is Good for You," *Consumers' Research* 79 (3[March 1996]): 10–15. Interestingly, a recent study of French eating habits found that only 4 percent of those surveyed got less than 10 percent of their calories from saturated fats, yet the French have a much lower rate of heart disease than do Americans; see Drewnowski et al., "Diet Quality and Dietary Diversity in France," 663–69. This is not proof in and of itself that saturated fat is not a factor in heart disease, but it does clearly show that it is only a player at best.

Second, Omega-3 fat (of which fish is an excellent source, along with canola oil) is probably actually good for your heart, though again calorically it is the same as any other fat and if you eat enough of it so that it contributes to your becoming obese, that's not good. See David S. Siscovick et al., "Dietary Intake and Cell Membrane Levels of Long-Chain n-3 Polyunsaturated Fatty Acids and the Risk of Primary Cardiac Arrest," *Journal of the American Medical Association* 724 (17[1 November 1995]): 1363–67.

Third, as far as cooking oils go, you can't do any better than olive oil. Olive oil, the central part of the much-touted Mediterranean diet, is one reason researchers like Harvard's Willett think Greeks and other Mediterranean-area peoples have such low rates of heart disease. "I think olive oil is the best and safest from all we know," says Willett. "But we still need some source of Omega-3." (Personal telephone communication with Walter Willett, M.D., 25 April 1996). Eat less meat (especially of the fatty kind), eat more fish, and if you use oil, use that from olives. Nuts are also a good source of Omega-3. And keeping watching the papers for the latest in this confusing field.

63. HHS, *Healthy People 2000*, 95.
64. CNN *Morning News*, "Non-Fat Foods Offer Consumers Tasty Alternatives," 18 April 1994, Transcript No. 582, Segment No. 8, p. 1.
65. Glenn Collins, "Ya-hooo! A Marketing Coup," *New York Times*, 30 May 1995, p. C3.
66. Food Marketing Institute and *Prevention* magazine, *Shopping for Health* (Washington, D.C.: Food Marketing Institute and *Prevention* magazine, 1996): p. 23; for frequency of use, see p. 24.
67. Karen Riley, "No Fear of Frying," *Washington Times*, 14 January 1996, p. A14.
68. Betsy Spethmann, "SnackWell's, SnackWell's Everywhere," *Brandweek*, 27 May 1996, p. 1.
69. CNN, *CNN Presents*, "Food to Die For," May 1995.
70. CNN *Morning News*, "Non-Fat Foods," p. 1.
71. Laura Fraser, "Fat-Free but Getting Fatter," *Vogue* 181 (1[January 1995]): 90.
72. Ibid., 92.
73. See Jeremy Iggers, *The Garden of Eating* (New York: HarperCollins, 1996), 107.

74. Nanci Hellmich, "A Hot Potato: Snackers Gobble Up Low-Fat Baked Lay's Crisps," *USA Today*, 5 March 1996, p. 4D.

75. See "Healthy Junk," *Nutrition Action Healthletter* 23 (8[October 1996]): 9.

76. Advertisement in *Woman's Day* 59 (13[6 August 1996]): 158.

77. Bonnie Liebman, "The Weighting Game," *Nutrition Action Healthletter* 22 (4[May 1995]): 7.

78. Kristine Napier, "Pasta Is Not Poison," *Harvard Health Letter* 20 (9[July 1995]): 1.

79. Nanci Hellmich, "Conquering the Scales for Good," *USA Today*, 3 January 1995, p. 3D.

80. O'Neill, "Eating Pasta," B7.

81. NPR's *All Things Considered*, "Bad News for Pasta Dieters," 8 February 1995, Transcript No. 1752, Segment No. 5, p. 1.

82. Traci Watson and Corrina Wu, "Are You Too Fat?" *U.S. News & World Report* 120 (1[8 January 1996]): 56.

83. Florence A. Caputo and Richard D. Mattes, "Human Dietary Responses to Perceived Manipulation of Fat Content in a Midday Meal," *International Journal of Obesity* 17 (9[April 1993]): 237–40.

84. Two other researchers, David Shide and Barbara Rolls, both of Pennsylvania State University, gave female subjects yogurt before dinner and then invited them to eat at dinner whatever they wished. Some of the women were told their yogurt was high in fat and some were told it was low in fat. Regardless of the actual fat content of their yogurt, the women who were told they had eaten low-fat stuff ate more at dinner than the women who were under the impression they had eaten the high-fat yogurt. See David J. Shide and Barbara Rolls, "Information about the Fat Content of Preloads Influences Energy Intake in Healthy Women," *Journal of the American Dietetic Association* 95 (9[September 1995]): 993–98.

85. FMI/PM, *Shopping for Health*, 24.

86. Tarkan, "How a Low-Fat Diet Can Make You Fat," 145.

87. "Sweets to Die For," *Nutrition Action Healthletter* 23 (5[June 1996]): 6.

88. "FTC Weighs in on Häagen-Dazs Fat Claims," *St. Petersburg Times*, 22 November 1994, p. 1E.

89. Fraser, "Fat-Free," 92.

90. Kristin Von Kreisler, "Diet Experts' Guide to Fat and Calories," *Readers' Digest* 147 (883[November 1995]): 44.

91. Shapiro, "A Food Lover's Guide," 54.

92. ABC, *Good Morning America*, "Low-Fat Foods," 12 September 1995, Show No. 2413, transcript p. 8.

93. Rosie Daly, *In the Kitchen with Rosie* (New York: Knopf, 1994).

94. Hellmich, "Conquering," 3D.

95. Elaine Moquette-Magee, *Fight Fat and Win* (Minneapolis: Chronimed/DCI Publishing, 1994), 101–2.

96. Robert Greene, "Fat Intake Dips but Not Pounds," *Denver Post*, 17 January 1996, p. A5.; Kim Painter, "Fatty Diets on Steady Decline," *USA Today*, 25 February 1994, p. 1D.

97. G. B. Haber, K. W. Heaton, and D. Murphy, "Depletion and Disruption of Dietary Fibre," *The Lancet* 2 (8040[1 October 1977]): 679–82.

98. Lauren Lissner, "Dietary Fat and the Regulation of Energy Intake in Human Subjects," *American Journal of Clinical Nutrition* 46 (6[December 1987]): 886–92. In another study, researchers at the University of Alabama in Birmingham set up an experiment in which ten subjects were given foods of high-energy density and ten subjects foods of low-energy density. The high-density food had larger amounts of fat and sugar. The low-energy-density food had less fat, less sugar, and consequently half as many calories per gram and seven times as much fiber. Those eating the low-density diet ended up eating only 1,570 calories a day on average versus an average of 3,000 calories a day for those eating the high-energy-density food. The researchers theorized that this may have been due to the sheer bulk of the diet and the fact that this bulk stretched out the eating time for those eating the low-energy dense food. Even though, calorically speaking, they took in only half what their counterparts took in, it took the low-energy-density eaters a third longer to consume their food. See Karen H. Duncan et al., "The Effects of High- and Low-Energy-Density Diets on Satiety, Energy Intake, and Eating Time of Obese and Nonobese Subjects," *American Journal of Clinical Nutrition* 37 (5[May 1983]): 763–67.

99. Anne Kendall et al., "Weight Loss on a Low-Fat Diet: Consequences of the Imprecision of the Control of Food Intake in Humans," *American Journal of Clinical Nutrition* 53 (5[May 1991]): 1124–29.

100. See Bonnie Liebman, "Food Labels: Made with Real Tricks," *Nutrition Action Healthletter* 22 (4[May 1995]): 9.

101. Advertisement, *Self* 17 (1[January 1995]): 48.

4. Give Us This Day Our Daily Half Pound of Sugar

1. Edwin Bayrd, *The Thin Game* (New York: Newsweek Books, 1978), p. 44.

2. Janice Finch, "Overweight Britons Getting Fatter," United Press International, 28 February 1983.

3. Geoffrey Cannon and Hetty Einzig, *Dieting Makes You Fat* (New York: Simon & Schuster, 1985), 82–83.

4. William Dufty, *Sugar Blues* (New York: Warner, 1975).

5. Ibid., 214.

6. Ibid., 213.

7. Ibid., 74.

8. Ibid., 211.

9. *Shopping for Health* (Washington, D.C.: Food Marketing Institute and *Prevention* magazine, 1996), p. 16.

10. U.S. Bureau of the Census, *Statistical Abstract* (Washington, D.C., 1995): 147, table 225.

11. Ibid.

12. Nancy Kalish, "Meals That Really Keep You Healthy," *McCall's* 121 (12[September 1994]): E10.

13. R. E. Hodges and W. A. Krehl, "The Role of Carbohydrate in Lipid Metabolism," *American Journal of Clinical Nutrition* 17 (5[November 1965]): 334, as cited in K. W. Heaton, "Food Fibre As an Obstacle to Energy Intake," *The Lancet* 2 (7843[22 December 1973]): 1418–21.

14. Marcia Mogelonsky, "Americans Are Sweet on Goodies," *Denver Post,* 11 October 1995, p. G1.

15. Michele Meyer, "Hidden Sugar," *Self* 17 (2[February 1995]): 66.

16. Paula J. Geiselman, "Sugar-Induced Hyperphagia: Is Hyperinsulinemia, Hypoglycemia, or Any Other Factor a 'Necessary' Condition?" *Appetite* 11 (supp. 1 [1988]): 26–34.

17. A. Sclafani and A. L. Kirchgessner, "Influence of Taste and Nutrition on the Sugar Appetite of Rats," *Nutrition and Behavior* 3 (1[1986]): 57–74.

18. See Geiselman, "Sugar-Induced Hyperphagia," 26–34; B. K. Anand in *Obesity Symposium,* W. L. Burland and J. Yudkin Samuel, eds. (Edinburgh: 1974): 116, as cited in Haber et al., "Dietary Fibre," 679–82.

19. See G. Harvey Anderson, "Sugars, Sweetness, and Food Intake," *American Journal of Clinical Nutrition* 62 (1supp.[July 1995]): 195S–202S.

20. For example, J. F. Richardson, "Sugar Intake of Businessmen and Its Inverse Relationship with Relative Weight," *British Journal of Nutrition* 27 (1972): 449–60.

21. Personal telephone communication with Marion Nestle, 24 April 1996.

22. Uncle Sam also must share the blame. In the new government-mandated information labels, there is only a space for simple sugars. Complex sugars, which make up two thirds of the sugar in corn syrup, for example, are not to be listed there. But when eaten, they turn into the very simple sugars that must be listed.

23. Caroline Lees and Tim Rayment, "New Sugar Warning On Diet," *Sunday Times* (London), 16 June 1991.

24. Meyer, "Hidden Sugar," 66.

25. J. E. Blundell and A. J. Hill, "Paradoxical Effects of an Intense Sweetener (Aspartame) on Appetite," *The Lancet* 1 (8489[10 May 1986]): 1092–93.

26. Barbara J. Rolls, "Effects of Intense Sweeteners on Hunger, Food Intake, and Body Weight: A Review," *American Journal of Clinical Nutrition* 53 (4[April 1991]): 872–78. Another study purporting to show that aspartame increases hunger—Michael G. Tordoff and Annette M. Alleva, "Oral Stimulation with Aspartame Increases Hunger," *Physiology and Behavior* 47 (3[March 1990]): 555–59—suffered the same defect.

27. Ibid.

28. David J. Canty and Mabel M. Chan, "Effects of Consumption of Caloric versus Noncaloric Sweet Drinks on Indices Hunger and Food Consumption in Normal Adults," *American Journal of Clinical Nutrition* 53 (5[May 1991]): 1159–64. This is also the case when the sweetener is put in a food, as in a 1994 study in which aspartame was mixed into a creamy white cheese product and fed to both lean and obese French women. These obese French women did end up eating almost twice as much as the lean ones, but this is simply because fat people eat more than thin ones, not because their appetite had been especially stimulated. The report concluded, "Aspartame did not increase hunger or promote food consumption." See Adam Drewnowski et al., "The Effects of Aspartame versus Sucrose on Motivational Ratings, Taste Preferences, and Energy Intakes in Obese and Lean Women," *International Journal of Obesity* 18 (8[August 1994]): 570–78.

29.   Rolls, "Effects of Intense Sweeteners," 872–78.
30.   Bonnie Liebman, "A Dozen Do's & Don'ts," *Nutrition Action Healthletter* 23 (5[May 1996]): 13.

5. Big Fat Myths That Make Us Fatter

1.   Center for Media and Public Affairs, "Food for Thought," *Media Monitor* 9 (6[November–December 1995]): 2.
2.   "Chubby? Blame Those Genes," *Time* 135 (23[4 June 1990]): 80.
3.   Claude Bouchard et al., "The Response to Long-Term Overfeeding in Identical Twins," *New England Journal of Medicine* 322 (21[24 May 1990]): 1477–82.
4.   Albert J. Stunkard, et al., "The Body Mass Index of Twins Who Have Been Reared Apart," *New England Journal of Medicine* 322 (21[24 May 1990]): 1483–88; Albert J. Stunkard et al., "An Adoption Study of Human Obesity," *New England Journal of Medicine* 314 (4[23 January 1986]): 193–98; Thorkild I. A. Sørensen, Claus Holst, and Albert J. Stunkard, "Childhood Body Mass Index: Genetic and Familial Environmental Influences Assessed in a Longitudinal Adoption Study," *International Journal of Obesity* 16 (9[September 1992]): 705–14.
5.   David B. Allison et al., "Race Effects in the Genetics of Adolescents' Body Mass Index," *International Journal of Obesity* 18 (6[June 1994]): 363–68.
6.   Claude Bouchard, "Current Understanding of the Etiology of Obesity: Genetic and Nongenetic Factors," *American Journal of Clinical Nutrition* 53 (6(supp.[June 1991]): 1561S–1565S.
7.   A. Astrup and A. Raben, "Obesity: An Inherited Metabolic Deficiency in the Control of Macronutrient Balance?" *European Journal of Clinical Nutrition* 46 (9[September 1992]): 611–20.
8.   Thorkild I. A. Sørenson and Albert J. Stunkard, "Does Obesity Run in Families Because of Genes?" *Acta Psychiatry Scandinavia* 87 (370(supp. 370[1993]): 67–72.
9.   Institute of Medicine, *Weighing the Options* (Washington, D.C.: National Academy Press, 1995): 53.
10.   Anne M. Fletcher, *Thin for Life* (Shelburne, Vermont: Chapters, 1994), p. 31.
11.   Astrup and Raben, "Inherited Metabolic Deficiency," 611–20.
12.   Personal telephone communication with Paul Williams, 24 June 1996.
13.   Timothy J. Rink, "In Search of a Satiety Factor," *Nature* 372 (6505[1 December 1994]): 406–7.
14.   Natalie Angier, "Researchers Link Obesity in Humans to Flaw in a Gene," *New York Times*, 1 December 1994, p. A1.
15.   Sally Smith, "Editorial: Setpoint or Set-up," *NAAFA Newsletter* 25 (5[March–April 1995]): 10.
16.   Daniel Pinkwater, "Portly's Complaint," *Omni* 17 (7[April 1995]): 103.
17.   Philip Elmer-DeWitt et al., "Fat Times," *Time* 145 (2[16 January 1995]): 63.
18.   "Fat Genes," *Courier-Journal* (Louisville, Kentucky), 4 December 1994, p. 2D.
19.   Associated Press, "Scientists Find Genetic Flaw that Spurs Obesity, Diabetes," *Washington Times*, 10 August 1995, p. A8.
20.   Ibid.

21. JoAnn E. Manson et al., "Body Weight and Mortality Among Women," *New England Journal of Medicine* 333 (11[11 September 1995]): 677–85.

22. Elizabeth Widén et al., "Association of Polymorphism in the β3-Adrenergic-Receptor Gene with Features of Insulin Resistance Syndrome in Finns," *New England Journal of Medicine* 333 (6[10 August 1995]): 348–51.

23. Gary D. Foster, Thomas A. Wadden, and Renee A. Vogt, "Resting Energy Expenditure in Obese African-American and Caucasian Women," *Obesity Research* 5 (1[January 1997]): 1–8, table 1.

24. Personal telephone communication with G. Ken Goodrick, 19 March 1996.

25. CNN *Morning News*, "Obesity Gene Still Plagues Americans," Transcript No.905, Segment No.12, 13 March 1995, p. 1.

26. Lisa Grunwald, Anne Hollister, and Miriam Bensimhon, "Do I Look Fat to You?" *Life* 18 (2[February 1995]): 64.

27. Gina Kolata, "Fat-Signaling Hormone Is Clue to Weight Control," *New York Times*, 1 August 1995, p. B8.

28. W. C. Knowler et al., "Diabetes Incidence and Prevalence in Pima Indians: A Nineteenfold Greater Incidence than in Rochester, Minnesota," *American Journal of Epidemiology* 108 (6[17 December 1978]): 497–505.

29. Russell Rising et al., "Racial Difference in Body Core Temperature Between Pima Indian and Caucasian Men," *International Journal of Obesity* 19 (1[January 1995]): 1–5.

30. Anne Marie Fontvielle, John Dwyer, and Eric Ravussin, "Resting Metabolic Rate and Body Composition of Pima Indian and Caucasian Children," *International Journal of Obesity* 16 (8[August 1992]): 535–42.

31. Eric Ravussin et al., "Reduced Rate of Energy Expenditure as a Risk Factor for Body-Weight Gain," *New England Journal of Medicine* 318 (8[25 February 1988]): 467–72.

32. Anne Marie Fontvielle, Andrea Kriska, and Eric Ravussin, "Decreased Physical Activity in Pima Indian Compared with Caucasian Children," *International Journal of Obesity* 17 (8[August 1993]): 445–52.

33. Russell Rising et al., "Determinants of Total Daily Energy Expenditure: Variability in Physical Activity," *American Journal of Clinical Nutrition* 59 (4[April 1994]): 800–4.

34. Eric Ravussin et al., "Effects of a Traditional Lifestyle on Obesity in Pima Indians," *Diabetes Care* 17 (9[September 1994]): 1067–74.

35. One of the photographs, showing two men and a woman, appeared in the *New Yorker* 72 (19[15 July 1996]): 15.

36. A. M. Hodge et al., "Dramatic Increase in the Prevalence of Obesity in Western Samoa Over the Thirteen-Year Period 1978–1991," *International Journal of Obesity* 18 (6[June 1994]): 419–28.

37. Ivan G. Pawson and Craig Janes, "Massive Obesity in a Migrant Samoan Population," *American Journal of Public Health* 71 (5[May 1981]): 508–13.

38. Tom Wolfe, *Radical Chic and Mau-Mauing the Flak Catchers* (New York: Farrar, Straus and Giroux, 1970), p. 107.

39. Pawson and Janes, "Massive Obesity," 510.

40. Stephen T. McGarvey, "Obesity in Samoans and a Perspective on Its Eti-

ology in Polynesians," *American Journal of Clinical Nutrition* 53 (6(supp.[June 1991]): 1586S–1594S.

41. J. David Curb and Ellen B. Marcus, "Body Fat and Obesity in Japanese-Americans," *American Journal of Clinical Nutrition* 53 (6 supp.[June 1991]): 1552S–1555S.

42. Lucile L. Adams-Campbell et al., "Obesity, Body Fat Distribution, and Blood Pressure in Nigerian and African-American Men and Women," *Journal of the National Medical Association* 86 (1[January 1994]): 60–64.

43. Ibid.

44. Personal telephone communication with John Foreyt, 3 January 1996.

45. Carrie Hemenway, "Celebrating Our Fat Culture," in Sally Smith, ed., *Size Acceptance and Self-Acceptance*, 2nd ed. (Sacramento: National Association for the Advancement of Fat Acceptance, 1994), p. 34.

46. Emily Harrison, "The Morality of Fat," letter in *The New York Times Magazine*, 31 March 1996, p. 10.

47. Mara E. Levison, "Fat or Thin, Accept People the Way They Are," letter in *USA Today*, 21 March 1995, p. 8A.

48. Gilbert A. Leveille, *The Setpoint Diet* (New York: Ballantine, 1985).

49. Robert Greene, "Survey: Less Fat, but Lots of Snacks and Soft Drinks," Associated Press, 17 January 1996.

50. Gina Kolata, "Metabolism Found to Adjust to a Body's Natural Weight," *New York Times*, 9 March 1995, p. A1.

51. Joan Beck, "Think You'll Ever Be Slim Again? Fat Chance!," *Denver Post*, 11 March 1995, p. 2D.

52. Christopher Mumma, "Even the Best Dieters May Be Doomed; Study Bolsters Setpoint Theory," *The Record*, 9 March 1995, p. A1.

53. "Dieting Won't Be of Much Help to the Obese; Body Weight Not Voluntary, Authors of New Study Say," *St. Louis Post-Dispatch*, 9 March 1995, p. 3A.

54. Rudolph L. Leibel, Michael Rosenbaum, and Jules Hirsch, "Changes in Energy Expenditure Resulting from Altered Body Weight," *New England Journal of Medicine* 332 (10[19 March 1995]): 626.

55. Ibid., 623–24.

56. ABC, *Day One*, "Why You Can't Lose Weight by Dieting," 12 April 1995, Transcript No.186, p. 6.

57. "Why Those Lost Pounds Keep Coming Back," *U.S. News & World Report* 118 (11[20 March 1995]): 19.

58. NPR's *All Things Considered*, "Battle of the Bulge May Be a Lost Cause," 11 March 1995, Transcript No. 1783, Segment No. 4, p. 1.

59. Deepak Chopra, *Perfect Weight* (New York: Harmony Books, 1994).

60. CNN *Morning News*, "Doctor Says Speed Up Metabolism to Lose Weight," 19 December 1994, Transcript No. 818, p. 1. For more on one of the master hucksters of the 1990s, see Matt Labash, "The End of History and the Last Guru," *The Weekly Standard* 1 (41[1 July 1996]): 18.

61. Glenn A. Gaesser, *Big Fat Lies* (New York: Ballantine, 1996), p. 119.

62. Leveille, *Setpoint Diet*, cover.

63. *Charlie Rose*, "Metabolism and Weight Change," 9 March 1995, Transcript No.1330, p. 4.

64. Dawn Margolis, "When Weight Loss Stalls," *American Health* 14 (9[November 1995]): 32.

65. Personal telephone communication with Steven Heymsfield, M.D., 22 February 1996.

66. Thomas A. Wadden et al., "Long-Term Effects of Dieting on Resting Metabolic Rate in Obese Outpatients," *Journal of the American Medical Association* 264 (6[8 August 1990]): 707–11. Similarly, a 1992 study of children and adolescents who had lost weight on a controlled diet found that after three weeks resting metabolic rate had declined from burning an average of 1,793 calories a day at the beginning of the diet to burning only 1,464 a day at the end of the diet. But from there the metabolic rate climbed so much that by twelve months after the diet's end, the resting metabolic rate was 2,047, far *higher* than it had been at the beginning. To be sure, some of this was because the kids were still growing. They were taller, hence their metabolisms had gone up to provide more energy for the added height. But let's look at the kids on a per-pound basis. Before the diets they burned on average 45 calories per kilogram (2.2 pounds) of fat-free mass while afterward it was exactly the same. Their metabolisms had completed readjusted. Further, the diet had been a successful one. At the twelve-month postdiet point they had 5 percent less fat than before they began dieting. See Karl F. M. Zwiauer, Thomas Mueller, and Kurt Widhalm, "Resting Metabolic Rate in Obese Children Before, During, and After Weight Loss," *International Journal of Obesity* 16 (1[January 1992]): 11–16.

   Other studies have found no reduction in metabolic rate other than that caused by losing the weight itself (again, the big car–small car analogy). One study in the *American Journal of Clinical Nutrition* stated, "When adjusted for either total body weight or more specifically calculated in relation to the fat-free mass, the post-obese group had a normal" basal metabolic rate. In W. Philip T. James, Michael E. J. Lean, and Geraldine McNeill, "Dietary Recommendations After Weight Loss: How to Avoid Relapse of Obesity," *American Journal of Clinical Nutrition* 45 (supp. 45[May 1987]): 1135–41. Another study, which lasted nine months, concluded, "Total calories needed to maintain body weight at the end of this program were slightly, though not significantly, *higher* than at baseline [emphasis added]," despite an average loss of more than twelve pounds for those who had become fat as children and more than seven pounds for those who had become fat as adults. In Jane M. Moore, William E. Oddou, and James E. Leklem, "Energy Need in Childhood and Adult-Onset Obese Women Before and After a Nine-Month Nutrition and Education and Walking Program," *International Journal of Obesity* 14 (5[May 1991]): 337–44.

67. Covert Bailey, *The New Fit or Fat* (Boston: Houghton Mifflin, 1991), pp. 7–8.

68. Joel Gurin, "Leaner, Not Lighter," *Psychology Today* 23 (6[June 1989]): 40.

69. Diane Epstein and Kathleen Thompson, *Feeding on Dreams* (New York: Avon, 1994), p. xx).

70. Dale Atrens, *Don't Diet* (New York: William Morrow and Company, Inc., 1988), p. 77.

71. Ibid., 75.

72. Dawn Atkins, "Genetics, Fat, and Weight," in Sally Smith, ed., *Size Acceptance & Self-Acceptance*, 2nd ed. (Sacramento: NAAFA,: 1994), p. 13.

73. See, for example, Valerie George et al., "Further Evidence for the Presence of 'Small Eaters' and 'Large Eaters' Among Women," *American Journal of Clinical Nutrition* 53 (2[February 1991]): 425–26; Marie-Françoise Rolland-Cachera and France Bellisle, "No Correlation Between Adiposity and Food Intake: Why Are Working Class Children Fatter?" *American Journal of Clinical Nutrition* 44 (6[December 1986]): 779–87.

74. Steven W. Lichtman et al., "Discrepancy Between Self-Reported and Actual Caloric Intake and Exercise in Obese Subjects," *New England Journal of Medicine* 327 (27[31 December 1992]): 1893–98.

75. CNN *World News*, "Failing Dieters Often Don't Admit to All They Eat," 30 December 1993, Transcript No.232, Segment No.4, p. 1.

76. Lichtman et al., "Discrepancy Between Self-Reported and Actual Caloric Intake and Exercise in Obese Subjects," 1893–98.

77. CNN's *Daybreak*, "Obesity Study Shows Misguided Attempts to Lose Weight," 3 January 1993, Transcript No. 257, Segment No. 5, p. 1.

78. Rosemary Green, *Diary of a Fat Housewife* (New York: Warner, 1995), p. 271.

79. Beth Donahue, *This Is Insanity!* (Fort Worth: The Summit Group, 1994), 10.

80. Terry Nicholetti Garrison and David Levitsky, M.D., *Fed Up!: A Woman's Guide to Freedom from the Diet/Weight Prison* (New York: Carroll & Graf, 1993), pp. 187–88.

81. Lisa J. Martin et al., "Comparison of Energy Intakes Determined by Food Records and Doubly Labeled Water in Women Participating in a Dietary-Intervention Trial," *American Journal of Clinical Nutrition* 63 (4[April 1996]): 483–90.

82. Berit Lilienthal Heitmann and Lauren Lissner, "Dietary Underreporting by Obese Individuals: Is It Specific or Non-Specific?" *British Medical Journal* 311 (7011[14 October 1995]): 986–89.

83. George A. Bray et al., "Eating Patterns of Massively Obese Individuals," *Journal of the American Dietetic Association* 72 (1[January 1978]): 24–27.

84. David Lansky and Kelly D. Brownell, "Estimates of Food Quantity and Calories: Errors in Self-Report Among Obese Patients," *American Journal of Clinical Nutrition* 35 (4[April 1982]): 727–32.

85. M. Prentice et al., "High Levels of Energy Expenditure in Obese Women," *British Medical Journal* 292 (6526[12 April 1986]): 983–87; W. P. T. James et al., "Elevated Metabolic Rates in Obesity," *The Lancet* 1 (8074[27 May 1978]): 1122–25; Jacques Fricker et al., "A Positive Correlation Between Energy Intake and Body Mass Index in a Population of 1,312 Overweight Subjects," *International Journal of Obesity* 13 (5[October 1989]): 673–81.

86. Stephen Welle et al., "Energy Expenditure Under Free-Living Conditions in Normal-Weight and Overweight Women," *American Journal of Clinical Nutrition* 55 (1[January 1992]): 14–21.

87. Personal telephone communication with Steven Heymsfield, M.D., 22 February 1996.

88. Ibid.

89. Ibid.

90. Gilbert B. Forbes, "Diet and Exercise in Obese Subjects: Self-Report Versus Controlled Measurements," *Nutrition Reviews* 51 (10[October 1993]): 296–300.

91. Elliot Danforth Jr. and Ethan A. H. Sims, "Obesity and Efforts to Lose Weight," *New England Journal of Medicine* 327(27[31 December 1992]): 1947–48.

92. Rand Stoneburner, M.D., as quoted in Michael Fumento, *The Myth of Heterosexual AIDS*, 2nd ed. (Washington, D.C.: Regnery Gateway, 1993), p. 91.

93. Ami Laws, "Actual versus Self-Reported Intake and Exercise in Obesity," letter in *New England Journal of Medicine* 328 (20[20 May 1993]): 1494–95.

94. George V. Mann, "The Influence of Obesity on Health," *New England Journal of Medicine* 291 (4[25 July 1974]): 178–85.

95. "Survey on Employment Discrimination," in Sally Smith, ed., *Size Acceptance & Self-Acceptance*, 2nd ed. (Sacramento: NAAFA, 1994), p. 93, table 1.

96. John Sedgwick, "America Is Fat!" *Self* 17 (1[January 1995]): 83.

97. *NAAFA Newsletter* 25 (5[March–April 1995]): 4.

98. ". . . You Have Nothing to Lose but Your Scales," *The American Enterprise* 6 (1[January–February 1995]): 10.

99. Laura Blackmon, "The 'A' Word," *NAAFA Newsletter* 25(5[March–April 1995]): 3.

100. Harry Gossett, "A Big Man's Fashion Statement," in Sally Smith, ed., *Size Acceptance & Self-Acceptance*, 2nd ed. (Sacramento: NAAFA, 1994), p. 39.

101. Pinkwater, "Portly's Complaint," 103.

102. NPR's *All Things Considered*, "Daniel Pinkwater Decries Anti-Fat Movement," 24 November 1994, Transcript No. 1676, Segment No. 4, p. 1.

103. CNN, *CNN News*, "Guests Discuss Findings Connecting Genetics and Obesity,"1 December 1994, Transcript pp. 824–25.

104. As quoted in Debra Gordon, "Cajun Chef Hears the Siren Call of Low-Fat," *Virginia Pilot* (Norfolk), 12 October 1995, p. F1.

105. Marian Burros, "Eating Well: Low Fat and Lots of It from Prudhomme," *New York Times*, 13 October 1993, p. C1.

106. Garrison and Levitsky, *Fed Up*, 200.

107. Remarks of John Garrow, "Symposium: Exploding the Myths of Obesity," at Robin Brook Centre, St. Bartholomew's Hospital, 22 November 1995.

108. Dale M. Atrens, *Don't Diet* (New York: William Morrow & Co., 1988), back flap.

109. Ibid., 54–55, 68.

110. Gaesser, *Big Fat Lies*, back cover.

111. Mike Sager, "Big," *GQ* 65 (6[June 1995]): 183.

112. Richard Klein, *Eat Fat* (New York: Pantheon, 1996).

113. Laura Fraser, *Losing It* (New York: Dutton, 1997).

114. Gaesser, *Big Fat Lies*, 4.

115. Ibid., 13.

116. Ibid., 76.

117. Ibid., 77.

118. Ibid., 153.

119. Ibid., 135.

120. Sager, "Big," 183.

121. Ibid., 215.

122. Laura Fraser, "The Office F Word," *Working Woman* 19 (6[June 1994]): 90.
123. "Verbatim," *Time* 148 (5[22 July 1996]): 19.
124. Susan Spillman, "Hollywood Is Falling for Hefty Heroes," *USA Today*, 8 February 1995, p. 10D.
125. *Heavyweights*, Buena Vista, 1995, Steven Brill, director.
126. Spillman, "Hollywood," 10D.
127. Cathy Miller, "Video Review: Fat Chance: The Big Prejudice," *NAAFA Newsletter* 25 (5[March–April 1995]): 2.
128. See William J. Fabrey, "Big News," *Radiance* 44 (Fall 1995):17.
129. "Lyons Educates Kaiser Permanente," *NAAFA Newsletter* 25 (5[March–April 1995]): 6.
130. Ken Hecht, "Oh, Come On Fatties!" *Newsweek* 116 (10[3 September 1990]): 8.
131. Susan Estrich, "Thin Feminists Drive Me Crazy," *USA Today*, 12 October 1995, p. 11A.
132. Green, *Diary of a Fat Housewife*, 322.
133. CNN, *CNN Presents*, "Food to Die For," May 1995.
134. Colleen S. W. Rand and Alex M. C. Macgregor, "Successful Weight Loss Following Obesity Surgery and the Perceived Liability of Morbid Obesity," *International Journal of Obesity* 15 (9[September 1991]): 577–79.
135. Charles Sykes, *A Nation of Victims* (New York: St. Martin's Press, 1992), p. 7.
136. Mike Royko, "A Discrimination Charge Hits Bottom," *Chicago Tribune*, 22 May 1991, as cited in Sykes, *A Nation of Victims*, p. 7.
137. "Only in America (Cont'd.)" *Fortune*, 5 November 1990, as cited in Sykes, *A Nation of Victims*, 7–8.
138. "Across the USA: News from Every State," *USA Today*, 10 February 1995, p. 11A.
139. J. Paul Leigh and Mark C. Berger, "Effects of Smoking and Being Overweight on Current Earnings," *American Journal of Preventive Medicine* 5 (1[January–February 1989]): 8–14.
140. C. T. Miller et al., "Social Interactions of Obese and Non-Obese Women," *Journal of Personality* 58(2[June 1990]): 365–80.
141. John Foreyt and G. Ken Goodrick, *Living Without Dieting* (New York: Warner Books, 1992), p. 64.
142. Geoffrey Cowley and Karen Springer, "The Biology of Beauty," *Newsweek* 127 (23[3 June 1996]): 65–66.
143. See Colleen S. W. Rand and John M. Kuldau, "The Epidemiology of Obesity and Self-Defined Weight Problem in the General Population: Gender, Race, Age, and Social Class," *International Journal of Eating Disorders* 9 (3[May 1990]): 329–43; Deborah A. Dawson, "Ethnic Differences in Female Overweight: Data from the 1985 National Health Interview Survey," *American Journal of Public Health* 78 (10[October 1988]): 1326–29; Sharon M. Desmond et al., "Black and White Adolescents' Perceptions of Their Weight," *Journal of School Health* 59 (8[October 1989]): 353–58; Shiriki Kumanyika, Judy F. Wilson, and Marsha Guilford-Davenport, "Weight-Related Attitudes and Behaviors of Black Women," *Journal of the American Dietetic Association* 93 (3[April 1993]): 416.

144. Robert W. Jeffrey et al., "Correlates of Weight Loss and Its Maintenance over Two Years of Follow-up Among Middle-Aged Men," *Preventive Medicine* 13 (2[March 1984]): 155–68.

145. James Langton, "The Right Stuff," *Sunday Telegraph*, 28 January 1996, Review, p. 1.

146. Dinesh D'Souza, *The End of Racism* (New York: Free Press, 1995), pp. 499–501.

147. Carol Johnson, *Self-Esteem Comes in All Sizes* (New York: Doubleday, 1995).

148. Philip Elmer-DeWitt et al., "Fat Times," *Time* 145(2[16 January 1995]): 65.

149. William Langley, "Size Is Everything," *Sunday Telegraph* (London), 13 November 1994, p. 1.

150. Rebecca Freligh, "The Weighty Politics of Size," *Cleveland Plain Dealer*, 19 September 1995, p. 1E.

151. NPR's *All Things Considered*, "Daniel Pinkwater Decries Anti-Fat Movement," Transcript No.1676, Segment No.4, 24 November 1994, p. 1.

152. Karen A. Wilson and Jean Libman Block, "Why Big Isn't Beautiful," *Good Housekeeping* 222 (3[March 1996]): 62–63.

153. Ibid., 66.

154. Ibid.

155. Jean Garton, "Who Broke the Baby?" *Living* (8[Fall 1995]): 5.

6. The Profiteers

1. Marketdata Enterprises, "Diet Drugs Now Hottest Segment of Slow-Growth, Competitive U.S. Weight-Loss Industry," press release of 21 March 1996. p. 3.

2. Advertisement, *New York Times Book Review*, 29 September 1996, p. 4.

3. Bonnie Liebman, "Carbo-Phobia," *Nutrition Action Healthletter* 23 (6[July–August 1996]): 3.

4. Susan Gilbert, *Medical Fakes and Frauds* (New York: Chelsea House Publishers, 1989), 297–98.

5. Ibid., 33.

6. Ibid., 46.

7. This appears to be an imitation of a device sold during the late 1960s called the Relax-A-Cisor, which the manufacturer promised would help people lose weight by delivering a mild electric shock. The FDA pulled it off the market, but not before 400,000 Americans shelled out for it. See ibid., 17, citing a report of the House of Representatives Select Committee on Aging, Subcommittee on Health and Long-Term Care.

8. Advertisement, *Profiles* 9 (8[August 1996]): unnumbered page.

9. Jean Antonello, *How to Become Naturally Thin by Eating More* (New York, Avon Books, 1989); Dean Ornish, *Eat More, Weigh Less* (New York: Harper-Collins, 1993); Cliff Sheats and Maggie Greenwood-Robinson, *Lean Bodies: The Revolutionary New Approach to Losing Bodyfat by Increasing Calories* (New York: Warner Books, 1992); Elaine Moquette-Magee, *Fight Fat and Win: How to Eat a Low-Fat Diet Without Changing Your Lifestyle* (Minneapolis: Chronimed/DCI, 1990).

10. Martin Schiff, M.D., *Dr. Schiff's Miracle Weight-Loss Guide* (West Nyack, New York: Parker, 1974).

11. Adele Puhn, *The Five-Day Miracle Diet* (New York: Ballantine, 1996).
12. Earl F. Updike, *The Miracle Diet: Fourteen Days to New Vigor and Health* (Phoenix: Best Possible Health, 1995).
13. Susan Powter, *Stop the Insanity!* (New York: Simon & Schuster, 1993).
14. Rachael F. Heller and Richard F. Heller, *The Carbohydrate Addict's Diet* (New York: Dutton, 1991), p. 85.
15. Barry Sears and William Lawren, *The Zone* (New York: HarperCollins, 1995).
16. For a good critique of this dumb book, see Liebman, "Carbo-Phobia," p. 3.
17. Abraham I. Friedman, *How Sex Can Keep You Slim* (Englewood Cliffs, New Jersey: Prentice Hall, 1972).
18. Robert F. Joseph, M.D., *The Chocolate Lovers' Diet* (Rancho Mirage, CA: Noble Porter Press, 1995); Debra Waterhouse, *Why Women Need Chocolate* (New York: Hyperion, 1995).
19. Debbie Johnson, *How to Think Yourself Thin* (Portland, Oregon: Deborah Johnson Publishing, 1994), p. 70.
20. Ibid., 113.
21. Suzanne Mantell, *Publishers Weekly* 243 (9[26 February 1996]): 72.
22. Martin Katahn, *The T-Factor Diet* (New York: W. W. Norton, 1989), back cover.
23. Herman Taller, *Calories Don't Count* (New York: Simon & Schuster, 1961).
24. Edwin Bayrd, *The Thin Game* (New York: Newsweek Books, 1978), p. 58.
25. Donald Dale Jackson, "The Art of Wishful Shrinking Has Made a Lot of People Rich," *The Smithsonian* 25 (8[November 1994]): 154.
26. Stillman, *The Doctor's Quick Weight-Loss Diet.*
27. Robert C. Atkins, *Dr. Atkins' Diet Revolution* (New York: Bantam, 1973).
28. Geoffrey Cannon and Hetty Einzig, *Dieting Makes You Fat* (New York: Simon & Schuster, 1985), p. 121.
29. United Artists, *Sleeper*, Woody Allen, director, 1973.
30. Richard Mackarness, *Eat Fat, Grow Slim* (New York: Pocket Books, 1962), 73.
31. Jane E. Brody, *Jane Brody's Good Food Book* (New York: W. W. Norton, 1985).
32. Wendy Marston, "The New Diet Food," *Health* 10 (5[September 1996]): 102.
33. Ibid.
34. Joel Herskowitz, *The Popcorn Plus Diet* (New York: Pharos Books, 1987); Judy Moscovitz, *The Rice Diet Report* (New York: G. P. Putnam's Sons, 1986).
35. Edwin McDowell, "Behind the Best-Sellers," *New York Times*, 23 August 1981, Section 7, p. 26.
36. Judy Mazel, *The New Beverly Hills Diet* (Deerfield Beach, Florida: Health Communications, Inc., 1996).
37. Harvey and Marilyn Diamond, *Fit for Life* (New York: Warner, 1987), cover. They also penned a sequel, Harvey and Marilyn Diamond, *Fit for Life II: Living Health* (New York, Warner, 1987).
38. Stephen Barrett and the editors of *Consumer Reports, Health Schemes, Scams, and Frauds* (Mount Vernon, New York: Consumers Union, 1990), p. 135.
39. As quoted in Ibid., 137.
40. Stuart Berger, M.D., *The Southampton Diet* (New York: Avon, 1983); Stuart Berger, M.D., *Forever Young: Twenty Years Younger in Twenty Weeks* (New York: Avon, 1990).

41. Stuart Berger, M.D., *The Immune Power Diet* (New York: Signet, 1985), pp. 4–5.
42. Ira Mortimer, "One Doctor Offers a Diet Cure for Everything from Asthma to Obesity, but Others Are Skeptical," *Chicago Tribune*, 12 February 1986, p. 23.
43. Allan Hall, "Death of the Diet Myth," *Daily Mirror* (London), 23 March 1995, p. 4.
44. Berger, *Immune Power Diet*, 4.
45. Ibid., 19.
46. Ibid., 31.
47. Nathan D. Schultz et al., *The Best Guide to Allergy* (Totowa, New Jersey: Humana Press, 1994), 113.
48. Ibid., 55.
49. Mary Voboril, "Of Chickens, Condoms, and a Con Man," *Newsday*, 15 May 1994, p. A26.
50. Powter, *Stop the Insanity!*, 87.
51. Ibid., 126.
52. Sharon Churcher, "Living Off the Fat of the Land," *Mail on Sunday* (London), 7 November 1994, p. 40.
53. Robinson G. Clark, "No More Fat City," *St. Louis Post-Dispatch*, 30 January 1994, p. 1E.
54. Powter, *Stop the Insanity!*, 153–54.
55. Ibid., 127.
56. Ibid., 132.
57. Ibid., 147.
58. As quoted in Laura Fraser, *Losing It* (New York: Dutton, 1997), 76.
59. Ibid., 107.
60. Ibid., 97.
61. Churcher, "Living Off the Fat of the Land," 40.
62. Nanci Hellmich, "Fitness Buff Powter's Battle of Bankruptcy," *USA Today*, 10 January 1995, p. 2D.
63. Nanci Hellmich, "Bringing Powter to the People," *USA Today*, 6 June 1995, p. 6D.
64. Cliff Sheats and Maggie Greenwood-Robinson, *Lean Bodies: The Revolutionary New Approach to Losing Bodyfat by Increasing Calories.*
65. Ibid., 2.
66. Ibid., 3.
67. Patrick Pasquet et al., "Massive Overfeeding and Energy Balance in Men: The *Guru Walla* Model," *American Journal of Clinical Nutrition* 56 (3[September 1992]): 483–90.
68. Patrick Pasquet and Marian Apfelbaum, "Recovery of Initial Body Weight and Composition After Long-Term Massive Overfeeding in Men," *American Journal of Clinical Nutrition* 60 (6[December 1994]): 861–63; Tracy J. Horton et al., "Fat and Carbohydrate Overfeeding in Humans: Different Effects on Energy Storage," *American Journal of Clinical Nutrition* 62 (1[July 1995]): 19–29; see also, Erik O. Diaz et al., "Metabolic Response to Experimental Overfeeding in Lean and Overweight Health Volunteers," *American Journal of Clinical Nutrition* 56 (4[October 1992]): 641–55; Angelo Tremblay et al., "Overfeeding and Energy Expenditure in Humans," *American Journal of Clinical Nutrition* 56 (5[November 1992]): 857–62.

69. "Metabolism Does Not Change to Prevent Weight Gain During Over-feeding, USDA Study finds," *Journal of the American Dietetic Association* 90 (11[November 1990]): 1556.

70. Neal Barnard, *Foods that Cause You to Lose Weight: The Negative Calorie Effect* (McKinney, Texas: Magni Group, Inc., 1992).

71. Judy Jameson, *Fat-Burning Foods and Other Weight Loss Secrets* (Chicago: Contemporary Books, 1994).

72. Sheats and Greenwood-Robinson, *Lean Bodies*, 176.

73. Ibid., 10.

74. Cliff Sheats and Maggie Greenwood-Robinson, *Lean Bodies Total Fitness* (New York: Summit, 1995).

75. Richard and Rachael Heller, *Healthy for Life* (New York: Dutton, 1995).

76. O'Neill, "So It May be True After All: Eating Pasta Makes You Fat," *New York Times*, 8 February 1995, p. A1.

77. Nanci Hellmich, "A Plate Full of Reasons for Eating Your Pasta," *USA Today*, 8 March 1995, p. 7D.

78. Ibid.

79. Yes, I'm just kidding. Please don't sue me, Pepsico.

80. Kristine Napier, "Pasta Is Not Poison," *Harvard Health Letter* 20 (9[July 1995]): 1.

81. Ibid., 2.

82. Heller and Heller, *Carbohydrate Addict's Diet*, 11.

83. Sears and Lawren, *The Zone*, 11.

84. Heller and Heller, *Carbohydrate Addict's Diet*, 54.

85. Ibid., 105.

86. Ibid., 11.

87. Ibid., 53.

88. Ibid., 84.

89. Ibid., 85.

90. John P. Foreyt and G. Ken Goodrick, *Living Without Dieting* (New York: Warner, 1994).

91. Jane Brody, *Jane Brody's Good Food Book* (New York: W. W. Norton, 1985).

92. James M. Ferguson, *Habits Not Diets* (Palo Alto: Bell Publishing Company, 1988).

93. Morton H. Shaevitz, *Lean and Mean* (New York: G. P. Putnam's Sons, 1993).

94. Wayne Callaway, *The Callaway Diet* (New York: Bantam, 1990).

95. Rosemary Green, *Diary of a Fat Housewife* (New York: Warner, 1994).

96. Anne M. Fletcher, *Thin for Life* (Shelburne, Vermont: Chapters, 1994).

97. Evelyn Tribole and Elyse Resch, *Intuitive Eating* (New York: St. Martin's Press, 1995).

98. Daniel S. Kirschenbaum, *Weight Loss Through Persistence* (Oakland: New Harbinger Publications, Inc., 1994).

99. C. J. S. Thompson. *The Quacks of Old London* (New York: Barnes & Noble Books, 1993), 346.

100. Gilbert, *Medical Fakes and Frauds*, 29.

101. Brigid Schulte, "Losing Battle of the Bulge," *Albany Times Union*, 6 December 1994, p. A6.

102. Revenue data from personal telephone communication with John LaRosa of 25 June 1996. Other information adapted from Leslie Vreeland, "Lean Times in Fat City," *Working Woman* 20 (7[July 1995]): 73, and current to that date. For another quick summary, see Institute of Medicine, *Weighing the Options* (Washington, D.C.: National Academy Press, 1995), 66–80, table 3-1.

103. New York City Department of Consumer Affairs, *A Weighty Issue: Dangers and Deceptions of the Weight Loss Industry* (New York: Department of Consumer Affairs, June 1991), 9.

104. Diane Epstein and Kathleen Thompson, *Feeding on Dreams* (New York: Avon, 1994), p. 72.

105. Personal telephone communication with Leila Farzan, 19 June 1996.

106. "Rating the Diets," p. 354.

107. Testimony of William Vitale, M.D., before the U.S. House of Representatives, 7 May 1990, as cited in NYC Consumer Affairs, *Weighty Issue,* 24–25.

108. Personal telephone communication with John LaRosa, 2 July 1996.

109. Beth Donahue, *This Is Insanity!* (Ft. Worth, Texas: Summit Group, 1994), p. 16.

110. Epstein and Thompson, *Feeding on Dreams,* 5.

111. Personal telephone communication with John LaRose, 2 July 1996.

112. Personal telephone communication with Leila Farzan, 10 June 1996.

113. Brian O'Reilly and Susan Caminiti, "Diet Centers Are Really in Fat City," *Fortune* 112 (5[5 June 1989]): 140.

114. "Rating the Diets," *Consumer Reports* 58 (6[June 1993]): 353.

115. Joanne Kenen, "Consumer Group Seeks Disclosure of Weight-Loss Centers' Full Costs," *Philadelphia Inquirer,* 30 May 1996, p. A12.

116. Center for Science in the Public Interest (CSPI), "Weight-Loss Firms Keep Consumers in the Dark about Prices, Effectiveness" (press release), 29 May 1996.

117. CSPI, "Statement of Bruce Silverglade, Director of Legal Affairs, on Petition to the FTC to Prohibit Unfair and Deceptive Practices by Commercial Weight-Loss Centers," 29 May 1996, pp. 1–2.

118. Ibid., 332.

119. CNN *Morning News,* "Dieters Have to Work Hard to Keep Their Weight Off," 1 December 1993, Transcript No. 467, Segment No. 4, p. 1.

120. "Weight Watchers Drops Lawsuit," Associated Press, 9 September 1991.

121. Joanne Silberner, "War of the Diets," *U.S. News & World Report* 112 (4[3 February 1992]): 56.

122. CNN *Sonya Live,* "Diet Business," 24 May 1994, Transcript No. 554, p. 1.

123. Laura Fraser, "The Death of Dieting," *Vogue* 183 (5[May 1994]): 293.

124. Maggie Garb, "Will Diet Debate Thin Ranks of Office Plans? Doctors Reassess Own Programs as Industry Scrutinized," *American Medical News* 33 (26[6 July 1990]): 17–21.

125. David S. Hilzenrath, "Liquid-Diet Firms Must Back Claims; FTC, Three Companies Settle Ad Charges," *Washington Post,* 17 October 1991, p. A1.

126. Marvin A. Kirschner et al., "An Eight-Year Experience with a Very Low Calorie Formula Diet for Control of Major Obesity," *International Journal of Obesity* 12 (1[February 1988]): 69–80.

127. Schulte, "Losing Battle of the Bulge," A6.

128. "Rating the Diets," 353.
129. Ibid., 357.
130. Ibid., 354.
131. Andrew Leckey, "Diet Industry Is Falling on Lean Times," *Baltimore Sun*, 3 February 1995, p. 9C.
132. Personal telephone communication with Marion Nestle, 19 June 1996.
133. "Rating the Diets," 355.
134. NYC Consumer Affairs, *Weighty Issue*, 7.
135. *Overeaters Anonymous* (Torrance, California: Overeaters Anonymous, 1980).
136. Epstein and Thompson, *Feeding on Dreams*, 23.
137. *Wall Street*, Twentieth Century Fox, Oliver Stone, director, 1987.

7. Diets Don't Work—Except When They Do

1. Bob Schwartz, *Diets Don't Work* (Houston: Breakthru Publishing, 1982).
2. Albert J. Stunkard, "The Management of Obesity," *New York State Journal of Medicine* 58 (part 1[1 January 1958]): 79–87, as cited in Thomas A. Wadden, "Treatment of Obesity by Moderate and Severe Caloric Restriction," *Annals of Internal Medicine* 119 (7[1 October 1993]): 688–93.
3. Wadden, "Treatment of Obesity," 688–93.
4. Jane E. Brody, "Panel Criticizes Weight-Loss Programs," *New York Times*, 2 April 1992, p. D22. An edited summary of the report appears as NIH Technology Assessment Conference Panel, "Methods for Voluntary Weight Loss and Control," *Annals of Internal Medicine* 119 (7[1 October 1993]): 764–70. It doesn't actually contain the 90 to 95 percent figure, however.
5. Lisa Grunwald, Anne Hollister, and Miriam Bensimhon, "Do I Look Fat to You?" *Life* 18 (2[February 1995]): 62.
6. Ibid.
7. "Rating the Diets," *Consumer Reports* 58 (6[June 1993]): 354.
8. Jonathan I. Robison et al., "Obesity, Weight Loss, and Health," *Journal of the American Dietetic Association* 93 (4[April 1993]): 445–49.
9. Alan S. Levey and Alan W. Heaton, "Weight Control Practices of U.S. Adults Trying to Lose Weight," *Annals of Internal Medicine* 119 (7[1 October 1993]): 661–66.
10. Robert W. Jeffrey et al., "Correlates of Weight Loss and Its Maintenance over Two Years of Follow-up Among Middle-Aged Men," *Preventive Medicine* 13 (2[March 1984]): 155–68.
11. F. Matthew Kramer et al., "Long-Term Follow-up of Behavioral Treatment for Obesity: Patterns of Weight Regain Among Men and Women," *International Journal of Obesity* 13 (2[April 1989]): 123–36.
12. G. A. Marlatt and J. R. Gordon, "Determinants of Relapse: Implications for the Maintenance of Behavior Change," in P. O. Davidson and S. M. Davidson, eds., *Behavioral Medicine: Changing Health Lifestyles* (New York: Brunner/Mazel, 1980), 410–52; G. A. Marlatt and J. R. Gordon, eds., *Relapse Prevention: Maintenance Strategies in Addictive Behavior Change* (New York: Guilford, 1985), as cited in Susan Kayman, William Bruvold, and Judith S. Stern, "Maintenance and Relapse after Weight Loss in Women: Behavioral Aspects," *American Journal of Clinical Nutrition* 52 (5[November 1990]): 800–807.

13. Cliff Sheats and Maggie Greenwood-Robinson, *Lean Bodies: The Revolutionary New Approach to Losing Bodyfat by Increasing Calories* (New York: Warner Books, 1995), p. 14.

14. Debra Waterhouse, *Outsmarting the Female Fat Cell* (New York: Warner Books, 1993), p. 20.

15. Diane Epstein and Kathleen Thompson, *Feeding on Dreams* (New York: Avon, 1994), pp. 28–29.

16. Grunwald et al., "Do I Look Fat to You?" 64.

17. Thomas A. Wadden et al., "Effects of Weight Cycling on the Resting Energy Expenditure and Body Composition of Obese Women," *International Journal of Eating Disorders* 19 (1[January 1996]): 5–12.

18. A review of the entire weight cycling literature in the *International Journal of Obesity* in 1995 also found that, "Except for one study of non-obese women, cross-sectional studies of both nonobese and obese subjects have not shown differences in body composition between cyclers and noncyclers." Further, "these studies found little evidence that weight cycling affects resting energy expenditure," in Erik Muls et al., "Is Weight Cycling Detrimental to Health? A Review of the Literature in Humans," *International Journal of Obesity* 19 (Supp. 3[September 1995]): S46–S50. Due to an annual "hungry season," women in the African country of Gambia cycle 50 to 60 percent of their fat stores each year, yet "This natural weight cycling does not have a detrimental effect on lean body mass," reported a research team, in Andrew M. Prentice et al., "Effects of Weight Cycling on Body Composition," *American Journal of Clinical Nutrition* 56 (supp.[July 1992]): 209S–216S.

19. Glenn A. Gaesser, *Big Fat Lies*, (New York: Pantheon, 1996), p. 163.

20. Muls et al., "Is Weight Cycling?" S46–S50.

21. Rena R. Wing et al., "A Prospective Study of Effects of Weight Cycling on Cardiovascular Risk Factors," *Archives of Internal Medicine* 155 (13[10 July 1995]): 1416–22.

22. Lawrence Hardy, "Yo-Yo Dieting Doesn't Raise Heart Risk," *USA Today*, 25 July 1995, p. D1.

23. National Task Force on the Prevention and Treatment of Obesity, "Weight Cycling," *Journal of the American Medical Association* 272 (15[19 October 1994]): 1196–1202.

24. Wayne Callaway, *The Callaway Diet* (New York: Bantam, 1990), pp. 34–35.

25. Ibid., 36.

26. Kathleen Keough, "Weight Loss: Find the Weight That's Right for You," *The Ethnic Newswatch, Heart & Soul*, 38.

27. Thomas A. Wadden et al., "Less Food, Less Hunger: Reports of Appetite and Symptoms in a Controlled Study of a Protein-Sparing Modified Fast," *International Journal of Obesity* 11 (3[March 1987]): 239–49.

28. David J. Laporte and Albert J. Stunkard, "Predicting Attrition and Adherence to a Very Low Calorie Diet: A Prospective Investigation of the Eating Inventory," *International Journal of Obesity* 14 (3[March 1990]): 197–206.

29. Albert J. Stunkard, "Conservative Treatments for Obesity," *American Journal of Clinical Nutrition* 45 (5[May 1987]): 1142–54.

30. Gary D. Foster et al., "Controlled Trial of the Metabolic Effects of a Very

Low Calorie Diet: Short- and Long-Term Effects," *American Journal of Clinical Nutrition* 51 (2[February 1990]): 167–72.

31. Barbara Graham, "The Incredible Expanding American Portion," *Self* 18 (9[September 1996]): 101.

32. Evelyn Tribole and Elyse Resch, *Intuitive Eating* (New York: St. Martin's Press, 1995), p. 72.

33. Jeremy Iggers, *Garden of Eating* (New York: HarperCollins, 1996) p. 161.

34. Ibid., 214–15.

35. A. J. Blair, V. J. Lewis, and D. A. Booth, "Does Emotional Eating Interfere with Success in Attempts at Weight Control?" *Appetite* 15 (2[October 1990]): 151–57.

36. David G. Schlundt et al., "Obesity: A Biogenetic or Behavioral Problem," *International Journal of Obesity* 14 (9[September 1990]): 815–28.

37. John P. Foreyt and G. Ken Goodrick, "Factors Common to Successful Therapy for the Obese Patient," *Medicine and Science in Sports and Exercise* 23 (3[March 1991]): 292–97.

38. Ornish, *Eat More, Weigh Less*, 65.

39. Susie Orbach, *Fat Is a Feminist Issue* (New York: Berkeley, 1994).

40. Susie Orbach, *Hunger Strike* (New York: W. W. Norton & Co., 1986), 63.

41. Orbach, *Feminist Issue*, 6.

42. Ibid.

43. As quoted on the cover of Orbach, *Feminist Issue*.

44. Susie Orbach, *Fat Is a Feminist Issue II* (New York: Berkeley, 1982).

45. G. R. Leon and L. Roth, "Obesity: Psychological Causes, Correlations, and Psychological Speculations," *Psychology Bulletin* 84 (1[January 1977]): 117–39.

46. Schlundt et al., "Obesity: A Biogenetic or Behavioral Problem," 815–28.

47. CNN *Morning News*, "Women's Love for Chocolate May Be Biological," 1 May 1995, Transcript No. 3928, Segment No. 10.

48. J. Gormally et al., "The Assessment of Binge Eating Severity among Obese Persons," *Addictive Behaviors* 7 (1[1982]: 47–55; A. D. Loro and C. S. Orleans, "Binge Eating in Obesity: Preliminary Findings and Guidelines for Behavioral Analysis and Treatment," *Addictive Behaviors* 6 (2[1981]): 155–66; M. D. Marcus, R. R. Wing, and D. M. Lamparksi, "Binge Eating and Dietary Restraint among Obese Patients," *Addictive Behaviors* 10 (2[1985]): 163–68.

49. Gladys Witt Strain, Richard J. Hershcopf, and Barnett Zumoff, "Food Intake of Very Obese Persons: Quantitative and Qualitative Aspects," *Journal of the American Dietetic Association* 92 (2[February 1992]): 199–203.

50. Personal telephone communication with Marion Nestle, 24 April 1996.

51. "Just the Facts," *Nutrition Action Healthletter* 19 (3[April 1992]): 2.

52. Lisa R. Young and Marion Nestle, "Food Labels Consistently Underestimate the Actual Weights of Single-Serving Baked Products," *Journal of the American Dietetic Association* 95 (10[October 1995]): 1150–51.

53. CNN *News*, "Some 'Healthy' Food Products Dangerously Mislabeled," 9 June 1994, Transcript No. 742-6, pp. 1–2.

54. Nestle, personal telephone communication, 24 April 1996.

55. John M. de Castro and Sara Orozco, "Moderate Alcohol Intake and Spontaneous Eating Patterns of Humans: Evidence of Unregulated Supplementation," *American Journal of Clinical Nutrition* 52 (2[August 1990]): 246–53.

56. Graham A. Colditz et al., "Alcohol Intake in Relation to Diet and Obesity in Women and Men," *American Journal of Clinical Nutrition* 54 (1[July 1991]): 49–55.

57. Martha L. Slattery et al., "Associations of Body Fat and Its Distribution with Dietary Intake, Physical Activity, Alcohol, and Smoking in Blacks and Whites," *American Journal of Clinical Nutrition* 55 (5[May 1992]): 943–49.

58. Charles S. Lieber, "Perspectives: Do Alcohol Calories Count?" *American Journal of Clinical Nutrition* 57 (6[December 1991]): 976–82; William R. Rumpler et al., "Energy Value of Moderate Alcohol Consumption by Humans," *American Journal of Clinical Nutrition* 64 (1[July 1996]): 108–14.

59. Michele Stacey, *Consumed* (New York: Simon & Schuster, 1994), p. 212.

60. Data from National Snack Food Association, Alexandria, Virginia.

61. *National Survey of American Attitudes on Substance Abuse II: Teens and Their Parents* (New York: National Center on Addiction and Substance Abuse at Columbia University, September 1996), 24.

62. Alan Geliebter et al., "Reduced Stomach Capacity in Obese Subjects After Dieting," *American Journal of Clinical Nutrition* 63 (2[February 1996]): 170–73.

63. As quoted in Cathy Perlmutter and Michele Stanten, "Shrink Your Stomach," *Prevention* 48 (7[July 1996]): 86.

64. Ibid.

65. Ibid.

66. Rachel Schemmel, Olaf Mickelson, and J. L. Gill, "Dietary Obesity in Rats: Body Weight and Fat Accretion in Seven Strains of Rats," *Journal of Nutrition* 100 (1970): 1041–48.

67. Anthony Sclafani and Steven Xenakis, "Sucrose and Polysaccharide Induced Obesity in the Rat," *Physiology and Behavior* 32 (2[February 1984]): 169–75.

68. Barbara J. Rolls, P. M. Van Duijenvoorde, and Edward A. Rowe, "Variety in the Diet Enhances Intake in a Meal and Contributes to the Development of Obesity in the Rat," *Physiology and Behavior* 31 (1[July 1983]): 21–27.

69. Barbara J. Rolls, Edward A. Rowe, and E. T. Rolls, "How Flavor and Appearance Affect Human Feeding," *Proceedings in Nutritional Sociology* 41 ([1982]): 109–17.

70. Barbara Ehrenreich, "A Nation Playing with Its Food," *Time* 145 (2[9 January 1995]): 78.

71. Iggers, *Garden of Eating*, 2.

72. Patricia Long, "Winning at Losing Weight," *Health* 10 (1[January–February 1996]): 64.

73. Nanci Hellmich, "Conquering the Scales for Good," *USA Today*, 3 January 1995, p. 3D.

74. Long, "Winning at Losing," 63–64.

75. Fletcher, *Thin for Life*, 136.

76. Ibid., 17.

77. Susan Kayman, William Bruvold, and Judith S. Stern, "Maintenance and Relapse after Weight Loss in Women: Behavioral Aspects," *American Journal of Clinical Nutrition* 52 (5[November 1990]): 800–807.

78. Ibid.
79. Pamela S. Haines, David K. Guilkey, and Barry M. Popkin, "Trends in Breakfast Consumption of U.S. Adults Between 1965 and 1991," *Journal of the American Dietetic Association* 96 (5[May 1996]): 464–70.
80. Kayman, Bruvold, and Stern, "Maintenance and Relapse," 800–807.
81. Fletcher, *Thin for Life*, 235.
82. Carol A. Johnson, *Self-Esteem Comes in All Sizes* (New York: Doubleday, 1985).

8. The Fiber Factor

1. Denis P. Burkitt and Gene A. Spiller, "Dietary Fiber: From Early Hunter-Gatherers to the 1990s," in Gene A. Spiller, ed, *CRC Handbook of Dietary Fiber in Human Nutrition*, 2nd ed. (Boca Raton, Florida: CRC Press, 1992), p. 3.
2. Audrey Eaton, *The F-Factor Diet* (New York, Crown Publishers, Inc.: 1982).
3. "Position of the American Dietetic Association: Health Implications of Dietary Fiber," *Journal of the American Dietetic Association* 92 (12[December 1993]): 1446–7.
4. See Ruth McPherson, "Dietary Fiber: A Perspective," in Gene A. Spiller, ed., *CRC Handbook of Dietary Fiber in Human Nutrition*, 2nd ed. (Boca Raton, Florida: CRC Press, 1993), p. 7.
5. Council on Scientific Affairs, "Dietary Fiber and Health," *Journal of the American Medical Association* 262 (4[28 July 1989]): 542–46.
6. Beatrice Trum Hunter, "You Asked for It," *Consumers' Research* 79 (2[February 1996]): 9; see also Jane G. Muir and Kerin O'Dea, "Measurement of Resistant Starch: Factors Affecting the Amount of Starch Escaping in Vitro," *American Journal of Clinical Nutrition* 56 (1[July 1992]): 123–27.
7. D. H. Staniforth et al., "The Effects of Dietary Fiber on Upper and Lower Gastrointestinal Transit Times and Fecal Bulking," *The Journal of International Medical Research* 19 [3(May–June 1991]): 228–33.
8. Alexander R. P. Walker, "Disease Patterns in South Africa as Related to Dietary Fiber Intake," in Gene A. Spiller, ed., *CRC Handbook of Dietary Fiber in Human Nutrition*, 2nd ed., 491–95.
9. Ibid.
10. Council on Scientific Affairs, "Dietary Fiber and Health," 542–46.
11. See McPherson, "Dietary Fiber," 8.
12. A. J. M. Brodribb, "Dietary Fiber in Diverticular Disease of the Colon," in Gene Spiller and Ruth McPherson Kay, eds., *Medical Aspects of Dietary Fiber* (New York: Plenum Publishing Corp., 1980), p. 60.
13. J. C. Brocklehurst, *Gerontologica Clinica* 2 (1969), 293, as cited in David Reuben, *The Save Your Life Diet* (New York: Ballantine, 1975), p. 31.
14. Sharon E. Fleming, Mark D. Fitch, and Michael W. Chansler, "High-Fiber Diets: Influence on Characteristics of Cecal Digesta Including Short-Chain Fatty Acid Concentrations and pH," *American Journal of Clinical Nutrition* 50 (1[July 1989]): 93–99.
15. Council on Scientific Affairs, "Dietary Fiber and Health," 542–46.
16. For an exhaustive, early review of studies on the effect of fiber on diabetes, see James W. Anderson and Carol A. Bryant, "Dietary Fiber: Diabetes and Obesity," *American Journal of Gastroenterology* 81 (10[October 1986]): 898–906.

17. Eric Rimm et al., "Vegetable, Fruit, and Cereal Fiber Intake and Risk of Coronary Heart Disease among Men," *Journal of the American Medical Association* 275 (6[14 February 1996]): 447–51.

18. Bonnie Liebman, "Fiber: Separating Fact from Fiction," *Nutrition Action Healthletter* 21 (7[September 1994]): 5.

19. Council on Scientific Affairs, "Dietary Fiber and Health," 542–46.

20. James W. Anderson and Janet Tietyen-Clark, "Dietary Fiber: Hyperlipidemia, Hypertension, and Coronary Heart Disease," *American Journal of Gastroenterology* 81 (10[October 1986]): 907–8.

21. Center for Media and Public Affairs, "Food for Thought," *Media Monitor* 9 (6[November–December 1995]): 2.

22. O. C. Gruner, "A Treatise on the Canon of Medicine of Avicenna Incorporating a Translation of the First Book" (London: Luzac, 1930), as cited in George A. Bray, "Obesity: Historical Development of Scientific and Cultural Ideas," *International Journal of Obesity* 19 (11[November 1990]): 909–26.

23. For example, Britta Hylander and Stephan Rössner, "Effects of Dietary Fiber Intake before Meals on Weight Loss and Hunger in a Weight-Reducing Club," *Acta Medica Scandinavia* 213 (1[1983]): 217–20; Robin S. Shearer, "Effects of Bulk-Producing Tablets on Hunger Intensity in Dieting Patients," *Current Therapeutic Research* 19 (4[April 1976]): 433–41.

24. Carlene C. Hamilton and James W. Anderson, "Fiber and Weight Management," *Journal of the Florida Medical Association* 79 (6[June 1992]): 379–81.

25. Ibid.

26. K. W. Heaton, "Food Fibre As an Obstacle to Energy Intake," *The Lancet* 2(7843[22 December 1973]): 1418–21.

27. R. A. McCance, K. M. Prior, and E. M. Widdowson, "A Radiological Study of the Rate of Passage of Brown and White Bread through the Digestive Tract of Man," *British Journal of Nutrition* 7 ([1953]): 98, as cited in Heaton, "Food Fibre," 1418–21.

28. D. A. T. Southgate and J. V. G. A. Durnin, "Calorie Conversion Factors: An Experimental Reassessment of the Factors Used in the Calculation of the Energy Value of the Human Diets," *British Journal of Nutrition* 24 (1970): 517.

29. R. A. McCance et al., "The Chemical Composition of Wheat and Rye and of Flours Derived Therefrom," *Biochemical Journal* 39 (2[1945]): 213.

30. Heaton, "Food Fibre," 1418–21.

31. See also Patrick Borel et al., "Wheat Bran and Wheat Germ: Effect on Digestion and Intestinal Absorption of Dietary Lipids in the Rat," *American Journal of Clinical Nutrition* 49 (6[June 1989]): 1192–1202.

32. D. S. Grimes and C. Gordon, "Satiety Value of Wholemeal and White Bread," letter in *The Lancet* 2 (8080[8 July 1978]): 106.

33. Wayne C. Miller et al., "Dietary Fat, Sugar, and Fiber Predict Body Fat Content," *Journal of the American Dietetic Association* 94 (6[June 1994]): 612–15.

34. Stephan Rössner et al., "Weight Reduction with Dietary Fibre Supplements," *Acta Medica Scandinavia* 222 (1[1987]): 83–88.

35. Allen S. Levine et al., "Effect of Breakfast Cereals on Short-Term Food Intake," *American Journal of Clinical Nutrition* 50 (6[December 1989]):

1303–7. Similar results came in a study in which two groups of undergraduate men, one lean and one obese, were given two roast beef sandwich halves containing either high or low amounts of fiber and told there was more to come. After eating their sandwiches, the meal was interrupted as had been planned, although the test subjects didn't know it had been planned. Thirty-five to forty minutes later they were allowed to resume eating. While the amount of fiber did not affect the subsequent consumption of the lean men, the obese men who ate the high-fiber bread ate considerably less than the obese men who ate the low-fiber bread. See Katherine Porikos and Susan Hagamen, "Is Fiber Satiating? Effects of a High Fiber Preload on Subsequent Food Intake of Normal-Weight and Obese Young Men," *Appetite* 7 (2[June 1986]): 153–62.

36.   June Stevens et al., "Effect of Psyllium Gum and Wheat Bran on Spontaneous Energy Intake," *American Journal of Clinical Nutrition* 46 (4[October 1987]): 812–17.

37.   Liebman, "Fiber: Separating Fact from Fiction," 6.

38.   Ken Resnikow, "The Relationship Between Breakfast Habits and Plasma Cholesterol Levels in School Children," *Journal of School Health* 61 (2[February 1991]): 81–85.

39.   James W. Anderson and Susan R. Bridges, "Dietary Fiber Content of Selected Foods," *American Journal of Clinical Nutrition* 47 (March 1988]): 440–47.

40.   Ann M. Albertson and Rosemary C. Tobelmann, "Consumption of Grain and Whole-Grain Foods by an American Population During the Years 1990 to 1992," *Journal of the American Dietetic Association* 95 (6[June 1995]): 703–4.

41.   *Shopping for Health*, (Washington, D.C.: Food Marketing Institute and *Prevention* magazine, 1996), p. 9.

42.   Reuben, *Save Your Life Diet*, 16–17.

43.   Ibid.

44.   Leila G. Saldanha, "Fiber in the Diet of U.S. Children: Results of National Surveys," *Pediatrics* 95 (5(supp.[November 1995]): 994–97, table 1.

45.   Theodor Seuss Geisel, *How the Grinch Stole Christmas* (New York: Random House, 1957), unpaginated.

46.   L. A. Barness, ed., *Pediatric Nutrition Handbook*, 3rd ed. (Elk Grove Village, Illinois: American Academy of Pediatrics, 1993): 100–106.

47.   Christine L. Williams, "Importance of Dietary Fiber in Childhood," *Journal of the American Dietetic Association* 95 (10[October 1995]): 1140–46.

48.   Ibid.

49.   Ibid.

50.   *Blazing Saddles*, Warner Brothers, 1974, Mel Brooks, director.

51.   Council on Scientific Affairs, "Dietary Fiber and Health," 542–46.

52.   Bruce N. Ames, Mark K. Shigenaga, and Tory M. Hagen, "Oxidants, Antioxidants, and the Degenerative Diseases of Aging," *Proceedings of the National Academy of Sciences* 90 (17[1 September 1993]): 7915–22. See also Rebecca Voelker, "Ames Agrees with Mom's Advice: Eat Your Fruits and Vegetables," *Journal of the American Medical Association* 273 (14[12 April 1995]): 14.

53.   Personal telephone communication with Ruth Kava, 27 August 1996.

54. As quoted in Wendy Marston, "The New Diet Food," *Health* 10 (5[September 1996]): 102.

55. Ruth Kava, "When Is a Vegetable Not a Vegetable? When It's a Pill!" *Priorities* 7 (4[1995]): 35.

56. Susan M. Krebs et al., "Fruit and Vegetable Intakes of Children and Adolescents in the U.S.," *Archives of Pediatric Medicine* 150 (1[January 1996]): 81–86.

57. *The Public Enemy*, Warner, 1931, William A. Wellman, director.

9. Exercise: Move It and Lose It

1. John Dryden, "Epistle to John Driden of Chesterton," as quoted in John Bartlett, *Familiar Quotations*, Emily Morison Beck, ed. (Boston: Little, Brown and Company, 1980), 306.

2. Health Education Authority London: Sports Council, The Allied Dunbar National Fitness Survey (London: Sports Council, 1992), as cited in Avril Blamey, Nanette Mutrie, and Tom Aitchison, "Health Promotion by Encouraged Use of Stairs," *British Medical Journal* 311 (7000[29 July 1995]): 289–90.

3. U.S. Department of Health and Human Services, *Physical Activity and Health: A Report of the Surgeon General* (Atlanta: U.S. Department of Health and Human Services, 1996): 85–86.

4. See Susan Brink, "Smart Moves," *U.S. News & World Report* 118 (19[May 1995]): 76–84.

5. For example, Peter Davis and Stephen Phinney, "Use of Exercise for Weight Control," in George L. Blackburn and Beatrice S. Kanders, eds., *Obesity: Pathophysiology, Psychology, and Treatment* (New York: Chapman & Hall, 1994), 219.

6. Grant Gwinup, "Weight Loss Without Dietary Restriction: Efficacy of Different Forms of Aerobic Exercise," *American Journal of Sports Medicine* 15 (3[May–June 1987]): 275–79.

7. As quoted in John Ritter, "Swim Yourself Thin," *American Health* 15 (6[July–August 1996]): 76.

8. Ibid.

9. Claude Bouchard, et al., "Long-term Exercise Training with Constant Energy Intake," *International Journal of Obesity* 14 (1[January 1990]): 57–73.

10. In another study along these lines, consider five formerly obese Canadian runners who after a lengthy period of time lost anywhere from 132 to 161 pounds and kept the weight off. While three runners reduced food intake, two claimed to have kept eating as before. See Angelo Tremblay, Jean-Pierre Després, and Claude Bouchard, "Adipose Tissue Characteristics of Ex-Obese Long-Distance Runners," *International Journal of Obesity* 8 (6[April 1984]): 641–48.

11. Abby C. King and Diane L. Tribble, "The Role of Exercise in Weight Regulation in Non-Athletes," *Sports Medicine* 11 (5[May 1991]): 331–49.

12. J. Dahlkoetter, E. J. Callahan, and J. Linton, "Obesity and the Unbalanced Energy Equation: Exercise Versus Eating Habit Change," *Journal of Consulting and Clinical Psychology* 47 (1979): 898–905, as cited in King and Tribble, "The Role of Exercise," 331–49.

13. James O. Hill et al., "Evaluation of an Alternating-Calorie Diet With and Without Exercise in the Treatment of Obesity," *American Journal of Clinical Nutrition* 50 (2[August 1989]): 248–54.

14. M. F. Ball, J. J. Canary, and L. H. Kyle, "Comparative Effects of Caloric Restriction and Total Starvation on Body Composition in Obesity," *Annals of Internal Medicine* 67 (1967): 60–61; and E. R. Buskirk et al., "Energy Balance of Obese Patients During Weight Reduction: Influence of Diet Restriction and Exercise," *Annals of the New York Academy of Sciences* 110 (1963): 918–40, as cited in Douglas L. Ballor et al., "Resistance Weight Training During Caloric Restriction Enhances Lean Body Weight Maintenance," *American Journal of Clinical Nutrition* 47 (1[January 1988]): 19–25.

15. Jack H. Wilmore, "Body Composition in Sport and Exercise: Directions for Future Research," *Medicine and Science in Sports and Exercise* 15 (1[1983]): 21–31.

16. Robert H. Colvin and Susan B. Olson, "A Descriptive Analysis of Men and Women Who Have Lost Significant Weight and Are Highly Successful at Maintaining the Loss," *Addictive Behaviors* 8 (3[1983]): 287–95.

17. K. N. Pavlou, S. Krey, and W. P. Steffee, "Exercise As an Adjunct to Weight Loss and Maintenance in Moderately Obese Subjects," *American Journal of Clinical Nutrition* 49 (5 supp.)[May 1989]: 1115–23.

18. King and Tribble, "The Role of Exercise," 331–49.

19. Martha L. Skender et al., "Comparison of Two-Year Weight-Loss Trends in Behavioral Treatments of Obesity: Diet, Exercise, and Combination Interventions," *Journal of the American Dietetic Association* 96 (4[April 1996]): 342–46.

20. Julia Califano, "Lose Weight for Life," *American Health* 14 (1[January–February 1995]): 54–55.

21. Personal telephone communication with John Foreyt, 3 January 1996.

22. Lisa Grunwald, Anne Hollister, and Miriam Bensimhon, "Do I Look Fat to You?," *Life* 18 (2[February 1994]): 66.

23. Califano, "Lose Weight for Life," 55.

24. See, for example, Colleen R. McGowan et al., "The Effect of Exercise on Nonrestricted Caloric Intake in Male Joggers," *Appetite* 7 (1[1986]): 97–105, and Rosy Woo, John S. Garrow, and F. Xavier Pi-Sunyer, "Voluntary Food Intake During Prolonged Exercise in Obese Women," *American Journal of Clinical Nutrition* 36 (3[September 1982]): 478–84.

25. David C. Nieman, Leann M. Onasch, and Jerry W. Lee, "The Effects of Moderate Exercise Training on Nutrient Intake in Mildly Obese Women," *Journal of the American Dietetic Association*, 90 (11[November 1990]): 1557–62.

26. Donahue, *This Is Insanity*, 143.

27. Bailey, *Fit or Fat?*

28. Ibid., 1; Covert Bailey, *The New Fit or Fat* (Boston: Houghton Mifflin, 1991), p. 7.

29. Ibid., 34.

30. Bailey, *Fit or Fat?*, cover.

31. Ibid., 38.

32. Ibid., 39.

33. Ibid., 33.

34. Ibid.

35. "TV's Exercise Riders: Hits in the Ratings?" *Consumer Reports* 61 (1[January 1996]): 16–17.

36. "Fit Facts" (flyer) distributed by the National Exercise for Life Institute, P.O. Box 200, Excelsior, Minnesota.

37. Waterhouse, *Outsmarting the Female Fat Cell*, 118.

38. Daniel S. Kirschenbaum, *Weight Loss Through Persistence* (Oakland: New Harbinger Publications, Inc., 1994), 144.

39. J. M. Jakicic et al., "Prescribing Exercise in Multiple Short Bouts versus One Continuous Bout: Effects on Adherence, Cardiorespirator Fitness, and Weight Loss in Overweight Women," *International Journal of Obesity* 19 (12[December 1995]): 893–901.

40. Mark Golin and Michele Stanten, "Walk Pounds Away Forever," *Prevention* 47 (10[October 1995]): 101 and 104.

41. Ibid., 104–5.

42. Ibid., 101.

43. Steve Lohr, "An Exercise High that Lasts," *New York Times Magazine*, 2 October 1994, sec. 6, p. 68.

44. Diane Medved, *The Case Against Divorce* (New York: Donald I. Fine, 1989).

45. John P. Foreyt and G. Ken Goodrick, *Living Without Dieting* (New York: Warner Books, 1992), 92.

46. David Sharp, "So Many Lists, So Little Time," *USA Weekend*, 15–17 March 1996, p. 4.

47. Anne I. Zeni et al., "Energy Expenditure with Indoor Exercise Machines," *Journal of the American Medical Association* 275 (18[8 May 1996]): 1424–27.

48. Linda Omichinski, *You Count, Calories Don't* (Winnipeg, Canada: Tamos Books, Inc., 1993), 72.

49. Angelo Tremblay, Jean-Aime Simoneau, and Claude Bouchard, "Impact of Exercise Intensity on Body Fatness and Skeletal Muscle Metabolism," *Metabolism* 43 (7[July 1994]): 814–18. As such, the study contradicted an earlier, less well-controlled study by the same main author. See Tremblay et al., "Effect of Intensity," 153–57.

50. See Jerry Adler, "Bye-Bye, Suburban Dream," *Newsweek* 25 (20[15 May 1995]): 46–53.

51. See James Howard Kunstler, "Home from Nowhere," *The Atlantic Monthly* 278 (3[September 1996]): 43.

52. Carol Lawson, "Disney's Newest Show Is a Town," *New York Times*, 16 November 1995, p. B6.

53. Dirk Johnson, "Town Sired by Autos Seeks Soul Downtown," *New York Times*, 7 August 1996, p. A7.

54. Avril Blamey, Nanette Mutrie, and Tom Aitchison, "Health Promotion by Encouraged Use of Stairs," *British Medical Journal* 311 (7000[29 July 1995]): 289–90.

55. Jane Brody, "How to Experience the Health Benefits of Regular Exercise Without Working Up a Sweat," *New York Times*, 8 February 1995, p. B7.

56. Dave Barry, "Go Ahead, Feel My Jelly Belly," *The Times* (Tampa–St. Petersburg), 23 June 1996, p. 8F.
57. Tom Kuntz, "Cashing In on the Abs Obsession," *New York Times*, 9 June 1996, sec. 4, p. 6.
58. Ibid.
59. Advertisement in *USA Today*, 9 August 1996, p. 15B.
60. James Rippe, *Fit Over Forty* (New York: Morrow, 1996).
61. Joe Urschel, "Good Abs: More than Just Sitting Up," *USA Today*, 21 May 1996, p. 4D.
62. Suzanne Painter-Supplee, "Beating the Spread," *Arizona Republic*, 16 May 1996, p. 4D.
63. Sharon Doyle Driedger, "The Joy of Being Fat Free," *Maclean's* 109 (28[8 July 1996]): 42.
64. Edwin Bayrd, *The Thin Game* (New York: Newsweek Books, 1978), p. 44.
65. Personal telephone communication with Paul Gardner, 30 August 1996.
66. Personal telephone communication with Charles Billington, 30 August 1996.
67. S. M. Garthwaite et al., "Aging, Exercise, and Food Restriction: Effects on Body Composition," *Mechanisms of Aging and Development* 36 (1986): 187–96; S. P. Tzankoff and A. H. Norris, "Effect of Muscle Mass Decrease on Age-Related BMR Changes," *Journal of Applied Physiology* 43 (6[December 1977]): 1001–6.
68. Nanci Hellmich, "Aging Boomers Lose the Battle of the Bulge," *USA Today*, 2 January 1996. p. D2.
69. Ballor et al., "Resistance Weight Training," 19–25.
70. Califano, "Lose Weight for Life," p. 56.
71. Wayne C. Campbell et al., "Increased Energy Requirements and Changes in Body Composition with Resistance Training in Older Adults," *American Journal of Clinical Nutrition* 60 (2[August 1994]): 167–75.
72. M. S. Treuth et al., "Effects of Strength Training on Total and Regional Body Composition in Older Men," *Journal of Applied Physiology* 77 (2[August 1994]): 614–20.
73. Devera Pine, "Better Body Building: Less Is More," *Longevity* 8 (2[January 1996]): 12.
74. Trevor Smith, "Older People Need Strength Training Too," *Consumers' Research* 79 (2[February 1996]):19.
75. See Kirschenbaum, *Weight Loss Through Persistence*, 148.

10. Pill Talk

1. Personal telephone communication with G. Ken Goodrick, 19 March 1996.
2. Marketdata Enterprises, "Diet Drugs Now Hottest Segment of Slow-Growth, Competitive U.S. Weight Loss Industry," press release of 21 March 1996, p. 2.
3. George A. Bray, "Use and Abuse of Appetite-Suppressant Drugs in the Treatment of Obesity," *Annals of Internal Medicine* 119 (7[1 October 1993]): 707–13.
4. Ibid.
5. Jeffrey T. Wack and Judith Rodin, "Smoking and Its Effects on Body Weight

and the Systems of Caloric Regulation," *American Journal of Clinical Nutrition* 35 (2[February 1982]): 366–80; David R. Jacobs and Sara Gottenborg, "Smoking and Weight: The Minnesota Lipid Research Clinic," *American Journal of Public Health* 71 (4[April 1981]): 391–6; U.S. Public Health Service, "The Health Benefits of Smoking Cessation: A Report of the Surgeon General (Washington, D.C.: DHHS Publication No. (CDC) 90-8416, 1980); David F. Williamson et al., "Smoking Cessation and Severity of Weight Gain in a National Cohort," *New England Journal of Medicine* 324 (11[14 March 1991]): 739–45.

6. Robert C. Klesges and Lisa M. Klesges, "Cigarette Smoking as a Dieting Strategy in a University Population," *International Journal of Eating Disorders* 7 (3[May 1988]): 413–19.

7. David Hill and Nigel Gray, "Australian Patterns of Tobacco Smoking and Related Beliefs in 1983," *Community Health Studies* 8 (3[1984]): 307–16; K. Biener, "Women Who Have Stopped Smoking," *Münchener Medizinscher Wochenschrift* 123 (25[19 June 1981]): 1035-38.

8. See, for example, Kenneth A. Perkins et al., "Acute Effects of Tobacco Smoking on Hunger and Eating in Male and Female Smokers," *Appetite* 22 (2[April 1994]): 149–58.

9. Jacobs and Gottenberg, "Smoking and Weight," 391–6; B. A. Stamford et al., "Cigarette Smoking, Physical Activity, and Alcohol Consumption Relationship to Blood Lipids and Lipoproteins in Premenopausal Females," *Metabolism* 33 (2[July 1984b]): 585–590; Stamford et al., "Cigarette Smoking," 585–90; Judith Rodin, "Weight Change Following Smoking Cessation: The Role of Food Intake and Exercise," *Addictive Behavior* 12 (4[April 1987]): 303–17.

10. Janet E. Audrain et al., "The Individual and Combined Effects of Cigarette Smoking and Food on Resting Energy Expenditure," *International Journal of Obesity* 15 (12[December 1991]): 813–21.

11. Angela Hofstetter et al., "Increased Twenty-four-Hour Energy Expenditure in Cigarette Smokers," *New England Journal of Medicine* 314 (2[9 January 1986]): 79–82.

12. Kenneth A. Perkins et al., "Acute Effects of Nicotine on Resting Metabolic Rate in Cigarette Smokers," *American Journal of Clinical Nutrition* 50 (3[September 1989]): 545–50; Kenneth A. Perkins et al., "The Effects of Nicotine on Energy Expenditure During Light Physical Activity," *New England Journal of Medicine* 320 (14[6 April 1989]): 898–903.

13. Peter Hajek, Paul Jackson, and Michael Belcher, "Long-Term Use of Nicotine Chewing Gum," *Journal of the American Medical Association* 260 (11[16 September 1988]): 1593–96.

14. Robert C. Lesges et al., "The Effects of Phenylpropanolamine on Dietary Intake, Physical Activity, and Body Weight After Smoking Cessation," *Clinical Pharmacological Therapy* 47 (6[June 1990]): 747–54.

15. Bonnie Spring, Regina Pingitore, and Kenneth Kessler, "Strategies to Minimize Weight Gain After Smoking Cessation: Psychological and Pharmacological Intervention with Specific Reference to Dexfenfluramine," *International Journal of Obesity* 16 (supp.3[December 1992]): S19–S23.

16. For example, Laura Fraser, *Losing It* (New York: Dutton, 1997), p. 96. Fraser also calls PPA "useless," p. 117. Such are the perils of an author who eschews the medical literature in favor of interviews with people who themselves have not read the medical literature.

17. For example, Arne Astrup, "Enhanced Thermogenic Responsiveness During Chronic Ephedrine Treatment in Man," *American Journal of Clinical Nutrition* 42 (1[July 1985]): 83–94.

18. Søren Toubro et al., "Safety and Efficacy of Long-Term Treatment with Ephedrine, Caffeine, and an Ephedrine/Caffeine Mixture," *International Journal of Obesity* 17 (supp. 1[February 1993]): S69–S72.

19. T. E. Graham and L. L. Spriet, "Performance and Metabolic Responses to a High Caffeine Dose During Prolonged Exercise," *Journal of Applied Physiology* 71 (6[December 1991]): 2292–8. See also "Ban Caffeine at Olympics, Scientists Urge," *Toronto Star*, 23 March 1993, p. D1.

20. A. G. Dulloo et al., "Normal Caffeine Consumption: Influence on Thermogenesis and Daily Energy Expenditure in Lean and Postobese Human Volunteers," *American Journal of Clinical Nutrition* 49 (1[January 1989]): 44–50.

21. Jane Brody, "The Latest on Coffee? Don't Worry. Drink Up," *New York Times*, 13 September 1995, p. B1.

22. As quoted in Randy Blaun, "How to Eat Smart," *Psychology Today* 29 (3[May 1996]): 42.

23. P. A. Daly, "Ephedrine, Caffeine, and Aspirin: Safety and Efficacy for Treatment of Human Obesity," *International Journal of Obesity* 17 (supp. 1[February 1993]): S73–S78.

24. Leif Berum et al., "Companions of an Ephedrine/Caffeine Combination and Dexfenfluramine in the Treatment of Obesity: A Double-Blind Multi-Center Trial in General Practice," *International Journal of Obesity* 18 (2[February 1994]): 99–103.

25. Arne Astrup et al., "Pharmacology of Thermogenic Drugs," *American Journal of Clinical Nutrition* 55 (supp. 1[January 1992]): 246S–48S.

26. Renato Pasquali and Francesco Casimirri, "Clinical Aspects of Ephedrine in the Treatment of Obesity," *International Journal of Obesity* 17 (supp. 1[February 1993]): S65–S68.

27. See, for example, Bruce Lambert, "Long Island County to Ban Sale of Drug Tied to Death," *New York Times*, 17 April 1996, p. B12.

28. "Beware of 'Energy Boosters,' " *Dallas Morning News*, 18 March 1996, p. 3C.

29. Michael A. Males, "U.S. Drugs: Officials Watch Pot-Smoking Teens, Skip Real Crisis," *Inter Press Service*, 25 September 1995.

30. For a longer discussion of this, see Larry S. Hobbs, *The New Diet Pills* (Irvine, California: Pragmatic Press, 1995), 114–15.

31. Marielle Rebuffé-Scrive, Per Marin, and Per Björntorp, "Short Communications: Effect of Testosterone on Abdominal Adipose Tissue in Men," *International Journal of Obesity* 15 (4[November 1991]): 791–95.

32. Personal telephone communication with John Foreyt, 23 January 1996; see also Madeleine L. Drent et al., "Orlisat (RO 1800647), a Lipase Inhibitor, in the Treatment of Human Obesity: A Multiple Dose Study," *International Journal of Obesity* 19 (4[April 1995]): 221–26; Madeleine L. Drent

and Eduard A. Van der Veen," Lipase Inhibition: A Novel Concept in the Treatment of Obesity," *International Journal of Obesity* 17 (4[April 1993]): 241–44.

33. See Marian Burros, "FDA Advisory Panel Backs Approval of a Fat Substitute," *New York Times*, 18 November 1995, sec. 1, p. 11.

34. Associated Press, "FDA OKs Fat Substitute," 25 January 1996.

35. For example, Robert E. Greenberg et al., "Mortality Association with Low Plasma Concentration of Beta Carotene and the Effect of Oral Supplementation," *Journal of the American Medical Association* 275 (9[6 March 1996]): 699–703.

36. Ibid.

37. Nanci Hellmich, "Fiber Tapped As No-Cal Fat Substitute," *USA Today*, 26 August 1996, p. D1.

38. Mary Ann Marrazzi, "Binge Eating Disorder: Response to Maltrexone," *International Journal of Obesity* 19 (2[February 1995]): 143–45.

39. Adam Drewnowski et al., "Naloxone, an Opiate Blocker, Reduces the Consumption of Sweet High-Fat Foods in Obese and Lean Female Binge Eaters," *American Journal of Clinical Nutrition* 61 (6[June 1995]): 1206–12.

40. Jeffrey A. Fisher, *The Chromium Program* (New York: Harper & Row, 1990).

41. Ibid.

42. S. P. Clancy et al., "Effects of Chromium Picolinate Supplementation on Body Composition, Strength, and Urinary Chromium Loss in Football Players," *International Journal of Sport Nutrition* 4 (2[June 1994]): 142–53; D. L. Hasten et al., "Effects of Chromium Picolinate on Beginning Weight Training," *International Journal of Sport Nutrition* 2 (4[December 1992]): 343–50; H. C. Lukaski et al., "Chromium Supplementation and Resistance Training: Effects on Body Composition, Strength, and Trace Element Status of Men," *American Journal of Clinical Nutrition* 63 (6[July 1996]): 954–65; L. K. Trent and D. Thieding-Cancel, "Effects of Chromium Picolinate on Body Composition," *Journal of Sports Medicine and Physical Fitness* 35 (4[April 1995]): 273–80.

43. Hallmark et al., "Effects of Chromium and Resistive Training on Muscle Strength and Body Composition," *Medicine and Science in Sports and Exercise* 28(1[January 1996]): 139–44.

44. See Hobbs, *The New Diet Pills*, 160–71.

45. L. S. Hirsch, "Controlling Appetite in Obesity," *Journal of Medicine* (Cincinnati) 20 (84[April 1939]): 84–85.

46. David E. Schteingart, "Effectiveness of Phenylpropanolamine in the Management of Moderate Obesity," *International Journal of Obesity* 16 (7[July 1992]): 487–93.

47. Frank L. Greenway, "Clinical Studies with Phenylpropanolamine: A Meta-analysis," *American Journal of Clinical Nutrition* 55 (1 supp. [January 1992]): 203S–5S.

48. See P. J. Collipp, "The Treatment of Exogenous Obesity by Medicated Benzocaine Candy: A Double-Blind Placebo Study," *Obesity and Bariatric Medicine* 10 (5[September–October 1981]): 123–25.

49. Schteingart, "Effectiveness," 487–93.

50. See, for example, David J. Goldstein, et al., "Fluoxetine: A Randomized Clinical Trial in the Maintenance of Weight Loss," *Obesity Research* 1 (2[March 1993]): 92–98.

51. G. Enzi et al., "Short-Term and Long-Term Clinical Evaluation of a Non-Amphetaminic Anorexiant (Mazindol) in the Treatment of Obesity," *Journal of International Medical Research* 4 (5[1976]): 305–18.

52. Steven Lamm and Gerald Secor Couzens, *Thinner at Last* (New York: Simon & Schuster, 1995).

53. Sheldon Levine, *The Redux Revolution* (New York: Morrow, 1996).

54. Ibid., 119.

55. Ibid., 207.

56. Ibid., 4.

57. Ibid., 107.

58. Ibid., 82–83 for eating and 119–20 for exercise.

59. John E. Blundell and Andrew J. Hill, "Serotoninergic Modulation of the Pattern of Eating and the Profile of Hunger-Satiety in Humans," *International Journal of Obesity* 11 (supp. 3[December 1987]): 141–55.

60. E. M. Goodall et al., "Ritapserin Attenuates Anorectic, Endocrine, and Thermic Responses to D-fenfluramine in Human Volunteers," *Psychopharmacology* 112 (4[1993]): 461–66; France Lafreniere et al., "Effects of Dexfenfluramine Treatment on Body Weight and Postprandial Thermogenesis in Obese Subjects: A Double-Blind Placebo-Controlled Study," *International Journal of Obesity* 17 (1[January 1993]): 25–30; Nicholas Finer, Susan Finer, and Rossitza P. Naumova, "Drug Therapy After Very Low-Calorie Diets," *American Journal of Clinical Nutrition* 56 (1[(supp.) July 1992]): 195S–198S.

61. B. Guy-Grand et al., "International Trial of Long-Term Dexfenfluramine in Obesity," *The Lancet* 2 (8672[11 November 1989]): 1142–45.

62. G. A. Ricaurte et al., "Dexfenfluramine Neurotoxicity in Brains of Non-human Primates," *The Lancet* 338 (8781[14 December 1991]): 1487.

63. Lamm and Couzens, *Thinner at Last*, 73–74.

64. Philip J. Hilts, "New Generation of Diet Pills Raises Some Old Questions about Safety," *New York Times*, 21 February 1996, p. B7.

65. Lucien Abenhaim et al., "Appetite-Suppressant Drugs and the Risk of Primary Pulmonary Hypertension," *New England Journal of Medicine* 335 (9[29 August 1996]): 609–16.

66. JoAnn E. Manson and Gerald A. Faich, "Pharmocoptherapy for Obesity: Do the Benefits Outweigh the Risks?" *New England Journal of Medicine* 335 (9[29 August 1996]): 659–60.

67. Levine, *The Redux Revolution*, 123.

68. Lamm and Couzens, *Thinner at Last*.

69. Bray, "Use and Abuse," 707–13.

70. Michael Weintraub, "Long-Term Weight Control: The National Heart, Lung, and Blood Institute Funded Multimodal Intervention Study: Introduction," *Clinical Pharmacological Therapy* 51 (5[May 1992]): 581–85; Bray, "Use and Abuse," 707–13.

71. Weintraub, "Long-Term Weight Control," 581–85.

72. Michael Weintraub, "A Double-Blind Clinical Trial in Weight Control," *Archives of Internal Medicine* 6 (144[June 1984]): 1143–48.

73. Michael Weintraub et al., "Long-Term Weight Control Study I (Weeks 0 to 34)," *Clinical Pharmacology and Therapeutics* 51 (5[May 1992]): 586–94.

74. Mary Murray, "Pill Seekers," *Allure* 5 (2[February 1995]): 103.

75. David J. Goldstein and Janet H. Potvin, "Long-Term Weight Loss: The Effect of Pharmacologic Agents,"*American Journal of Clinical Nutrition* 60(5 [November 1994]): 647–57.

76. Personal telephone communication with John Foreyt, 3 January 1996.

77. Gina Kolata, "Researchers Find Hormone Causes a Loss of Weight," *New York Times*, 27 July 1995, p. A1.

78. Mary Ann Pelleymounter et al., "Effects of the Obese Gene Product on Body Weight Regulation in ob/ob Mice," *Science* 269 (5223[28 July 1995]): 540–43.

79. "A Fabulous Flabless Future," editorial in *St. Petersburg Times*, 4 August 1996, p. 18A.

80. Robert V. Considine et al., "Evidence Against Either a Premature Stop Codon or the Absence of Obese Gene mRNA in Human Obesity," *Journal of Clinical Investigation* 95 (6[June 1995]): 2986–88.

81. Personal telephone communication with José Caro, 8 August 1995.

82. Gina Kolata, "New Research Dims Hopes for a Quick Fat Cure," *New York Times*, 30 August 1995, p. B6.

83. Bradford Hamilton et al., "Increased Obese mRNA Expression in Omental Fat Cells from Massively Obese Humans," *Nature Medicine* 1 (9[September 1995]): 953–56, and F. Lonnqvist et al., "Overexpression of the Obese (Ob) Gene in Adipose Tissue of Human Obese Subjects," *Nature Medicine* 1 (9[September 1995]): 950–53.

84. Kolata, "New Research," B6.

85. Robert W. Considine et al., "Serum Immunoreactive-Leptin Concentrations in Normal-Weight and Obese Humans," *New England Journal of Medicine* 334 (5[1 February 1996]): 292–S; Robert V. Considine et al., "The Hypothalmic Leptic Receptor in Humans," *Diabetes* 19 (7[July 1996]): 992–96.

86. Nanci Hellmich, "Some Use Fat Discoveries as License to Eat," *USA Today*, 10 August 1995, p. D1.

11. Defatting the Land

1. Actually, I later asked him about this. He said he originally tried that with this obese patients, but "You just lose them that way. They just go to another doctor."

2. Glenn A. Gaesser, *Big Fat Lies*; Richard Klein, *Eat Fat* (New York: Pantheon, 1996); Laura Fraser, *Losing It* (New York: Dutton, 1997).

3. Dale M. Atrens, *Don't Diet* (New York: Morrow, 1988), 176.

4. Ibid., 241.

5. Institute of Medicine, *Weighing the Options* (Washington, D.C.: National Academy Press, 1995), p. 168.

6. "Short shrift" is one of those expressions that almost all of us have used at

one time or another and have no idea what it means. Neither did I till I looked it up. It actually refers to being given only a little bit of time to make peace with God prior to being executed. Kind of ghoulish, huh?

7. Michael Fumento, *The Myth of Heterosexual AIDS* (Washington, D.C.: Regnery Gateway, 1993); Michael Fumento, *Science Under Siege* (New York; Morrow, 1993).

8. Ibid., 16.

9. Institute of Medicine, *Improving America's Diet and Health*, Paul R. Thomas, ed. (Washington, D.C.: National Academy Press, 1991), p. 23.

10. See Fumento, *Science Under Siege*, 19 and 27–31. The original *60 Minutes* report was " 'A' Is for Apple," 26 February 1989.

11. Martha Groves, "Schools' Action Widens the Apple Controversy," *Los Angeles Times*, 13 March 1989, p. 1.

12. IOM, *Improving America's Health*, 23.

13. Kim Painter, "Women in the Dark About Heart Risks," *USA Today*, 14 September 1995, p. ID.

14. ABC *Nightly News*, 13 September 1996.

15. See "Alar in Apples: Facts and Fantasies," *Consumer Reports* 54 (5[May 1989]): 288; See "Secondhand Smoke: Is It a Hazard?" *Consumer Reports* 60(1[January 1995]): 27; See "Radon: The Problem No One Wants to Face," *Consumer Reports* 54 (10[October 1989]): 623.

16. See Fumento, *Science Under Siege*, 19–24.

17. William Bennett and Joel Gurin, *The Dieter's Dilemma* (New York: Basic Books, 1982).

18. "Addicted to Tobacco Stories," *MediaNomics* 4 (7[July 1996]): 2. (Available from Media Research Center, 113 South West Street, 2nd Floor, Alexandria, Virginia 22314.)

19. Jim Sexton and Wayne Biddle, "The Pounding Is Intense," *USA Weekend*, 16–18 August 1996, p. 5.

20. Jeremiah Stamler, "Epidemic Obesity in the United States," *Archives of Internal Medicine* 153 (9[10 May 1993]): 1040–44.

21. IOM, *Weighing the Options*, 152.

22. "From There to Intolerance," *The Economist* 320 (7716[20 July 1991]): 15–16.

23. (I'm not kidding.) See Sherri Vazquez, "It's No Longer Lonely at the Top of the Class," *Rocky Mountain News*, 18 May 1996, p. 4A.

24. Karl Zinsmeister, "Doing Bad and Feeling Good," *American Enterprise* 7 (5[September–October 1996]): 48.

25. Steven Muller, "How to Restore Excellence in Society," *Cosmos* 4 (1994): 6.

26. Charles Sykes, *Dumbing Down Our Kids* (New York: St. Martin's Press, 1995), p. 49.

27. Carol Johnson, *Self-Esteem Comes in All Sizes* (New York: Doubleday, 1995).

28. See Mary Ann Scheirer and Robert Kraut, "Increasing Educational Achievement via Self-Concept Change," *Review of Educational Research* 49 (1[1979]): 131–49.

29. Personal telephone communication with Rosemary Green, 5 September 1996.

30. National Center on Addiction and Substance Abuse, *National Survey of American Attitudes on Substance Abuse II: Teens and Their Parents* (New York: National Center on Addiction and Substance Abuse at Columbia University, September 1996), 24.

31. Tim Friend, "Many Parents Resigned to Kids' Drug Use," *USA Today*, 10 September 1996, p. A2.

32. Nanci Hellmich, "School Lunches Start to Lighten Up," *USA Today*, 5 September 1996, p. 8D.

33. Personal e-mail communication from Daniel Lapin, 10 July 1996.

34. Linda Woodhead, "Learning to Love the Good in Community," in Digby Anderson, ed., *This Will Hurt* (London: Social Affairs Unit, 1996), 144.

35. As quoted in Gertrude Himmelfarb, "Preface," in Digby Anderson, ed., *This Will Hurt* (London: Social Affairs Unit, 1996), p. x.

36. Personal telephone communication with G. Ken Goodrick, 2 July 1996.

37. Laura Shapiro et al., "Is Fat That Bad?" *Newsweek* 129 (16[21 April 1997]): 48.

38. See Michael Fumento, "Fakery Against Fat," *Washington Times* 13 November 1996, A 15.

39. See Jennifer Bojorquez, "Who Will Smoke?" *Sacramento Bee*, 2 August 1996, p. SC1.

40. As quoted in Ibid.

41. IOM, *Improving America's Health*, 206.

42. U.S. Department of Health and Human Services, *Activity and Health: A Report of the Surgeon General* (Atlanta: U.S. Department of Health and Human Services, 1996), 229–30 and table 6-3.

43. IOM, *Improving America's Health*, 66.

44. See generally Sykes, *Dumbing Down Our Kids*.

45. Jacques Strinberg, "Why America's Ever-Fatter Kids Don't Go to Gym," *New York Times*, 25 August 1996, Sec. 4, p. 14.

46. Census Bureau, *1995 Statistical Abstract*, tables 1118 and 1378.

47. Kelly D. Brownell, "Get Slim with Higher Taxes," *New York Times*, 15 December 1995, p. A29.

48. "Final California Election Returns," *Los Angeles Times*, 5 November 1992, p. A9.

49. See Jeremy Iggers, *The Garden of Eating* (New York: HarperCollins, 1996), p. 107.

50. George A. Bray, M.D., "An Approach to the Classification and Evaluation of Obesity," in Per Björntorp and Bernard N. Brodoff, eds., *Obesity* (Philadelphia: J. D. Lippincott, 1992), 301.

51. See Ronald Bailey, ed., *The True State of the Planet* (New York: Free Press, 1995), 443–53.

52. U.S. Department of Health and Human Services, *Activity and Health*, table 217.

53. Philip Elmer-De Witt et al., "Fat Times," *Time* 145 (2[16 January 1995]): 65.

Index

abdomen exercisers, 133, 222–24
acarbose, 237
Acutrim, 233
adolescents, 17, 28, 53, 200
advertising, 42, 55, 132, 133, 158, 159
aging, 21, 24–25, 226, 237
Agricultural Research Service, 34
AIDS, 10, 114, 142, 168, 255, 256, 257
alcoholic drinks, 178–79
Alphin, Franca, 90
American Academy of Pediatrics Committee
    on Nutrition, 201
American Cancer Society study, 2, 12
American Council on Science and Health, 265
American Dietetic Association, 38, 59, 73, 162,
    187
American Health Foundation, 201
American Heart Association, 159, 191
American Medical Society Council on
    Scientific Affairs, 202
amphetamines, 231
anorexia nervosa, 9
anorexiants, 233, 242–43
antioxidants, 203
appetite, 171, 182, 195, 235, 262–63
appetite suppressants, 139–40, 184, 233, 235,
    242–43
"apple" shape, 19, 21
arteries, hardening of, 17, 69
arthritis, 13, 21, 22
artificial sweeteners, 83, 84, 88, 90–92, 239
aspartame, 90, 91, 92, 239
aspirin, 235, 236
Associated Press, 58, 96
Atkins, Dawn, 108–9
Atrens, Dale, 10, 108, 118, 119, 254–55
Australia, 36, 66
automobiles, 51–52, 271
Avicenna, 192

Bailey, Covert, 57, 108, 136, 212–14
Banting, William, 137, 138
Barnard, Neal, 147
Barrett, Stephen, 141
Barry, Dave, 222
BBW/Big Beautiful Women, 126, 129
Beck, Joan, 103
Belgium, 65
benzocaine, 243
Berenson, Gerald, 16
Berger, Stuart, 142–43, 150
Berkeley National Laboratory study, 95
beverage consumption, 35–36
Beverly Hills Diet, The (Mazel), 140
bicycling, 52, 207, 208, 218, 219
Big Fat Lies (Gaesser), 12, 19, 20, 23, 38, 105,
    119–20, 168
Billington, Charles, 225
binge eating, 174, 176–77, 240–41
Blackburn, George, 149, 169
blacks, 11, 28, 29, 37, 94, 97, 101, 127, 128,
    188–89, 265–66
Blair, Steven, 23, 24
blockers, 237–38
Bod Pod, 9
body fat: conversion of dietary fat to, 60–65;
    desirable percentages, 223–24; excessive
    (*see* obesity); liposuction, 224–25; losing,
    61–62 (*see also* weight loss); loss due to
    exercise, 208, 215, 219, 227; measuring,
    8–9; waist-to-hip ratios, 19–20; weight
    cycling effects, 168
Body Mass Index (BMI), 3, 4, 8, 14, 17, 20, 27,
    29, 36–37, 94, 97, 99, 122
Bogalusa Heart Study, 16
Bombeck, Erma, 41
Boswell, James, 108
Bouchard, Claude, 94
Bray, George, 96

Brazil, 36
bread, 193–94, 198–99, 200
breakfast, 175, 180, 185, 194, 195
breast cancer, 5, 12, 13, 21, 257
Brody, Jane, 43, 139, 151, 169, 221, 234
Brownell, Kelly, 131, 165, 210, 251, 270
Build and Blood Pressure studies, 1–2
bulimia, 177
Burke, Edmund, 263

caffeine, 233–36
Califano, Joseph, 262
Callaway, C. Wayne, 141, 151, 159, 169
Callaway Diet, The, 141, 151
calorie-restricted diets, 61–62, 139, 164,
    170–71; and exercise, 208–9, 210. See also
    low-calorie diets
calories: and body fat, 61–62; burned by
    exercise machines, 218; counting, 177–79;
    "don't count" claims, 58, 60, 66, 138, 145,
    146–48; food labels, 268; intake data,
    33–34, 84; recommended level for weight
    loss, 170–71
Calories Don't Count (Taller), 138
Canada, 36, 121
cancer, 5, 12–13, 17, 19, 21, 120, 129, 133, 168,
    188, 189, 190, 192, 257
candy bars, 46–47, 81
Caputo, Florence, 73
"carbohydrate addiction," 149–51
Carbohydrate Addict's Diet (Heller and Heller),
    135, 137
carbohydrates, 84, 85–86, 139; absorption
    blockers, 237; conversion to body fat,
    60–61; cravings for, 149–50, 173; fad diet
    prohibitions, 138, 139, 148–51; sugar,
    82–92
cardiovascular conditioning, 213, 215
Caro, José, 251
carotenoids, 239
Castelli, William, 4, 6
cataracts, 14
Celebration, Florida, 219
Center for Media and Public Affairs, 58, 93,
    191–92
Center for Science in the Public Interest
    (CSPI), 6, 45, 58, 148, 155, 157–58, 171,
    265
Centers for Disease Control and Prevention
    (CDC) surveys, 50
cereals, 194, 196, 200
children, 15–19, 28, 38, 50, 52–55, 195,
    199–200, 201, 204, 261–62, 269
China, 31, 52, 64, 66
chocolate, 71–72, 136, 240–41
cholesterol, 10, 12, 16, 20, 22, 68, 191, 194,
    195; dietary, 69, 271
Choose to Lose (Goor and Goor), 57
Chopra, Deepak, 105
chromium, 241–42
cigarette smoking, 4, 6, 117, 166, 231–33, 258,

    264, 265–66; weight gain after quitting,
    31, 232–33
clothes, 40–41, 43, 180–81, 184
CNN exposé, 178
Colditz, Graham A., 21
colon cancer, 5, 12, 17, 21, 25, 188, 189,
    190
Connolly-Schoonen, Josephine, 203
Consumer Alert, 265
Consumer Reports, 141, 155, 157, 160–61, 162,
    165, 214, 257
Consumers Union, 257
cookies, 46, 70–71, 79–80, 267
Cornell University studies, 54, 79, 116
Coronary Heart Mortality Risk Study, 10
Couzens, Gerald, 244, 247
cross-country ski machine, 214, 218

Daley, Rosie, 76
Danforth, Elliot Jr., 113, 114
Darm, Jerry, 1, 22
Dexatrim, 233
dexfenfluramine, 154, 233, 235, 243–47, 249
diabetes, 1, 2, 11–12, 21, 22, 90, 98, 100, 120,
    188, 189, 191, 237, 242, 250, 251
Diamond, Harvey and Marilyn, 141
Diary of a Fat Housewife (Green), 1, 110,
    123–24, 151, 261
Dick Gregory's Bahamian Diet, 153
Diet and Health report, 256
Dietary Goals for the United States (McGovern
    Report), 82
diet books, 57, 131–52, 185, 241;
    recommended titles, 151
Diet Center, 153, 154–55, 161
diet drinks, 152–53
Dieter's Dilemma, The (Gurin), 257
diet gurus, 132, 137–38, 142–51
diet industry, 152–63
"dieting," 38. See also weight loss
diet pills, 229–52
"diets don't work" claims, 164–68
Dietz, William, 53–54, 97
Dishman, Rod, 216
diverticular disease, 188, 189–90
Dr. Atkins Diet Revolution, 137, 138
Doctor's Quick Weight-Loss Diet, The (Stillman),
    138, 139
Dr. Schiff's Miracle Weight-Loss Guide, 135
Donahue, Beth, 110, 156, 212
Don't Diet (Atrens), 10, 108, 118, 254–55
doubly labeled water technique, 109
Drewnowski, Adam, 240, 241
Drinking Man's Diet, The, 138, 179
drug use, 166, 180, 262. See also weight-loss
    drugs
Dryden, John, 206
D'Souza, Dinesh, 128
Dufty, William, 82–83, 92
Duke University study, 119
Dybdahl, Tom, 76

Eat Fat (Klein), 119
Eat Fat and Grow Slim (Mackarness), 139
eating, 54, 171–77; effect of exercise on, 211–12. *See also* overeating
"eating clothes," 32, 181
eating disorders, 9, 38, 174, 176
eating-recall studies, 62, 109–10
Eat More, Weigh Less (Ornish), 57, 61, 73, 135, 224
Economist, The, 259
Eljaiek, Laura, 128
Elysee Electro Exercise System, 133
England, 36, 206
Entenmann's products, 73, 267
Environmental Protection Agency, 245
ephedrine, 233–36, 244
Epstein, Diane, 108, 155, 163, 167
Epstein, Leonard, 18
Estrich, Susan, 123
estrogen, 21
Europe, 36, 46, 52, 64, 65, 84, 176
Evans, Gary, 241
exercise, 23–24, 206–28; "ab" fad, 222–24; benefits, 206–7; compared to: weight loss, 23–24; weight-loss drugs, 230; in daily activities, 220–22; decline of, 48–52; effect on eating, 211–12; vs. liposuction, 224–25; "magic pill" promotions, 212–14; to maintain weight loss, 183, 184–85, 209–11; recommended frequency and amount, 214–17; recommended intensity, 218–19; resistance training, 226–28; and television viewing, 53, 54, 217; time of day, 216; and weight loss, 207–10
exercise machines, 213–14, 217, 218

Fabricant, Florence, 44
fad diets, 132, 134–51
Faich, Gerald, 246
Faludi, Susan, 175–76
Farzan, Leila, 155, 157
fast-food restaurants, 44, 45, 46, 47, 265
Fastin, 247
fasting, 184, 185
fat, dietary, 56–81, 83–84, 87; absorption blockers, 237–38; and body fat, 56, 60–65; consumption levels, 65–67; demonization of, 56–62, 82, 144–45, 191–92, 268; and heart disease, 68–69; *See also* cholesterol; high-fat diet; low-fat diets; low-fat foods
"fat," euphemisms for, 39, 41. *See also* body fat; obesity
fat acceptance movement, 12, 19, 20, 23, 39, 96, 102, 103–4, 105, 106, 110, 113, 115–30, 167, 186, 206, 207, 257, 260, 263–64
Fat Attack Plan (Natow and Heslin), 58, 66
fat blockers, 237–38
Fat Burner, 241
"fat-burning enzymes," 212–13
"fat-burning foods," 148
Fat Chance: The Big Prejudice (film), 121

Fat Counter (Natow and Heslin), 57, 58
fat-free foods, 70–77, 86, 87
"fat genes," 93–97, 123, 244–45, 259
Fat Is a Feminist Issue (Orbach), 175–76
fat substitutes, 238–40
Federal Trade Commission (FTC), 75, 157–58, 160
Fed Up! (Garrison and Levitsky), 117–18
Feeding on Dreams (Epstein and Thompson), 108, 155, 163, 167
fenfluramine, 154, 230, 244, 246, 247
Ferguson, James M., 151
fertility, and waist size, 126
fiber, 63, 78, 79, 187–205; content of various foods, 196–98; recommended amount, 200–203
fiber supplements, 192, 194, 195, 202
Fight Fat and Win (Moquette-Magee), 57, 77, 135
Finland, 65
Fischer, Jeffrey, 241
Fit for Life (Diamond and Diamond), 137, 141
Fit or Fat? (Bailey), 212–13
Five-Day Miracle Diet, The (Puhn), 135, 224
Flatt, Jean-Pierre, 62
Fletcher, Anne M., 151, 184, 186, 215
fluoxetine, 243
food(s): consumption data, 33–35; giant portions, 43–48; number available, 182; processed vs. unprocessed, 78–81, 85; removal of fiber from, 198–200; wasting, 267
food absorption: blockers, 237–38; effect of fiber, 193
food allergies, 142–43
Food and Drug Administration (FDA), 59, 71, 234, 236, 237, 238, 239, 244, 245, 246, 247, 248, 258
food-combining diets, 141, 150
food cravings, 88–89, 171–75, 240
Food Guide Pyramid, 204, 268
food labels, 58–59, 89, 178, 198, 268
food logs, 110
Food Marketing Institute, 59, 70, 76, 179–80
Foods That Cause You to Lose Weight (Barnard), 147–48
Forbes, Gilbert B., 113
Foreyt, John P., 9, 17, 101, 126, 151, 152, 159, 160, 173, 210, 217, 237, 249
Framingham Heart Study, 4, 10
France, 65, 96–97
Frankel, Richard and Gerald, 144, 146
Franklin, Benjamin, 1
Fraser, Laura, 20, 119, 121, 160, 233
fruit juice sweeteners, 81, 85
fruits, 79, 198, 203–5, 257, 267, 269

Gaesser, Glenn, 12, 19, 20, 21, 23, 24, 38, 105, 119–20, 122, 168
gallbladder disease, 13, 21
Garden of Eating, The (Iggers), 172

Gardner, Paul, 225
Garrison, Terry Nicholleti, 117–18
Garrow, John, 22, 118
Garton, Jean, 130
Geliebter, Allan, 180
Germany, 36, 65
Gifford, K. Dun, 36
glaucoma study, 26
Glucobay, 237
gluttony, 25, 76, 113, 130, 264, 266
Godbey, Geoffrey, 217
Goodrick, G. Ken, 17, 97, 126, 151, 173, 217, 230, 246, 263
Gortmaker, Steven, 53–54
Gossett, Harry, 116
gout, 14
grains, 188, 200. *See also* cereals
grazing, 179–81
Green, Rosemary, 1, 110, 123–24, 129–30, 151, 261–62
Greenwood-Robinson, Maggie, 146–47, 148
Gurin, Joel, 108, 257
Guru Walla, 147
Gwinup, Grant, 207

Habits Not Diets (Ferguson), 151
Hallfrisch, Judith, 35
Hamilton, Bradford, 251
Hand, Michael, 40
Harrison, Emily, 102–3
Harris polls, 30–31
Harvard Health Letter, 149
Harvard University studies, 3–4, 17, 64. *See also* Nurses' Health Study
Harvey, William, 137
Healthline magazine, 159
Health Management Resources (HMR), 153, 157, 160, 161
HealthRider, 213–14
Health Schemes, Scams, and Frauds (Barrett and *Consumer Reports* eds.), 141
Healthy Choice foods, 71, 86, 87, 270
Healthy for Life (Heller and Heller), 148
Healthy People 2000 (DHHS), 70
heart disease, 1, 2, 10, 16, 17, 19, 20–21, 22, 23, 68–69, 120, 168, 188, 189, 191, 257
Heath, Gregory, 50
Heavyweights (film), 121
Hecht, Ken, 122–23
height-weight charts, 6–8, 23, 30
Heller, Richard and Rachael, 136, 148–51
Hemenway, Carrie, 102
Herbal Life, 153
Herskowitz, Joel, 140
Heymsfield, Steven, 34, 106, 110, 111–13
high blood pressure. *See* hypertension
high-carbohydrate diet, 139
high-density lipoprotein (HDL), 12, 191
high-fat diet, 63–64, 139
high-fiber diet, 187, 188–89, 190–92, 193–94, 200–201, 202, 203

high-protein, low-carbohydrate diets, 138–40
Hill, James, 183–84
Hippocratic texts, 1
Hirsch, Jules, 97, 106, 107, 182
Hispanics, 11, 28
Honolulu Heart Study, 10
How to Become Naturally Thin by Eating More (Antonello), 57, 135
How to Think Yourself Thin (D. Johnson), 136
Hungary, 65
hunger, 91, 170, 171–72, 173, 175, 176–77, 179, 192; symptoms, 172
Hurley, Jane, 171
hydroxycitric acid (HCA), 242
hypertension (high blood pressure), 1, 10–11, 16, 19, 20, 21, 22, 118, 189, 194
hypnosis, 185
hypoglycemic state, 88–89
hypothyroidism, 112
hysterectomy, 14

Iggers, Jeremy, 172
Immune Power Diet, The (Berger), 142
impulsive eating, 173
Institute for Standards Research, 41
Institute of Medicine (IOM), 21, 29, 30–31, 94–95, 152, 176, 255, 256, 259, 266, 267
insulin, 11, 88–89, 149–50, 191
insulin resistance, 148–49
intense sweeteners, 90–91
Internet users, 55
Intuitive Eating (Tribole and Resch), 76, 151, 171–73, 177
Ionamin, 247
Israel, 65
Italy, 66, 96

Jameson, Judy, 148
Jane Brody's Good Food Book, 139, 151
Japan, 52, 66, 100–101
Jarvis, William, 141
Jenkins, David, 195
Jenny Craig, 153, 155, 156–57, 158–59, 160, 161
Johns Hopkins University study, 245
Johnson, Carol A., 186
Johnson, Debbie, 136
Johnson, Samuel, 108, 115
Judelson, Debra, 257

Kaiser Permanente, 122, 264
Katahn, Martin, 57, 59–60, 62, 68, 64
Kaufman, Wendy, 42
Kava, Ruth, 203
Keating, Peggy, 210–11
Kessler, David, 258
ketosis, 139–40
King, Abby, 208, 210
Kirschenbaum, Daniel S., 151, 215
Klein, Calvin, 41
Klein, Richard, 119

knees, arthritis of, 13, 22
Koch, Ed, 152
Kolata, Gina, 69
Koop, C. Everett, 265
Kunstler, James Howard, 219
Kushi, Lawrence, 52, 64
Kushner, Robert, 72-73

Lamm, Steven, 244, 247
Lane Bryant, 40-41, 43
Langton, James, 32
Lasorda, Tommy, 152-53
Last Five Pounds, The (Pope), 57
Laval University studies, 208, 219
Lawren, Bill, 135
Lean and Mean (Shaevitz), 151
Lean Bodies (Sheats and Greenwood-
    Robinson), 135, 146-47, 148, 167
Lean Cuisine, 45
Lefavi, Robert, 241
legumes, 188, 197
Leibel, Rudolph, 104, 105, 106, 107
leptin, 250-51
Leung, Alexander, 18
Levine, Sheldon, 244, 247
Levitsky, David, 117-18
Lieberman, Harris, 245
Liebman, Bonnie, 148
Lipo Slim Briefs, 133
liposuction, 224-25
liquid-fast programs, 152, 160, 161
Lithium, 243
Little, Tony, 222
Living Without Dieting (Foreyt and Goodrick),
    126, 151, 230
Loewy, Michael, 40
Losing It (Fraser), 119, 233
low-calorie diets, 143, 170-71. See also calorie-
    restricted diets
low-cholesterol diet, 69
low-carbohydrate diets, 139
low-density eating, 78-81
low-density lipoprotein, 191
low-fat diets, 56-81, 83-84, 144-45, 191-92
low-fat foods, 65, 69-74, 80, 83, 86. See also fat-
    free foods; reduced-fat foods
low-fiber diet, 188, 189, 190, 192, 193, 194
low-roughage diet, 190
low-sugar diet, 202-3
Lyons, Pat, 119, 122

McCarthy, William, 216
McDonald's restaurants, 44, 46, 124-25, 265
McDougall Plan for Super Health and Life-Long
    Weight Loss, 57
McGovern Report, 82
Mackarness, Richard, 139
Maclean's magazine, 225
magazine articles, 56, 133
Maharam, Lewis G., 207
Ma Huang (ephedra), 233, 236

maintenance, 170, 183-86, 209-10
Mann, George, 114
Manson, JoAnn, 4, 5, 6, 21, 246
Marketdata Enterprises, 152, 156
Marlett, Judith, 191
Marrazzi, May Ann, 240
Mattes, Richard, 73, 75-76
Mayer, Jean, 152
Mayo Clinic, 25, 63
Mazanor, 243
Mazel, Judy, 140
mazindol, 243, 249
Media Research Center, 258
Medifast, Inc., 153, 155, 160, 161
Medved, Diane, 217
Meichenbaum, Donald, 26
menopause, 20-21
metabolism, 103-7, 109-110, 111-13, 115, 147,
    167, 170, 209, 226-27, 232, 233, 234
Metamucil, 192, 195, 202
Metropolitan Life Insurance Company, 1-2,
    30; height-weight tables, 6-8, 30
Mexican-Americans, 28
mindful eating, 172
Miracle Diet, The (Updike), 135
Mitchell, Tedd, 216
moderation, 76, 270
Moffitt Cancer Center and Research Institute
    study, 13
Moquette-Magee, Elaine, 77
Moscovitz, Judy, 140
muffins, 44, 46, 86, 88
Mullaly, Nyleen, 125
Muller, Steven, 260
muscle mass, 104, 167, 168, 170, 208-9, 226

naloxone, 240-41
naltrexone, 240
National Association for the Advancement of
    Fat Acceptance (NAAFA), 39, 40, 96, 105,
    108, 115-16, 117, 119, 120, 121, 122, 126,
    128, 129, 166
National Cancer Institute, 200, 204
National Center for Health Statistics survey, 50
National Center on Addiction and Substance
    Abuse, 262
National Consumers League survey, 178
National Exercise for Life Institute, 214
National Health and Nutrition Examination
    Survey (NHANES II), 12
National Institutes of Health, 98, 165, 168
National Research Council, 35
National Task Force on the Prevention and
    Treatment of Obesity, 168
National Weight Control Registry, 183
Nation of Victims, A (Sykes), 124-25
Native Americans, 11
native peoples, 98-102
Natural Resources Defense Council (NRDC),
    256-57
Nestle, Marion, 33-34, 35, 53, 74, 89, 162, 178

Nestlé's Sweet Success, 86, 87, 152
Netherlands, 3, 37, 52, 65
New Fit or Fat, The (Bailey), 108, 212
New York City Department of Consumer
　Affairs study, 154–55
New Zealand, 65
nicotine, 232
Nonas, Cathy, 73
NordicTrack, 52, 206, 214, 223
norepinephrine, 247
Norway, 3, 66
NPD Group, 39, 40, 53
Nurses' Health Study, 3, 4–5, 11–12, 13, 21, 97
NutraSweet (aspartame), 239
Nutri/System, 146, 153, 154, 155, 156, 157,
　158, 159, 161
nutrition activism, 264–65
NYPD Blue (TV series), 266

oat bran, 191, 202
obese persons: calorie intake, 177;
　discrimination against, 124–27; fat
　activism (*see* fat acceptance movement);
　metabolic rates, 111–13; understating of
　intake by, 89, 109–11, 114
obesity: American adjustment to, 38–43; annual
　costs, 21; biological prejudice against,
　126–27, 263; as a chronic disease, 166, 231,
　255; contagious nature of, 22, 254; deaths
　and mortality rates associated with, 1–6, 14;
　diseases and health problems associated
　with, 1, 10–16, 17, 19, 22, 127, 189;
　euphemisms for, 39; failure to publicize
　risks and mobilize against, 254–58; genetic
　vs. environmental factors, 94–102;
　incidence and trends, 27–31, 36–37; and
　lack of dietary fiber, 188–89, 194; as a
　national problem, 27–55, 99, 100–101,
　253–55; in other countries, 36–37; and
　physical activity, 50; reversing ill effects of,
　22–23; social and psychological problems
　associated with, 15, 17; societal and
　cultural problems contributing to, 252,
　259–64; and sugar consumption, 82, 83;
　suggestions for campaign against, 264–70;
　and television viewing, 53–55; traditional
　definition, 3, 27. *See also* body fat;
　overeating; weight gain
"obesity genes," 93–97, 123, 244–45, 259
obesity myths and fallacies: "Fat is a feminist
　issue" myth, 175–76; "It's a myth that fat
　people eat more than thin people" myth,
　108–11; "It's OK. I'm a 'pear' " myth,
　19–21; "not an independent cause"
　fallacy, 19; slow metabolism myth, 104,
　111–13; "95 percent" fallacy, 165–66;
　setpoint myth, 102–7; "20 percent" myth,
　3–6; "yo-yo" myth, 103–4, 166–71
O'Callahan, John, 246
Olean, 239
olestra, 238–40, 265

Oliver, Michael, 68–69
Olways Preservation and Exchange Trust, 36
one-food diets, 140, 182
O'Neill, Molly, 148–49
Optifast, 153, 155, 160, 161
Orbach, Susie, 175–76
Orlistat, 237
Ornish, Dean, 57, 58, 61, 73, 136, 173
Outsmarting the Female Fat Cell (Waterhouse),
　58, 136, 167, 215
Overeaters Anonymous (OA), 162–63
overeating, 24–25, 173–74, 176, 177, 181–82,
　265–66. *See also* binge eating
"overweight," 27–28. *See also* obesity

Paris Prospective Study, 10
"pear" shape, 19–21
pectin, 202
People magazine, 9
Pepper, John, 239
Perdiem, 192, 202
"phen/fen" combination, 244, 246–50
phentermine, 154, 244, 246–50
phenylpropanolamine (PPA), 232–33,
　242–43
physical activity, 48–55, 183, 220–22. *See also*
　exercise
physical education, 268–69
Physicians Weight Loss, 153, 154, 158, 161
phytochemicals, 203
Pierre, Colleen, 73
Pima Indians, 98–99, 118
Pinkwater, Daniel, 96, 116, 117, 128
Pi-Sunyer, Xavier, 165, 167
Playboy, 39
Pollock, Michael, 227
Pondimin, 247
popcorn, 44, 71, 74
Popcorn Plus Diet (Herskowitz), 140
Pope, Jamie, 57
portion sizes, 43–48, 156–57, 178, 267, 268
potato chips, 72, 76, 78–79, 239
potatoes, 78–79, 199
PowerBar, 81
Powter, Susan, 57, 68, 135, 136, 143–46, 152
President's Council on Physical Fitness and
　Sports, 50
Prevention magazine, 59, 70, 76
Price, Arlen, 95
processed foods, 78–81, 85
protein, 61, 139–40
Prozac, 243
Prudhomme, Paul, 117
psyllium, 191, 192, 195
Puhn, Adele, 135, 136

quackery, 132–34, 151–52

Raglin, John, 217
Ravussin, Eric, 98
Reaven, Gerald, 149

reduced-fat foods, 75, 76–77. *See also* low-fat
    foods
Redux, 243–47
relapse, after weight loss, 164, 165, 166,
    184–85
Resch, Elyse, 151, 171–73, 177
resistance training, 226–28
resistant starch, 188
restaurant servings, 44–45, 46, 267
Reward Meal, 150
Ricaurte, George, 245
Rice Diet Report (Moscovitz), 140
Rippe, James, 224
Robson, William, 18
Rockefeller University studies, 63–64, 103–6
Rolls, Barbara, 75, 91, 182
Rosenbaum, Michael, 18, 106, 107
Rosenbloom, Chris, 177
Rotation Diet, The (Katahn), 60, 137
Roth, George, 24
rowing machines, 218
Royal College of Physicians, 82
roughage (insoluble fiber), 188, 191, 192–93
Royko, Mike, 125
Rubens, Peter Paul, 126
running, 95, 208, 219

saccharin, 90–91, 239
Sager, Mike, 120–21
St. Luke's–Roosevelt Hospital studies, 109–10,
    113, 180
Samoans, 99–100
Sanders, Tom, 145
Sanorex, 243
Schaumburg, Illinois, 219
Schiff, Martin, 135
Scott, Willard, 152–53
Sears, Barry, 135
sedentary lifestyles, 48–55, 98, 220–22
Seiden, Lewis, 246
self-esteem, 186, 210–11, 259–61, 263
Self-Esteem Comes in All Sizes (C. Johnson), 128,
    186, 260
serotonin, 243, 246, 247
Setpoint Diet, The (Leveille), 103, 106
setpoint myth, 102–7
sex, and obesity, 15
Shaevitz, Morton H., 151
Shape Up America, 265
Sheats, Cliff, 136, 146–48, 167
Simmons, Richard, 52, 104
Simplesse, 238
Sims, Ethan A. H., 113, 114
Singh, Devendra, 126
size acceptance. *See* fat acceptance movement
Skinny Rolls, 178
skipping meals, 176–77, 180, 185, 195
Slim-Fast, 152, 153, 169
Slim Time Weight Loss Center, 153, 154
sloth, 49–50, 264, 266
Smith, Anna Nicole, 39

Smith, Sally, 96, 105, 106, 128
Snack Food Association, 70
snack foods, 70–71, 179–80, 270
snacks, 54, 185
SnackWell's products, 70–71, 74, 75, 76, 86
Snapple products, 42, 86
soft drinks, 35, 46, 47, 80, 91–92, 265
soluble fiber, 192, 195, 202
sorbitol, 90
Sosin, Elyse, 47
South African study, 187, 188–89
Spain, 66
stair machines, 218
Stamler, Jeremiah, 259
Stampfer, Meir, 6, 239
Stanford University, 159
stationary bicycles, 207, 208, 218, 219
Stillman, Irwin, 138, 139
stomach capacity, 180
Stop the Insanity! (Powter), 57, 135, 137,
    144–46
strength training, 226–28
stroke, 10, 11
Study of Men Born in 1913, 10
Stunkard, Albert, 94, 95, 164
sugar, 74, 78, 82–92, 150; words for on food
    labels, 89
Sugar Blues (Dufty), 82–83, 92
surgery, dangers of obesity, 13–14
Sweden, 3, 23–24, 37
swimming, 207–8
Switzerland, 63, 66
Sykes, Charles, 124–25

Take It Off! Keep It Off! (Ulene), 58
Take Off Pounds Sensibly (TOPS), 162
Taller, Herman, 138, 150
target weight, 9
television viewing, 52–55, 217, 264, 271
testosterone, 237
tetrahydrolipstatin, 237
T-Factor Diet, The (Katahn), 57, 59–60, 137
thermogenic agonists, 233
Thin for Life (Fletcher), 151, 184
Thin Game, The (Bayrd), 25
Thinner at Last (Lamm and Couzens), 247
thinness, 3–4, 9, 37–38, 40
Thomas, Dave, 42, 211
Thomas Jefferson Medical Center study, 251
Thompson, C. J. S., 151–52
Thompson, Kathleen, 108, 155, 163, 167
thyroid, 109
trauma, 14
treadmills, 218
treatment adherence, 25–26, 164–65
Tribble, Diane, 208, 210
Tribole, Evelyn, 76, 151, 171–73, 177
triglycerides, 12, 22
Tucker, Larry, 53
Turk, Dennis, 26
twin studies, 94–95

ulcerative colitis, 189
Ulene, Art, 58, 136
Ultra Slim-Fast products, 86, 87, 152
undernutrition, 24
underweight, and mortality, 2, 4
United Kingdom, 66, 177
United States: adjustment to obesity, 38–43;
    effect of diet on other peoples, 36–37,
    98–102; fat consumption as a percent of
    calories, 66–67; food and beverage
    consumption, 33–36; incidence of obesity,
    27–33, 37; self-reported eating habits, 38
United Weight Control Corporation, 153
University of Florida study, 227
University of Hawaii study, 101
University of Minnesota study, 54
University of Pennsylvania studies, 94, 95, 107,
    170, 182
University of Pittsburgh studies, 168, 183
urban planning, 220
U.S. Department of Agriculture, 33, 34–35, 36,
    66, 147; Food Guide Pyramid, 204, 268
U.S. Department of Health and Human
    Services, 70

Vanderbilt University study, 64
Van Dyke, Charles, 119, 120–21
Van Itallie, Theodore, 98
variety, and overeating, 181–82
vegetable capsules, 203–4
vegetables, 196–97, 203–5, 267, 269
Verdon, Ray, 70
Veronis, Suhler & Associates, 53
victimization, cult of, 259, 263
Virella, Mike, 129

Wadden, Thomas, 184
waist-to-hip ratios, 19–21, 126
walking, 52, 183, 207, 219
Wallace, John, 265–66
Walpole, Sir Robert, 132
Walt Disney Company, 219
Ward, Elizabeth, 162
water diet, 140–41
Waterhouse, Debra, 58, 136, 167, 215
water loss, 169
Weighing the Options (IOM), 21, 94–95, 255, 259
weight: averages, 32; ideal, 6–9; and mortality,
    3–6; "natural," 128; understatement of,
    28; target, 9
weight-control methods, 171, 183–86, 192–95;
    exercise, 209–10, 214–15
weight cycling ("yo-yoing"), 166–71
weight gain: after quitting smoking, 31,
    232–33; effect on mortality, 5; health risks,

    11, 13; relapse after weight loss, 164, 165,
    166, 184; small, reversing, 184
weight loss: and attitudes toward obesity, 127;
    contagious nature, 22–23; dietary fat
    studies, 62–65; dieter success rates,
    157–62, 164–66; and exercise, 207–10;
    and fiber intake, 193–94, 195; in Hawaiian
    study, 101; health benefits, 12, 22, 23–24,
    119–20; maintaining, 183–86, 209–10;
    metabolic effects, 103–7, 167, 170, 209;
    rapid vs. slow, 169–71
weight-loss centers, 152–63
weight-loss devices, 133, 134
weight-loss drugs, 24, 154, 229–52. *See also
    entries for specific substances*
weight-loss programs: at diet centers, 153–54;
    self-administered, 165–66, 184
weight-loss support groups, 162–63
Weight Loss Through Persistence (Kirschenbaum),
    215, 151
weight tables, 6–8
Weight Watchers, 86, 153, 155, 156, 157, 158,
    159, 161, 162, 183, 185
Weintraub, Michael, 248
Wendy's restaurants, 42, 211, 265
Westcott, Wayne, 226
Western Samoa, 99–100
wheat bran, 188, 191
White, Frances, 117
White, Philip, 140
whole-grain foods, 201
Why Women Need Chocolate (Waterhouse), 136,
    224
Willett, Walter, 13, 64, 69
Williams, Paul, 95
Wilmore, Jack, 226
Wilson, Karen, 129
Winfrey, Oprah, 40, 76
Wing, Rena R., 168, 183
Wolfe, Tom, 100
Woodhead, Linda, 262
workplace fitness programs, 267
World Health Organization, 90

Xenical, 237
xylitol, 90

You Count, Calories Don't (Omichinski), 219
Young, Lisa, 178
"yo-yo" dieting, 103–4, 166–71

Zandl, Irma, 47
Zone, The (Sears and Lawren), 135, 137, 149
Z-Trim, 239–40

35674053087590

CPSIA information can be obtained at www.ICGtesting.com
Printed in the USA
LVOW121429100513

333274LV00014B/409/P

9 780140 261448